Parental Mental Health and Child Development

Parental Mental Health and Child Development

Guest Editors

Dimitrios Papadopoulos
Katerina Maniadaki

MDPI

Basel • Beijing • Wuhan • Barcelona • Belgrade • Novi Sad • Cluj • Manchester

Guest Editors
Dimitrios Papadopoulos
Department of Early Years
Learning and Care
University of Ioannina
Ioannina
Greece

Katerina Maniadaki
Department of Social Work
University of West Attica
Athens
Greece

Editorial Office
MDPI AG
Grosspeteranlage 5
4052 Basel, Switzerland

This is a reprint of the Special Issue, published open access by the journal *Children* (ISSN 2227-9067), freely accessible at: https://www.mdpi.com/journal/children/special_issues/42KF55XIWF.

For citation purposes, cite each article independently as indicated on the article page online and as indicated below:

Lastname, A.A.; Lastname, B.B. Article Title. *Journal Name* **Year**, *Volume Number*, Page Range.

ISBN 978-3-7258-7320-3 (Hbk)
ISBN 978-3-7258-7321-0 (PDF)
https://doi.org/10.3390/books978-3-7258-7321-0

Contents

About the Editors

Dimitrios Papadopoulos

Dimitrios Papadopoulos is an Assistant Professor of Developmental Psychology in Early Childhood at the University of Ioannina, Greece. He has conducted postdoctoral research at the intersection of developmental psychology and developmental psychopathology, focusing on parental mental health and child behavior in families of children with autism, integrating developmental and applied perspectives.

His academic work focuses on early childhood development and family processes, with particular emphasis on giftedness and the social–emotional needs and psychosocial adjustment of gifted children, as well as parental functioning and mental health, alongside evidence-based interventions for children with neurodevelopmental differences and their families. He has published in international peer-reviewed journals and serves as a reviewer for scientific journals in child development. In 2025, he received the University of Ioannina Excellence Award for Research.

He has completed clinical training in the assessment of infant and child development, as well as in evidence-based interventions, such as Cognitive Behavioral Therapy (CBT) and psychoanalytic approaches to working with infants, children, and adolescents, including psychoanalytic infant observation and training at the Anna Freud Centre and the Tavistock Clinic. He has extensive clinical experience in mental health and child development services.

Katerina Maniadaki

Katerina Maniadaki is a Professor of Developmental Psychopathology and Director of the Research Laboratory of Counseling, Psychosocial Support and Community Interventions at the Department of Social Work, University of West Attica, Greece. She has also served as Head of the Department. She is a clinical psychologist with extensive experience in the assessment and treatment of developmental and mental health disorders, and her academic work focuses on developmental psychopathology across the lifespan, with particular emphasis on ADHD. Her research interests include early identification, secondary prevention, and evidence-based interventions for neurodevelopmental disorders. She has an extensive publication record that includes academic books, edited volumes, book chapters, and numerous papers in international peer-reviewed journals, as well as a significant number of conference presentations. She has also contributed as a reviewer and editorial board member in several international scientific journals. In addition, she has coordinated and delivered numerous specialized training programs on neurodevelopmental disorders for mental health professionals and educators, contributing substantially to professional development and knowledge transfer in the field.

Preface

Parental mental health has been increasingly recognized as a key factor influencing children's development and wellbeing. A growing body of research has shown that parental stress, depression, anxiety, and broader psychosocial challenges may affect parenting practices, family functioning, and children's emotional, behavioral, and developmental outcomes. At the same time, particular attention has been given to families raising children with atypical developmental trajectories, including children with neurodevelopmental disorders such as Autism Spectrum Disorder, Attention-Deficit/Hyperactivity Disorder, and related developmental conditions.

This Reprint brings together contributions that explore different aspects of the relationship between parental mental health and child development. The included papers address topics such as parental stress, family functioning, parenting practices, and the broader psychosocial environments in which children grow and develop. Some contributions also examine families raising children with neurodevelopmental disorders and discuss how family-centered and evidence-based interventions may support both parental wellbeing and children's adjustment in these contexts.

The aim of this Reprint is to provide an overview of current perspectives in this field and to highlight the importance of supporting parental mental health as a pathway for promoting positive child development. By integrating empirical research and theoretical perspectives, this Reprint emphasizes the need for multidisciplinary approaches that address both parental wellbeing and children's developmental needs. The contributions included offer insights that may be valuable for researchers, clinicians, psychologists, educators, and policymakers interested in strengthening the wellbeing and developmental outcomes of both parents and children.

Dimitrios Papadopoulos and Katerina Maniadaki
Guest Editors

children

MDPI

Article

Effects of Mindfulness-Based Cognitive Therapy on Parental Mental Health and Child Behavior in Families of Children with Autism Spectrum Disorder: A Randomized Controlled Trial

Dimitrios Papadopoulos [1,2,*] and Katerina Maniadaki [1]

1 Department of Social Work, University of West Attica, 12244 Athens, Greece; maniadaki@uniwa.gr
2 Department of Early Years Learning and Care, University of Ioannina, 45500 Ioannina, Greece
* Correspondence: d.papadopoulos@uoi.gr

Highlights

What are the main findings?

- Mindfulness-Based Cognitive Therapy (MBCT) adapted with mindful parenting components produced substantial reductions in parental depression, anxiety, and stress, alongside increases in positive affect and life satisfaction at post-intervention and at one month follow-up compared with a waitlist control group.
- Parents who received MBCT reported parent perceived reductions in the severity of their children's behavior problems at post-treatment and at one-month follow-up, despite children receiving no direct intervention.

What are the implications of the main findings?

- Integrating MBCT with mindful parenting principles in both group and individual practice represents a feasible and acceptable family-centered approach for enhancing the mental health of parents raising a child with ASD and for supporting children's behavioral adjustment.
- Early screening for parental depression, anxiety, and stress should be integrated into ASD services, to facilitate timely, practical, and cost-effective mental health interventions.

Abstract

Background/Objectives: Caring for a child with Autism Spectrum Disorder (ASD) is often associated with elevated psychological distress and reduced life satisfaction. Mindfulness-based interventions may offer substantial benefits by enhancing emotion regulation, reducing maladaptive cognitive patterns, and strengthening mindful parenting. This randomized controlled trial (RCT) examined the effectiveness of an eight-week Mindfulness-Based Cognitive Therapy (MBCT) program, enriched with mindful parenting practices, delivered to parents of children with ASD. The primary aim was to improve parental mental health, while secondary analyses explored potential indirect, parent-perceived changes in child behavior outcomes. **Methods**: Fifty-six parents of children with ASD were randomly assigned to an MBCT intervention group (n = 30) or a waitlist control group (n = 26). Parents completed assessments at baseline (T0), post-intervention (T1), and at one-month follow-up (T2), including the Depression Anxiety Stress Scales–21 (DASS-21), the Positive and Negative Affect Schedule (PANAS), and the Satisfaction With Life Scale (SWLS). They also rated the overall severity of their child's behavior problems to explore indirect treatment effects. **Results**: All parents receiving MBCT (100%) completed the program successfully and reported high acceptability. At baseline, no significant differences were observed between groups. At T1, the MBCT group demonstrated significant reductions

https://doi.org/10.3390/children13010053

in depression, anxiety, and stress, alongside increases in positive affect and life satisfaction. These improvements were maintained or strengthened at T2. However, the control group showed no significant changes over time. Additionally, parents in the MBCT group reported indirect improvements in their children's behavioral adjustment at T1 and T2. **Conclusions**: Findings demonstrate that MBCT constitutes an effective intervention for reducing parental psychopathology and indirectly supporting parent-perceived improvements in child behavior, emphasizing the importance of incorporating mindfulness and mindful parenting components into family-centered interventions for parents of children with ASD.

Keywords: Mindfulness-Based Cognitive Therapy (MBCT); mindful parenting; Autism Spectrum Disorder (ASD); parental mental health; parenting stress; child behavior; family; development; psychopathology

1. Introduction

1.1. Parental Mental Health of Children with Autism Spectrum Disorder

Autism Spectrum Disorder (ASD) is a multifactorial and lifelong neurodevelopmental disability that not only affects the individuals diagnosed but also imposes substantial and persistent mental health challenges on their families. The core features of ASD—difficulties in social communication and interaction, along with restricted and repetitive patterns of behavior—often lead to considerable limitations in functional independence and sustained caregiving demands across the lifespan [1,2]. As many individuals with ASD require ongoing specialized health, educational, and rehabilitation services, a substantial body of research has documented significant psychological consequences for caregivers, including diminished quality of life, emotional exhaustion, and increased social isolation [3–5].

Parenting, even under typical conditions, is an inherently challenging and emotionally complex process. Although most parents undertake this role with dedication and warmth, they often experience elevated parenting-related stress that is further intensified when either the parent or the child presents with symptoms of psychopathology, such as anxiety, depression, or behavioral dysregulation [6]. Developmental disability research consistently shows that approximately one-third of parents of children with ASD report notably elevated levels of stress, anxiety, and depressive symptoms compared to parents of neurotypical children [7–9]. In fact, Davis and Carter [10] found that 33% of mothers and 17% of fathers raising a child with ASD endorsed clinically significant depressive symptoms, while 6% in both groups reported clinically significant anxiety. Additionally, Carter et al. [11] found that maternal depressive symptoms among mothers of young children with ASD remained relatively stable over time, and that children's behavior problems emerged as a key predictor of subsequent increases in parental psychopathology. In this framework, parental depression has been consistently associated with disruptions in parent–child interactions, including increased intrusiveness and reduced emotional sensitivity [12], which in turn are linked to adverse developmental outcomes in children across emotional social, and cognitive domains [13–15] as well as reduced learning capacity [16].

Raising a child with ASD is a chronic and enduring source of parental stress, often exceeding the burden reported by caregivers of children with other developmental disabilities such as Down syndrome, ADHD, and impairments in intellectual and adaptive functioning [17–21]. Consistent with these findings, Chen et al. [22], in a large cross-sectional study of 1450 parents, demonstrated that caregivers of children with ASD experienced significantly greater mental health difficulties than parents of children with intellectual

https://doi.org/10.3390/children13010053

or sensory disabilities. More recently, Papadopoulos [23] found that parents of children with ASD experienced higher emotional burden compared to parents of children with ADHD or global developmental delay. Notably, the strongest predictors of parental psychopathology were lower socioeconomic status and dysfunctional child behaviors rather than ASD severity. These results align with extensive evidence showing that child behavioral dysregulation is one of the most potent and consistent contributors to parental stress, symptoms of depression, and emotional exhaustion in families of children with ASD [2,4]. Behavioral difficulties—such as irritability, aggression, tantrums, self-injury, and non-compliance—place sustained demands on caregivers, often exceeding the challenges associated with core ASD symptoms alone [24,25]. In this regard, previous studies have demonstrated that these behavior problems not only predict higher levels of parental stress and depression but also exacerbate feelings of helplessness, reduce parenting efficacy, and strain family functioning [26,27]. Moreover, child behavior problems are among the strongest predictors of caregiver burnout and service utilization, reflecting their pervasive and cumulative impact on daily routines and emotional well-being [28].

Psychological distress has also been associated with increased marital dissatisfaction and a higher likelihood of marital dissolution [29,30]. Research consistently shows that the chronic psychological burden of raising a child with ASD can strain partner relationships, contributing to higher conflict, reduced emotional intimacy, and lower perceived relationship quality [31,32]. Couples raising children with ASD often report more disagreements about parenting responsibilities, financial strain, and reduced time for shared activities, all of which predict poorer marital functioning [33,34]. Marital distress, in turn, can exacerbate parenting stress and diminish the emotional resources available for effective caregiving. For single parents, the absence of co-parenting support may further intensify the stress associated with ASD-related caregiving demands, heightening vulnerability to psychological distress and burnout.

Parental psychological well-being represents a central component of the family's developmental ecology [35]. Longitudinal research provides strong support for this transactional model, demonstrating that parental emotional functioning and child behavior dynamically influence each other over time [36,37]. A consistent bidirectional association has been documented between parenting stress and child behavior problems [38], forming a coercive and mutually reinforcing cycle of dysfunctional interaction. In this regard, higher levels of child behavior problems contribute to increased parental stress, which in turn predicts a subsequent exacerbation of behavioral difficulties. For example, Neece et al. [37] reported that parenting stress and child behavior problems significantly predicted one another through multiple developmental phases whereas elevated early parenting stress has been linked to poorer later child social skills [39,40].

Compared to parents of typically developing children, research suggests that parents of children with ASD exhibit distinct personality and socio-emotional profiles that may influence how they cope with the demands of caregiving. Li et al. [41] noted that these parents tend to show lower levels of novelty seeking and adaptability to change, as well as reduced social engagement, characteristics that may heighten stress vulnerability in unpredictable caregiving environments. Earlier work by Wolff et al. [42] also found that fathers of children with ASD displayed higher levels of schizoid traits relative to comparison groups, potentially reflecting broader familial patterns of social withdrawal or interpersonal detachment. More recent studies corroborate these observations, noting elevated levels of neuroticism, introversion, and reduced emotional stability among parents of children with ASD [43,44]. These personality characteristics have been associated with increased psychopathology, greater sensitivity to child behavior problems, and a tendency toward less flexible coping strategies. Conversely, protective traits such as emotional

https://doi.org/10.3390/children13010053

intelligence, resilience, conscientiousness, and extraversion have been linked to lower parenting stress and more adaptive responses to daily challenges [45,46]. Collectively, this literature suggests that parents' dispositional factors significantly shape their psychological adjustment and coping skills when raising a child with ASD.

1.2. Mindfulness and Parental Mental Health

Mindfulness—classified within the third wave of Cognitive–Behavioral Therapies (CBT) [47–49]—constitutes a set of practices aimed at cultivating present-moment awareness of thoughts, emotions, and bodily sensations with an attitude of openness and non-judgmental acceptance [50,51]. These characteristics render mindfulness a particularly practical and relevant avenue for caregivers who face persistent stressors, chronic emotional demands, and elevated caregiving burdens associated with raising a child with ASD. At the neurocognitive level, mindfulness practices have been linked to systematic changes in neural circuits involved in attentional control, emotional regulation, and self-referential processing, contributing to improvements in affect, well-being, and adaptive behavioral functioning [52,53].

A growing body of evidence demonstrates that mindfulness training can reduce parental stress and depressive symptoms, improve parents' perceptions of their interactions with their children, and decrease both internalizing and externalizing child behaviors [38,54,55]. MBCT originally developed as an eight-week relapse-prevention program for individuals with recurrent depression [56,57], integrates mindfulness meditation with cognitive therapy strategies to help individuals identify maladaptive cognitive patterns, interrupt ruminative thought cycles, and cultivate greater emotional flexibility. Research findings suggest that MBCT may also positively influence parenting by reducing emotional reactivity, promoting empathic attunement, and increasing constructive engagement in parent–child interactions [58].

Mindful Parenting, introduced by Kabat-Zinn and Kabat-Zinn [59], extends mindfulness principles into the parenting context by emphasizing intentional, present-centered, and compassionate engagement with both the child and the parenting experience. This relational framework highlights attunement, acceptance, emotional awareness, and non-reactivity as core mechanisms that support healthier family relationships. Empirical studies show that Mindful Parenting programs strengthen parent–child relationships, reduce parental preoccupation and parenting stress, enhance children's executive functioning, and promote more adaptive co-parenting interactions [60]. Importantly, Mindful Parenting has been associated not only with improvements in parental functioning but also in children's attention and behavioral regulation, especially among those with externalizing or attentional difficulties [54,61,62]. Moreover, studies suggest that parents of children with ASD who endorse elevated levels of dispositional mindfulness report lower levels of stress, anxiety, and depression, as well as fewer behavioral problems and ASD-related symptoms in their children [63,64].

In summary, mindfulness-based interventions appear theoretically well-grounded and clinically appropriate for parents of children with ASD, as well as for parents experiencing clinically significant depressive symptoms or heightened vulnerability to psychological distress. By fostering acceptance, emotional regulation, and present-focused awareness, mindfulness practices may help parents interrupt maladaptive cycles of experiential avoidance and reactive parenting while strengthening their capacity for attuned, sensitive, and compassionate caregiving. Nevertheless, further experimental research—particularly from diverse cultural contexts—is needed to clarify the direct and long-term effects of mindfulness interventions on parental well-being, parenting processes, and child developmental outcomes.

https://doi.org/10.3390/children13010053

1.3. Current Study

According to the above evidence, the aim of the present RCT was to evaluate the preliminary efficacy of MBCT for parents of children aged 4–17 years with ASD who reported at least mild symptoms of depression, anxiety, or stress. The intervention preserved the core structure of standard MBCT while integrating mindful parenting elements designed to enhance mindful awareness specifically with emphasis on reducing emotional reactivity, fostering acceptance and empathy, and strengthening parental engagement. Importantly, the program did not include explicit behavioral parenting strategies. In contrast, it focused on applying mindfulness principles to daily parenting challenges which are often characterized by heightened emotional fatigue and may contribute to the intergenerational transmission of depressive vulnerability.

The present study examined the effects of MBCT on parental mental health and explored potential indirect parent-perceived changes in child behavioral outcomes in an outpatient mental health care setting. We hypothesized that: (a) parents in the MBCT group would exhibit significant reductions in depressive, anxiety, and stress symptoms, as well as significant increases in positive affect and life satisfaction, both immediately post-intervention and at one-month follow-up, compared to parents in the waitlist control group; (b) parents in the MBCT group would demonstrate high intervention acceptability; and (c) children of parents in the MBCT group would show greater improvements in parent reported severity of child's behavior problems relative to those in the waitlist control group.

2. Materials and Methods

2.1. Study Design and Setting

The study used a two-arm RCT comparing an intervention group receiving MBCT with a waitlist-control group. Assessments were conducted at baseline (T0), immediately post-intervention (T1), and at one-month follow-up (T2) to evaluate both the immediate effects and short-term maintenance of treatment outcomes. Participants were randomly allocated to conditions using simple randomization procedures to minimize selection bias and ensure comparable groups. The study design followed key CONSORT recommendations—such as random allocation and clearly defined assessment timepoints; thereby, enhancing the methodological clarity and interpretability of the findings.

The study was conducted between February 2024 and April 2025 in an outpatient mental health clinic in Athens, Greece. This setting offered a structured, supportive, and therapeutically appropriate environment for family-focused interventions. All sessions and assessments were carried out in designated therapeutic rooms to ensure privacy, consistency, and adherence to professional standards.

This study was part of a postdoctoral research project and received ethical approval from the Ethics and Research Committee of the University of West Attica (Approval No. 8119/12-02-2024). Additional authorization for implementation of the intervention was granted by the administrative board of the collaborating mental health clinic (Approval No. 661/11-12-2023). All study procedures complied with the ethical principles outlined in the Declaration of Helsinki for research involving human participants.

2.2. Participants and Sample Size

A total of 78 Greek parents were initially screened for eligibility through multiple recruitment sources, including primary care settings, outpatient mental health clinics, parent associations in local primary schools, and community outreach initiatives (e.g., social media announcements, flyers, public advertisements). Eighteen individuals were excluded during screening due to insufficient DASS-21 symptom severity, concurrent psychotherapy participation, or refusal to provide informed consent. The remaining

60 eligible parents were enrolled and randomly assigned to either the MBCT intervention group (n = 30) or the waitlist-control group (n = 30). Figure 1 summarizes participant flow through the study following CONSORT guidelines.

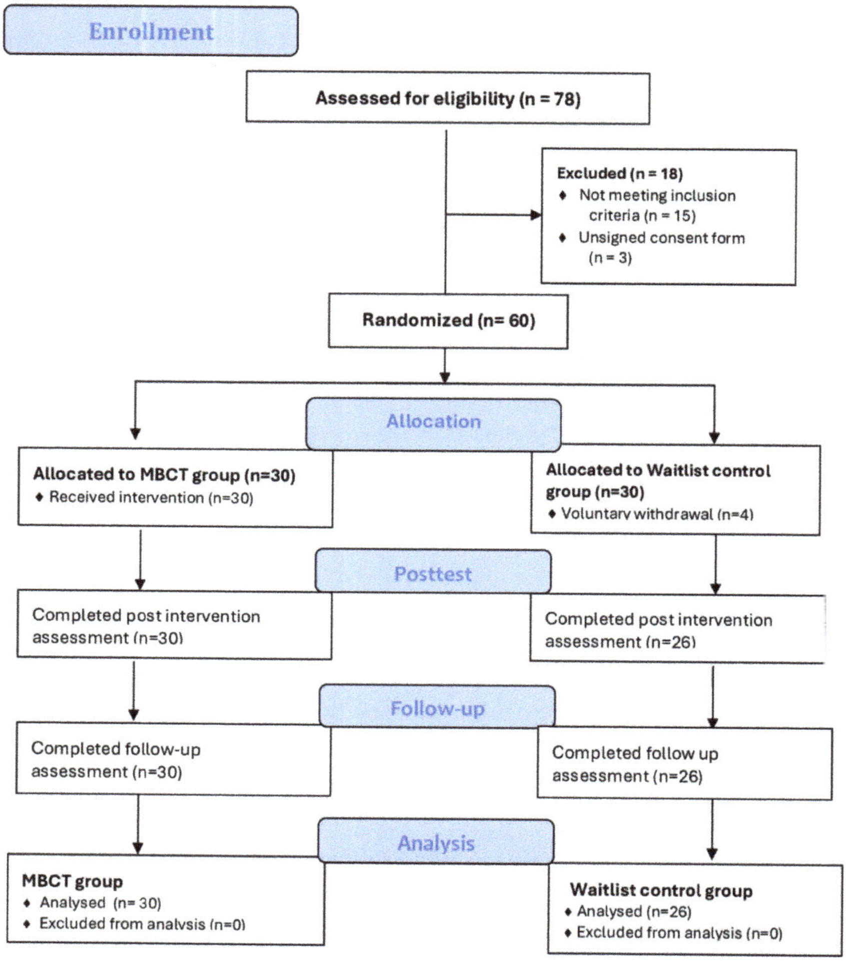

CONSORT flow diagram

Figure 1. Flow chart of the study.

An a priori power analysis was conducted using G*Power 3.1.9.4 [65] to determine the required sample size. The analysis was based on a repeated-measures ANOVA examining the group × time interaction (two groups; three assessment points: T0, T1, T2). Assuming a medium effect size (f = 0.25), α = 0.05, and desired power of 0.96, a minimum of 46 participants was required. Due to potential attrition, we sought to recruit at least 20% more participants, targeting an overall sample of 56 parents.

2.3. Inclusion and Exclusion Criteria

To be included in the study, individuals were required to meet the following criteria: (a) be a parent and primary caregiver aged ≥18 years and have at least one child diagnosed with ASD, aged 4 to 17 years, living in the same household; and (b) have sufficient fluency in Greek to understand instructions and complete all study procedures. To ensure parents

https://doi.org/10.3390/children13010053

most likely to benefit from the intervention, eligible participants were also required to present at least mild symptoms of depression, anxiety, or stress, based on the established DASS-21 cut-offs [66]: Depression $\geq$ 10, Anxiety $\geq$ 8, or Stress $\geq$ 15.

Exclusion criteria included participation in individual or group Cognitive Behavioral Therapy (CBT) within the previous 12 months, to maintain sample homogeneity and minimize confounding treatment effects. Participants were also required to attend at least 80% of MBCT sessions (i.e., $\geq$5 out of 8) to be included in post-intervention (T1) and follow-up (T2) assessments. However, the exclusion criterion based on attendance was not applied as no participants in the intervention group dropped out or failed to meet this attendance requirement.

2.4. Measures

2.4.1. Psychosocial and Demographic Questionnaire

Participants completed a sociodemographic questionnaire developed by the researchers to provide a comprehensive assessment of individual and family characteristics. The first section collected parent-related information, including gender, age, marital and employment status, as well as educational attainment. The second section concerned the child, gathering data such as gender, age, and time since diagnosis. Parents also rated their child's overall behavior using a four-point ordinal scale (0 = "no behavioral problems" to 3 = "severe behavioral problems"), a brief approach previously used in ASD research [28]. This rating reflected parents' impressions of the child's everyday behavioral functioning, considering common domains such as aggression, anxiety-related behaviors, regulatory difficulties, and non-compliance.

2.4.2. Parental Mental Health and Wellbeing

Depression Anxiety and Stress Scale (DASS-21) [66]

The DASS-21 is a self-report instrument comprising 21 items divided into three subscales: Depression, Anxiety, and Stress. Items are rated on a four-point Likert scale (0 = "Did not apply to me at all" to 3 = "Applied to me very much or most of the time"). Subscale scores are calculated by summing the relevant items and multiplying by two to ensure comparability with the full DASS-42. The DASS-21 has been widely used with parents of children with developmental disabilities [67,68] and has been validated in the Greek population [69]. In the present study, internal consistency coefficients (Cronbach's α) were α = 0.75 for Depression, α = 0.64 for Anxiety, and α = 0.82 for Stress, indicating acceptable to good reliability (see Table 1).

Satisfaction with Life Scale (SWLS) [70]

The SWLS assesses overall life satisfaction through five items rated on a seven-point Likert scale (1 = strongly disagree to 7 = strongly agree). Total scores range from 5 to 35, with higher scores indicating greater life satisfaction. Suggested interpretive categories include: 5–9 (extremely dissatisfied), 10–14 (dissatisfied), 15–19 (below average satisfaction), 20–24 (moderately satisfied), 25–29 (quite satisfied), and 30–35 (very satisfied). The Greek adaptation demonstrates satisfactory psychometric properties [71]. As shown in Table 1, Cronbach's α in the present study was 0.82, indicating good internal consistency.

Positive and Negative Affect Scale (PANAS) [72]

The PANAS consists of 20 items that measure the frequency of positive affect (10 items) and negative affect (10 items) on a five-point Likert scale (1 = very slightly or not at all to 5 = extremely). The instrument has been widely used in research involving parents of children with disabilities [73]. The scale has been translated and adapted into Greek with adequate

https://doi.org/10.3390/children13010053

psychometric properties [74]. Table 1 presents the internal consistency coefficients for the current study, which were α = 0.63 for Positive Affect and α = 0.77 for Negative Affect.

Table 1. Summary of instruments used in the study.

Instruments	Items/Subscales	Scoring and Interpretation	Cronbach's α (Present Study)
DASS-21 [66] (Depression, Anxiety, Stress)	21 3 subscales (7 items each)	4-point Likert scale (0–3); subscale scores multiplied by 2; higher scores indicate greater symptom severity.	Depression = 0.75, Anxiety = 0.64, Stress = 0.82
PANAS [70] (Positive–Negative Affect)	20; 2 subscales (10 items each)	5-point Likert scale (1–5); higher PA = greater positive affect, higher NA = greater distress.	Pos. = 0.63 Neg. = 0.77
SWLS [72] (Satisfaction with Life)	5	7-point Likert scale (1–7); higher total scores reflect greater life satisfaction.	Life satisfaction = 0.82

2.4.3. Intervention Acceptability

Acceptance of the intervention was assessed using a brief study-specific questionnaire developed by the researchers based on relevant literature on mindfulness interventions. Parents evaluated important program components (e.g., session structure, content relevance, home practice activities, facilitator support) on a five-point Likert scale (1 = strongly disagree, 5 = strongly agree). Participants were asked to provide qualitative feedback on their overall experience by responding to two more open-ended questions about the program's most and least beneficial elements.

2.5. Procedure

Parents who expressed interest in the study were contacted by email or telephone and completed an eligibility screening, which included confirmation of their child's ASD diagnosis. The study's objectives, methods, and procedure were thoroughly described to parents who met the inclusion criteria at an online or in-person briefing session. Informed consent was obtained prior to participation. The study followed CONSORT recommendations for RCTs.

After completing baseline assessments, participants were randomly allocated to the MBCT intervention group (n = 30) or the waitlist-control group (n = 30) using a com-puter-generated randomization sequence to minimize selection bias. Outcome measures were collected via self-administered questionnaires completed independently by par-ticipants, without direct interaction with the research team, reducing the likelihood of assessment bias related to awareness of group assignment. Data entry and dataset preparation were performed by a researcher blinded to group assignment to minimize analytic bias.

Participants allocated to the MBCT group proceeded to the intervention phase (described in Section 2.6). To maintain consistency and enhance group cohesion, the 30 participants allocated to the MBCT condition were organized into two fixed subgroups of 15 individuals each, which remained stable throughout the eight-week program. Participants in the waitlist-control group continued with treatment as usual.

Post-intervention assessments (T1) were conducted within one week following the final session, and follow-up assessments (T2) were administered four weeks later to examine short-term maintenance of treatment effects. All assessments were completed individually.

https://doi.org/10.3390/children13010053

All data were anonymized using unique identification codes and stored on encrypted, password-protected systems in accordance with GDPR requirements.

In the intervention group, all 30 parents initiated and completed the eight-week MBCT program without attrition and all participants satisfied the predefined ≥80% attendance criterion. In the waitlist control group, 26 of 30 parents completed both T1 and T2 assessments; four participants withdrew immediately after randomization and completed only the baseline assessment. Thus, the final analytic sample comprised 56 parents (MBCT: $n = 30$; control: $n = 26$). All exclusions were due solely to missing follow-up data rather than intervention-related reasons.

2.6. Intervention

The intervention followed the standard eight-week MBCT protocol [56,57], delivered in weekly two-hour group sessions. MBCT integrates cognitive therapy principles with mindfulness meditation practices to cultivate present-moment awareness, reduce automatic negative thinking, enhance emotional regulation, and strengthen self-compassion, thereby enabling participants to experience greater psychological wellbeing.

To ensure relevance for parents of children with ASD, the program incorporated established mindful parenting components [6,59,75], without altering the core MBCT curriculum. These additions emphasized applying mindfulness to real-time parenting challenges, including recognizing emotionally driven parenting reactions, increasing awareness of the parent–child relational dynamic, cultivating acceptance, and promoting nonreactive responding in high-stress caregiving situations.

Each session included guided mindfulness practices (e.g., body scan, sitting meditation, mindful movement), compassion-focused exercises toward self and child, cognitive-behavioral elements (identifying automatic thoughts, cognitive reactivity, and decentering), experiential activities, and structured group inquiry linking personal practice experiences to MBCT principles. Table 2 presents the program's structure and content. Participants were assigned 30–40 min of daily home practice supported by Greek-translated audio recordings and written materials. To encourage participation and skill consolidation, home practice was reviewed weekly.

Sessions were facilitated by the first author, an academic specializing in developmental psychology and developmental psychopathology with accredited training in mindfulness-based interventions and clinical psychotherapeutic practice. Attendance was recorded, with an expectation of ≥80% participation to ensure adequate exposure. Participants in the waitlist-control group continued treatment as usual and were offered the MBCT program after completing T2. Attendance was recorded to ensure adequate exposure and after completing T2, the MBCT program was offered to participants in the waitlist-control group who continued to receive standard treatment.

Table 2. Overview of the MBCT Intervention: Session-by-Session Protocol.

Week/Session	Core Theme	Primary Mindfulness Practices	MBCT/Mindful Parenting Components
Week 1	Awareness and Autopilot	Mindful eating (raisins task); Introduction to body scan	Recognizing automatic parenting reactions; introducing the program structure and group guidelines
Week 2	Facing Obstacles/A Different Way of Knowing	Body scan; Short mindful breathing	Distinguishing "doing" vs. "being" mode; observing difficult parenting thoughts/emotions as mental events

https://doi.org/10.3390/children13010053

Table 2. *Cont.*

Week/Session	Core Theme	Primary Mindfulness Practices	MBCT/Mindful Parenting Components
Week 3	Focusing the Scattered Mind	Extended mindful breathing; Mindful movement; 3-min breathing space	Applying attentional focus before/after challenging parent–child interactions
Week 4	Responding to Experience/Recognizing Aversion	Sitting meditation (breath, body, sounds, thoughts)	Noticing pleasant and unpleasant events in parenting; cultivating nonjudgmental awareness toward the child
Week 5	Allowing and Letting Be	Acceptance-focused meditation (observing difficult emotions)	Allowing parental emotions (guilt, frustration, sadness) to arise without avoidance or suppression
Week 6	Thoughts Are Not Facts	Sitting meditation emphasizing thought awareness	Decentering from self-critical thoughts (e.g., "I am not a good parent"); reframing automatic interpretations
Week 7	Self-Care and Relapse Prevention	Extended sitting meditation	Identifying personal stress triggers; developing a self-care and mindful parenting maintenance plan
Week 8	Maintaining and Extending New Learning	Review of core practices; Choice of preferred meditation	Creating individualized mindful parenting plans; integrating mindfulness into daily routines

2.7. Statistical Analysis

All statistical analyses were conducted using IBM SPSS Statistics (Version 25). Assumptions of normality were evaluated through skewness and kurtosis values, all of which fell within the acceptable ±2 range, supporting the use of parametric procedures [76,77]. This approach aligns with other RCTs in the mindfulness literature [78].

Descriptive statistics were computed for all sociodemographic and baseline clinical variables, and internal consistency (Cronbach's α) was examined for each psychometric instrument. Independent-samples t-tests for continuous variables and chi-square tests for categorical variables were used to evaluate baseline equivalence between the MBCT and waitlist-control groups.

Intervention effects were examined using repeated-measures ANOVAs with time (T0, T1, T2) as the within-subjects factor and group (MBCT vs. waitlist-control) as the between-subjects factor. The primary focus of inference was the group × time interaction. Partial eta squared ($\eta^2 p$) was reported as the effect size for ANOVA models. When significant interactions were detected, post hoc paired-samples t-tests evaluated within-group changes across time, and independent-samples t-tests compared groups at each assessment point. For within-group comparisons, effect sizes were calculated using Cohen's d for paired samples (d_z), whereas standard Cohen's d was used for between-group comparisons.

Changes in parent-reported child behavior problem severity over time and between groups were analyzed using chi-square tests, and effect sizes were measured using Cramer's V. Statistical significance was set at $\alpha = 0.05$ (two-tailed).

https://doi.org/10.3390/children13010053

3. Results

3.1. Sociodemographic and Clinical Characteristic

Table 3 presents the baseline sociodemographic characteristics of participating parents and their children. There were no statistically significant differences between the MBCT and waitlist-control groups on any demographic category (all $p > 0.05$), indicating appropriate baseline equivalence. Most parents (66.1%) were mothers and were married. Nearly half (42.9%) had received technical or technological education. The mean age of the parents was 40.67 years (SD = 6.45), and the two groups did not differ in age, gender distribution, or employment status. In terms of child characteristics, most children (80.4%) were males, with a mean age of 10.54 years and an average time since ASD diagnosis of 5.84 years. Similar to parental factors, no statistically significant between-group variations were found in child sociodemographic variables at baseline.

Baseline clinical outcomes are shown in Table 4. All mental health indicators showed no significant between-group differences (all $p > 0.05$). Parents were classified within mild to moderate symptom severity range on the DASS-21 ($M_{depression} = 17.32$; $M_{anxiety} = 13.00$, and $M_{stress} = 26.14$). Life satisfaction scores were low (M = 15.71) and fell into the category of "slightly dissatisfied". Similarly, PANAS scores across groups showed a clinically significant trend of increased negative affect (M = 22.80) and decreased positive affect (M = 27.79). At baseline (T0) ($p = 0.923$), parent-reported severity of child behavioral problems did not differ significantly between groups, suggesting that both groups had comparable clinical profiles at the start of the study. The homogeneity of the overall sample strengthens the methodological validity of subsequent between-group comparisons.

Table 3. Social and Demographic Characteristics of Participants.

Variables	Total Participants (n = 56)	MBCT Group (n = 30)	Waitlist Control Group (n = 26)	χ^2/t	p
Parental characteristics					
Gender, n (%)					
Male	19	9	10		
Female	37	21	16	0.445	0.505
Age in years (M/SD)	40.67	40.52	40.85	−0.194	0.846
Marital status, n (%)					
Married	42	22	20 (76.9%)		
Divorced	9	4	5		
Single parent	5	4	1	1.729	0.421
Education level, n (%)					
Secondary	10	3	7		
Technical/Technological	24	15	9		
University	22	12	10	3.011	0.222
Employment status, n (%)					
Public employee	16	7	9		
Private employee	27	15	12		
Self-employed	13	8	5	0.995	0.608
Child characteristics					
Gender, n (%)					
Boy	45	24	21		
Girl	11	6	5	0.005	0.942
Age in years (M/SD)	10.54	10.51	10.59	0.072	0.942

https://doi.org/10.3390/children13010053

Table 3. *Cont.*

Variables	Total Participants (n = 56)	MBCT Group (n = 30)	Waitlist Control Group (n = 26)	χ^2/t	p
Time since diagnosis (years) (M/SD)	5.84	5.78	5.9	−0.129	0.897
Severity of child's behavior problem, n (%)					
Mild	9 (16.1%)	5 (16.7%)	4 (15.4%)		
Moderate	20 (35.7%)	10 (33.3%)	10 (38.5%)		
Severe	27 (48.2%)	15 (50%)	12 (46.2%)	0.160	0.923

Table 4. Baseline Clinical Characteristics of Participants.

Indicators	Total Participants (n = 56)	MBCT Group (n = 30)	Control Group (n = 26)	t	p
	M/SD	M/SD	M/SD		
DASS-21					
Depression	17.32 ± 4.29	17.40 ± 4.85	17.23 ± 3.63	0.150	0.882
Anxiety	13.00 ± 2.70	12.93 ± 3.27	13.08 ± 1.90	−0.210	0.832
Stress	26.14 ± 4.73	26.13 ± 5.01	26.15 ± 4.49	−0.021	0.987
PANAS					
Positive Affect	27.79 ± 2.10	27.70 ± 2.45	27.88 ± 1.65	−0.334	0.746
Negative Affect	22.80 ± 2.70	23.03 ± 3.35	22.54 ± 1.70	0.710	0.485
SWLS					
Life satisfaction	15.71 ± 2.81	15.60 ± 3.16	15.85 ± 2.41	−0.340	0.739

3.2. Effect of the MBCT Program on Parental Mental Health Outcomes

3.2.1. Depression

Repeated-measures ANOVA revealed significant main effects of group (F = 22.950, $p < 0.001$, η^2p = 0.298) and time (F = 50.344, $p < 0.001$, η^2p = 0.482) on depressive symptoms. Importantly, a Group × Time interaction emerged (F = 64.126, $p < 0.001$, η^2p = 0.543). As presented in Table 5, within-group comparisons indicated substantial reductions in depression in the MBCT group from baseline to post-intervention and from baseline to follow-up suggesting continued symptomatic relief over time. In contrast, the waitlist control group showed no significant changes in depression levels across assessments. Figure 2 illustrates that, the MBCT group reported significant lower depressive symptoms than the control group at post-intervention, with this difference being even more pronounced at follow-up.

3.2.2. Anxiety

Repeated-measures ANOVA revealed significant main effects of group (F = 21.730, $p < 0.001$, η^2p = 0.287) and time (F = 18.462, $p < 0.001$, η^2p = 0.255), as well as a significant Group × Time interaction (F = 29.298, $p < 0.001$, η^2p = 0.352). As shown in Table 5, participants in the MBCT group exhibited marked reductions in anxiety from baseline to post-intervention, followed by additional improvements at follow-up. No additional change was observed between post-intervention and follow-up, indicating stability of treatment gains over time. Conversely, no comparable changes were observed in the control group. Be-tween-group comparisons further indicated that the MBCT group reported significantly lower anxiety levels than the control group at post-intervention, with anxiety levels continuing to decline at follow-up (see Figure 2).

3.2.3. Stress

A repeated-measures ANOVA revealed significant main effects of group ($F = 25.530$, $p < 0.001$, $\eta^2 p = 0.321$) and time ($F = 143.828$, $p < 0.001$, $\eta^2 p = 0.727$), as well as a significant Group × Time interaction ($F = 188.515$, $p < 0.001$, $\eta^2 p = 0.777$). As shown in Table 5, within-group analyses indicated substantial reductions in stress in the MBCT group from baseline to post-intervention. A smaller but statistically significant improvement was also observed between post-intervention and follow-up, suggesting continued symptom improvement over time. In comparison, the waitlist control group exhibited no significant changes in stress across any of the three assessment points. Between-group comparisons further supported the effectiveness of the intervention, with lower stress levels observed in the MBCT group compared to the control group at post-intervention and follow-up (see Figure 2).

3.2.4. Life Satisfaction

Repeated-measures ANOVA revealed significant main effects of group and time, as well as a robust Group × Time interaction (Fs = 62.429 and 87.903 respectively, ps < 0.001; interaction: $F = 132.156$, $p < 0.001$). According to Table 5, within-group analyses indicated substantial increases in life satisfaction in the MBCT group from baseline to post-intervention, followed by additional increases at follow-up. However, no significant changes emerged at any time point in the waitlist control group. Figure 2 shows that parents in the MBCT group reported higher levels of life satisfaction than those in the control group at post-intervention, with this difference remained evident at follow-up.

3.2.5. Positive and Negative Affect

For positive affect, analyses revealed a significant main effect of group ($F = 9.725$, $p = 0.003$, $\eta^2 p = 0.153$) and time ($F = 23.866$, $p < 0.001$, $\eta^2 p = 0.306$), as well as a significant Group × Time interaction ($F = 32.066$, $p < 0.001$, $\eta^2 p = 0.373$). As reported in Table 5, within-group analyses indicated that parents in the MBCT group showed marked increases in positive affect from baseline to post-intervention, with further gains maintained at follow-up. No significant changes over time were observed in the control group. Between-group comparisons further demonstrated that the MBCT group reported higher levels of positive affect than the control group at both post-intervention and follow-up assessments (see Figure 2).

As illustrated in Table 5, a significant main effect of group ($F = 7.292$, $p = 0.009$, $\eta^2 p = 0.119$) and time ($F = 14.189$, $p < 0.001$, $\eta^2 p = 0.208$), as well as a significant Group × Time interaction ($F = 25.267$, $p < 0.001$, $\eta^2 p = 0.319$), was revealed. Within-group analyses indicated that the MBCT group showed consistent reductions in negative affect from baseline to post-intervention and this effect remained evident at follow-up. In the control group, however, no significant changes were observed across the three assessment points. According to Figure 2, between-group comparisons (further demonstrated that the MBCT group reported significantly lower negative affect than the control group at post-intervention with the advantage persisting and strengthening at follow-up.

https://doi.org/10.3390/children13010053

Table 5. Comparisons of Parental Mental Health Outcomes by Group and Time.

Indicator	Group	M ± SD (T0)	M ± SD (T1)	M ± SD (T2)	T0 vs. T1	T0 vs. T2	T1 vs. T2	Group × Time Interaction (F, p)
Depression	MBCT	17.40 ± 4.85	11.77 ± 2.67	11.00 ± 2.39	$t(29) = 10.37$, $p < 0.001$, $d = 1.89$	$t(29) = 8.52$, $p < 0.001$, $d = 1.56$	$t(29) = 2.37$, $p = 0.020$, $d = 0.43$	$F = 64.126$, $p < 0.001$, $\eta^2p = 0.543$
	Control	17.23 ± 3.63	17.46 ± 3.28	17.69 ± 3.47	$t(25) = -1.14$, $p = 0.265$, $d = -0.22$	$t(25) = -1.54$, $p = 0.136$, $d = -0.30$	$t(25) = -0.90$, $p = 0.376$, $d = -0.18$	
Anxiety	MBCT	12.73 ± 3.50	9.40 ± 2.24	9.30 ± 2.09	$t(29) = 7.53$, $p < 0.001$, $d = 1.37$	$t(29) = 6.72$, $p < 0.001$, $d = 1.23$	$t(29) = 0.40$, $p = 0.687$, $d = 0.07$	$F = 29.298$, $p < 0.001$, $\eta^2p = 0.352$
	Control	12.92 ± 2.05	13.15 ± 2.05	13.46 ± 2.16	$t(25) = 1.14$, $p = 0.265$ $d = -0.22$	$t(25) = -1.54$, $p = 0.136$, $d = -0.30$	$t(25) = -0.90$, $p = 0.376$, $d = -0.18$	
Stress	MBCT	26.13 ± 5.01	18.93 ± 4.48	17.30 ± 4.09	$t(29) = 16.96$, $p < 0.001$, $d = 3.10$	$t(29) = 17.56$, $p < 0.001$, $d = 3.21$	$t(29) = 4.18$, $p < 0.001$, $d = 0.76$	$F = 188.515$, $p < 0.001$, $\eta^2p = 0.777$
	Control	26.15 ± 4.09	26.46 ± 4.09	26.85 ± 3.76	$t(25) = -0.39$, $p = 0.800$, $d = -0.05$	$t(25) = -1.17$, $p = 0.025$, $d = -0.23$	$t(25) = -0.65$, $p = 0.500$, $d = -0.13$	
Positive Affect	MBCT	27.70 ± 2.45	29.97 ± 2.34	30.43 ± 2.39	$t(29) = -6.38$, $p < 0.001$, $d = -1.16$	$t(29) = -6.46$, $p < 0.001$, $d = -1.18$	$t(29) = -2.45$, $p = 0.020$, $d = -0.45$	$F = 32.066$, $p < 0.001$, $\eta^2p = 0.373$
	Control	26.69 ± 3.96	27.88 ± 1.66	27.65 ± 1.65	$t(25) = -1.28$, $p = 0.211$, $d = -0.25$	$t(25) = -1.01$, $p = 0.323$, $d = -0.20$	$t(25) = 1.19$, $p = 0.247$, $d = 0.23$	
Negative Affect	MBCT	23.03 ± 3.35	20.83 ± 1.72	20.23 ± 1.92	$t(29) = 4.41$, $p < 0.001$, $d = 0.80$	$t(29) = 5.34$, $p < 0.001$, $d = 0.98$	$t(29) = 3.67$, $p = 0.001$, $d = 0.67$	$F = 25.267$, $p < 0.001$, $\eta^2p = 0.319$
	Control	22.54 ± 1.70	22.81 ± 1.90	22.96 ± 1.97	$t(25) = 0.97$, $p = 0.341$, $d = -0.19$	$t(25) = -1.53$, $p = 0.139$, $d = -0.30$	$t(25) = -1.69$, $p = 0.103$, $d = -0.33$	
Life Satisfaction	MBCT	15.60 ± 3.16	21.77 ± 2.97	23.07 ± 2.49	$t(29) = -12.50$, $p < 0.001$, $d = -2.29$	$t(29) = -14.80$, $p < 0.001$, $d = -2.71$	$t(29) = -4.71$, $p < 0.001$, $d = -0.86$	$F = 132.156$, $p < 0.001$, $\eta^2p = 0.710$
	Control	15.31 ± 1.69	15.12 ± 1.53	15.04 ± 1.93	$t(25) = 0.48$, $p = 0.638$, $d = 0.09$	$t(25) = 1.32$, $p = 0.199$, $d = 0.26$	$t(25) = 0.20$, $p = 0.844$, $d = 0.04$	

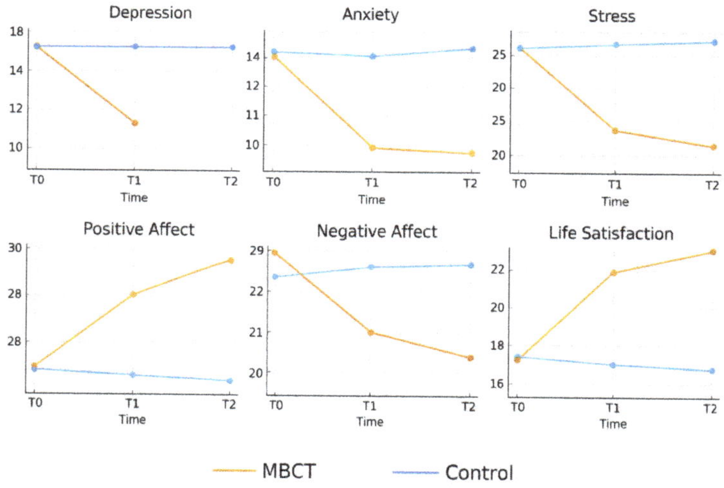

Figure 2. Changes in Parental Mental Health Outcomes Across Time by Group.

3.3. Intervention Acceptability

Parents receiving the MBCT intervention demonstrated very high levels of acceptability, with 96.4% reporting overall strong satisfaction with the program (M = 4.82, *SD* = 0.39). Regarding the structure and content of the intervention, 95.4% of participants indicated high satisfaction, reflecting strong approval of the program's organization, session flow, and

https://doi.org/10.3390/children13010053

relevance to their personal and family needs. Similarly, 97.4% rated their overall experience and the suitability of the program as highly positive, highlighting the supportive group atmosphere, the facilitator's guidance, and the practical usefulness of the skills taught. Open-ended responses also revealed that parents found the mindfulness practices highly appropriate for daily parenting and intended to continue using them beyond the program. The main obstacles identified were childcare needs and travel distance, while some parents suggested that future interventions could benefit from smaller group sizes to enhance interaction and personal sharing.

3.4. Child Behavioral Outcomes

Because no significant between-group differences were observed in parent-reported child behavioral problems at baseline (T0) ($p = 0.923$; see Section 3.1), subsequent analyses focused on changes in parent-perceived child behavior at post-intervention (T1) and follow-up (T2). At T1, a statistically significant between groups difference was observed ($\chi^2(3) = 18.262$, $p < 0.001$), corresponding to a large effect size (Cramer's $V = 0.57$). In the MBCT group, only 6.7% of children remained in the severe range while 13.3% were rated as having no behavioral problems. In contrast, in the waitlist-control group, 53.8% of children continued to exhibit severe behavioral difficulties and no child was rated as problem-free. This pattern was further strengthened at T2, where another significant group difference was revealed ($\chi^2(3) = 25.169$, $p < 0.001$; Cramer's $V = 0.67$). As shown in Figure 3, the proportion of children rated as having no behavioral difficulties increased to 20% in the MBCT group, while only 3.3% remained in the severe category. Conversely, 61.5% of children in the control group continued to present with severe problems, and none were rated as having no difficulties

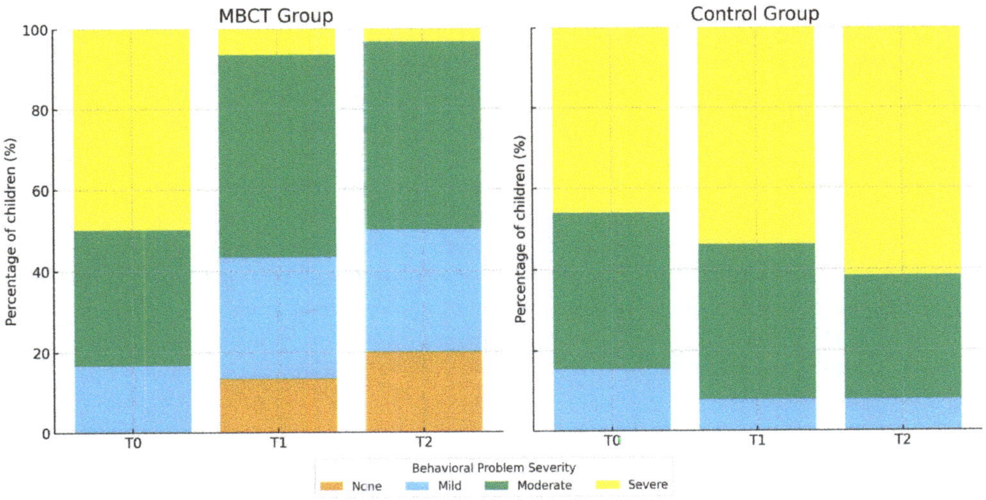

Figure 3. Comparison of Children's Behavioral Problems Across Time by Group.

4. Discussion

4.1. Preliminary Findings

At baseline, the two groups were comparable in terms of all sociodemographic and clinical factors, confirming the adequacy of randomization. More specifically, parents had significantly higher levels of depression, anxiety, and stress, accompanied by reduced life satisfaction. These scores fell within clinically relevant ranges across important mental health indices and were significantly higher than normal population norms [79]. Such find-

https://doi.org/10.3390/children13010053

ings have been consistently reported in previous studies which demonstrate the elevated psychological burden experienced by parents of children with ASD and underline the clinical relevance of evaluating interventions specifically targeting this population [73,80,81]. Moreover, this high level of initial distress provided substantial scope for therapeutic improvement.

4.2. Effectiveness of MBCT on Parental Mental Health

The current study's results suggest that the MBCT program was highly effective in reducing depressive symptoms, with parents in the MBCT group exhibiting significant gains both at immediately post-intervention and at follow-up. These findings align with a large body of research showing that MBCT reliable improves depressive symptoms and prevents relapse [56,57,82,83] while also enhancing psychological flexibility and resilience [84,85]. Depression is typically characterized by rigid negative schemas, ruminative thinking, and heightened attentional focus on distressing emotional states [86,87]. MBCT can reduce depressive symptomatology by interrupting the repetitive negative cognitive cycles that sustain emotional distress and depressive episodes; thereby fostering metacognitive awareness, cognitive flexibility, acceptance, and self-compassion. Accordingly, this cognitive shift enables individuals to cope with difficult situations with less automatic reactivity and greater psychological flexibility, functioning as a broad regulatory mechanism that yields downstream benefits across anxiety- and stress-related processes.

Within the context of parenting a child with ASD—an environment marked by chronic stressors and heightened emotional demands—these internal regulatory gains are likely further reinforced by the mindful parenting components embedded in the MBCT protocol. These practices foster present-moment awareness, emotional attunement, and compassion in parent–child interactions [60,75,88,89], which, in turn, help disrupt entrenched reactive patterns and reduce the likelihood that everyday challenges will elicit negative interpretations or self-critical rumination. Through this dual pathway—targeting both internal emotion-regulation processes and the interpersonal quality of parent–child exchanges—the combined MBCT and mindful parenting approach fosters a more regulated, attuned, and compassionate caregiving stance.

In terms of parental stress, the MBCT group showed both immediate post-intervention and long-term gains, with stress levels decreasing significantly from the severe range at baseline to the mild range at T1 and falling within the normative range by T2. These results are consistent with previous studies revealing that mindfulness-based interventions reliably reduce stress and enhance emotional functioning among caregivers of children with ASD [90–93]. Mindfulness may serve as a protective factor particularly for parents who must balance demanding caregiving responsibilities alongside professional pressures, financial strain, and persistent work–family conflict [94]. Parents receiving MBCT learn to interrupt automatic stress responses and shift attention toward more adaptive interpretations through practices that cultivate a non-judgmental present-moment stance, mindful disengagement from "autopilot", and greater sensitivity to internal cues [95]. This in turn expands their capacity to cope with daily challenges in more flexible and adaptive ways. Indeed, such cognitive–emotional shifts reduce reliance on fight-or-flight patterns—commonly associated with anxiety and heightened reactivity [96]—and foster more deliberate, emotionally regulated parenting behaviors.

Significant improvements in perceived positive affect and life satisfaction were observed among participants in the MBCT group, who shifted from "somewhat dissatisfied" at baseline to "somewhat satisfied" at post-intervention and follow-up. Such findings align with evidence indicating that mindfulness practice reduces self-criticism, enhances positive emotion, and supports broader psychological flourishing [97–99]. According to the Mindfulness-to-Meaning Theory [95], mindfulness contributes to psychological well-being through conscious emotion regulation and disengagement from habitual negative attentional patterns, facilitating metacognitive awareness. Mindfulness practices that cultivate decentering and broaden attentional scope may initiate an upward spiral of adaptive cognitive–affective processing that progressively transforms how individuals respond to stress. This shift enables individuals to engage in more constructive cognitive reappraisal and to flexibly reinterpret both internal and external experiences, thereby enhancing their capacity to cope with adversity with greater clarity, emotional calmness, and a strengthened sense of purpose. More specifically, these cognitive processes are linked to enhance well-being primarily through their influence on affective functioning, including increased positive affect and reduced negative affect [100].

For families raising a child with ASD, this process may represent a central pathway linking mindfulness practice to improved life satisfaction [101] as parents become more capable of re-experiencing positive emotions and evaluating daily life more favorably. In turn this may foster a more compassionate and meaningful stance toward their caregiving role while reducing automatic negative appraisals. such as guilt or self-blame, related to the child's disability and challenging behaviors. Within this framework, the Mindfulness-to-Meaning Theory helps conceptualize how mindfulness-based interventions may promote mindful parenting by interrupting automatic stress-driven reactions and fostering greater psychological flexibility [94]. Rather than reacting reflexively, parents may learn to pause, attend to present-moment experience, and broaden awareness to include alternative perspectives and coping options that may previously have been overlooked (e.g., identifying flexible strategies to manage work–family demands).

Several of the observed intervention effects were relatively large compared to those typically reported in psychosocial interventions, and this finding warrants careful consideration. One contributing factor may be the elevated levels of psychological distress observed at baseline, which likely provided greater scope for therapeutic improvement following intervention. Indeed, the present sample appeared to report increased psychological burden, reflecting the heightened vulnerability and unmet mental health needs of parents raising a child with ASD in Greece, a population that remains comparatively under-researched, and highlighting the chronic emotional demands associated with caregiving in this context [5,23]. Such elevated baseline distress may allow greater observable change following interventions focused on emotional regulation, reflecting heightened unmet support needs at treatment entry and increased receptivity to structured, practical therapeutic input [82]. In addition, observed intervention effects may reflect not only MBCT-specific techniques but also the influence of non-specific therapeutic factors. Participants in the intervention group received additional attention, structured group support, and regular engagement with facilitators and other parents sharing similar caregiving experiences. In constrast, these elements were not provided in the same form to the control group, which continued to receive individual support as usual. As a result, between-group differences may reflect the combined contribution of intervention-specific components and broader contextual and psychosocial factors that were not equally distributed across conditions.

Contemporary neuroscientific models describing the therapeutic mechanisms underlying mindfulness practice provide a coherent explanatory framework for understanding the treatment gains observed in the current study. Research evidence indicates that MBCT induces functional and structural neuroplastic changes in brain system supporting attentional and cognitive control, emotional regulation, and self-referential processing [102]. Indeed, mindfulness practice has been found to enhance activation in prefrontal and anterior cingulate regions, which are critical for top-down emotion regulation [53]. Additionally, it reduces amygdala reactivity, thereby improving threat sensitivity and strengthening emo-

https://doi.org/10.3390/children13010053

tional resilience [103,104]. In parallel, mindfulness practices modulate the hypothalamic–pituitary–adrenal (HPA) axis, contributing to reductions in cortisol levels [105,106] and counteracting the chronic stress dysregulation frequently reported among parents of children with ASD [107]. As these neurobiological processes unfold, they may support greater interoceptive awareness and regulatory flexibility, facilitating more sustained emotional regulation in the context of chronic caregiving stress.

Because the present study focused on intervening at the individual parent level, the effectiveness of the intervention can be interpreted in relation to broader contextual and cultural factors that may have shaped both treatment engagement and observed outcomes. Importantly, mindfulness-based interventions have not been widely implemented or established as evidence-based approaches within the Greek mental health care system. As a result, participants in the present study were largely unfamiliar with mindfulness practices prior to enrollment. This lack of prior exposure may have influenced both the perceived acceptability of the intervention and the magnitude of observed treatment effects, potentially contributing to substantial improvements from baseline to post-intervention that were maintained at the one-month follow-up. In this context, engagement with mindfulness practices may have represented a novel and meaningful psychological resource, particularly for parents with limited prior access to structured emotional regulation strategies.

In addition, broader socioeconomic conditions may have further shaped parents' responsiveness to the intervention. The prolonged economic crisis in Greece has disproportionately affected families raising children with autism, who often face increased financial burden related to ongoing therapeutic and educational needs [5,23]. Empirical evidence indicates that these financial pressures are associated with heightened parenting stress, anxiety, and a pervasive sense of insecurity, which may reduce parents' psychological availability and increase reliance on automatic, reactive parenting responses. Within this context, mindfulness-based interventions that cultivate present-moment awareness and emotional regulation may be particularly salient, offering parents psychological space to disengage from habitual stress-driven reactions. Overall, these contextual factors may have created conditions under which parents were particularly receptive to the intervention, thereby amplifying its perceived effectiveness. At the same time, they underscore the importance of considering how broader contextual influences interact with mindfulness-based interventions to shape acceptability, engagement, and treatment outcomes across diverse settings.

4.3. Acceptance of the Intervention

All 30 parents (100%) in the MBCT group completed the eight-week program and consistently attended sessions, engaged in daily mindfulness practice (30–45 min), and applied mindful parenting skills at home. Participants' consistent involvement throughout the program reflects high commitment and strong feasibility to the intervention protocol. Acceptability ratings were consistently positive with parents reporting that the program's structure, content, and relevance aligned closely with their needs. They also identified the supportive group environment and the facilitator's guidance as key strengths of the program. Open-ended responses further revealed the practical value of mindfulness practices for managing everyday parenting challenges. Reported obstacles were primarily associated with increased childcare demands and travel distance to and from the intervention setting. These findings align with international research demonstrating high satisfaction and strong engagement with mindfulness-based programs [73,108,109], confirming MBCT as a feasible and well-accepted intervention for ASD caregivers.

https://doi.org/10.3390/children13010053

4.4. Indirect Parent—Perceived Changes in Children's Behavior

Although children did not receive direct intervention, parent-reported assessments at post-intervention and follow-up indicated exploratory between-group differences in behavioral outcomes, with the MBCT group showing notable reductions in perceived problem severity. Given that child outcomes were assessed using a single parent-reported item, these findings should be interpreted as parent-perceived changes rather than objective behavioral improvement. Consistent with the transactional model of development [35] and with prior evidence [55,61,110] these parent-perceived gains in children's behavior may reflect improvements in parents' emotional regulation and increased use of adaptive parenting strategies. Reductions in parental stress may interrupt maladaptive parent–child transactional cycles and promote a calmer, more supportive caregiving environment that parents may experience as facilitating improvements in their child's self-regulation. As parents become more regulated, attentive, and responsive to their child's needs and behaviors, the parent child relationship may improve, and daily interactions may be perceived as less reactive and more supportive. In turn, parents are more able to create a caregiving environment characterized by emotional stability and consistency supporting changes in how child behavior is perceived and managed over time. Therefore, mindful parenting functions as a key mechanism through which parental well-being translates into changes in parents' perceptions of their child's behavioral adjustment, underscoring the reciprocal interplay between parental wellbeing and child behavior.

4.5. Strengths, Limitations, and Future Research

This study has several methodological strengths. The use of an RCT with an experimental and a waitlist-control group enhances the rigor of the study and supports robust conclusions about the effectiveness of MBCT on parental mental health. Importantly, there was no attrition in the MBCT group, indicating high acceptability, strong engagement, and good feasibility which are all critical factors for interventions targeting parents of children with ASD. Additionally, the inclusion of parents of children aged 4 to 17 years may enhance the applicability of the findings to a broad spectrum of ASD caregiving experiences.

Despite these strengths, several limitations need consideration. First, although the sample size exceeded a priori power criteria, it remained relatively modest, which may limit the precision of effect size estimates and the generalizability of the findings [111]. It should be noted, however, that similar sample sizes are commonly reported in clinical mindfulness-based intervention studies with parents of children with neurodevelopmental conditions, reflecting both the intensity of such interventions and the practical challenges associated with recruiting and retaining this population [58,78,82]. Future studies should recruit larger and more socioeconomically and geographically diverse samples, including families from rural settings and varied cultural backgrounds, to enhance the applicability of results [83]. Second, this study aimed to examine the short-term treatment effects of the MBCT intervention on parental psychopathology; therefore, conclusions regarding the long-term sustainability of treatment gains are limited by the one-month follow-up period [112]. Short-term follow-up assessments (e.g., one to two months) have also been used in pilot and early-stage randomized controlled trials of family mindfulness interventions to examine initial trajectories of change [94,113], as they allow evaluation of early maintenance of effects while minimizing attrition and participant burden before longer-term assessments become feasible. Nevertheless, future research should incorporate extended follow-up assessments spanning several months or years post-intervention in order to more accurately capture long-term trajectories of change. Given that mindfulness is not a stable personality trait but rather a trainable and dynamic capacity, accumulating evidence suggests that the

https://doi.org/10.3390/children13010053

effects of mindfulness-based interventions may not be static, but instead continue to evolve, consolidate, or even emerge more clearly over time [88,91,109].

An additional limitation concerns the absence of an active control condition and the potential influence of expectancy effects. Although the primary aim of the present trial was not to compare MBCT with another active psychological intervention, but rather to evaluate its effects relative to a condition that did not receive MBCT, participants in the control group continued to receive treatment as usual. While this design accounts for ongoing support and routine care [114], as is common in similar studies [38,82,94], improvements in parental mental health and parent-perceived child outcomes in the intervention group may still have been partly influenced by positive treatment expectations, increased attention, or other non-specific factors associated with participation in a structured program. This limitation is particularly relevant given the waitlist control design and the reliance on self-report measures.

Indeed, outcomes in the present study were assessed exclusively using quantitative self-report instruments. Although these measures demonstrate strong psychometric properties [66,70] and are sensitive to change, they may be influenced by cognitive reappraisal processes and positive expectancy effects following participation in a structured intervention. Moreover, self-report measures may not fully capture the subjective complexity of parents' lived experiences or provide detailed insight into how mindfulness skills are translated into everyday parenting practices. As such, reliance on self-report data may limit the depth with which underlying change processes can be understood.

Finally, child behavioral outcomes in the present study were assessed exclusively through parent-reported ratings, reflecting parents' perceptions of changes in their child's behavior over time. Although parent reports provide ecologically valid information about daily functioning, this approach may be influenced by expectancy effects and reporting biases, particularly in the context of psychosocial interventions targeting parental emotional regulation [115]. In addition, reliance on a single informant does not allow differentiation between perceived behavioral change and objective behavioral improvement, nor does it adequately account for the presence of co-occurring psychopathology (e.g., attention-deficit/hyperactivity disorder), which may independently shape children's behavioral presentations and trajectories [116]. Consequently, findings related to child behavior should be interpreted as preliminary and parent-perceived changes rather than definitive evidence of direct behavioral improvement. Future research would benefit from incorporating multi-informant assessment strategies (e.g., reports from teachers and clinicians), structured behavioral observations, and standardized assessment tools to enhance the validity and robustness of child outcome evaluation.

5. Conclusions

This RCT provides robust evidence that MBCT, combined with mindful parenting practices, is an effective and acceptable intervention for parents of children with ASD. Parents who received MBCT demonstrated significant improvements in overall mental health and wellbeing, with particularly notable reductions in parental psychopathology along with strong gains in positive affect and life satisfaction. These improvements were evident at post-intervention and either further increased or, in the case of anxiety, remained stable at follow-up, revealing both the direct impact and short-term durability of treatment gains. In contrast, the waitlist-control group showed no meaningful changes, underscoring both the efficacy of MBCT and the persistent psychological burden experienced by parents caring for a child with ASD.

Preliminary indications of parent-perceived changes in children's behavior suggest that improvements in parental emotional regulation may positively influence family dy-

https://doi.org/10.3390/children13010053

namics and parent–child relationships. These improvements are likely explained by gains in present-moment awareness, acceptance, and self-compassion all of which are central mechanisms cultivated through MBCT and mindful parenting. As a result, through these practices parents experience neurocognitive changes which interrupt maladaptive cognitive patterns and reduce emotional reactivity while enhancing prefrontal control processes involved in psychological flexibility and emotional regulation. Thus, these changes enable parents to respond to caregiving demands in a more adaptive and flexible manner rather than relying on habitual stress or emotional-driven reactions [6,117].

In clinical practice, MBCT represents a well-accepted intervention that can be integrated into individual therapy, group-based parent support, and broader psychoeducational programs. By strengthening parental mental health, MBCT has the potential to indirectly support children's positive behavioral, highlighting its value as a family-centered approach to promoting psychological well-being and healthier parent–child interactions.

Author Contributions: Conceptualization, D.P. and K.M.; methodology, D.P.; software, D.P.; validation, D.P. and K.M.; formal analysis, D.P.; investigation, D.P.; writing—original draft preparation, D.P.; writing—review and editing, K.M. and D.P.; supervision, K.M. All authors have read and agreed to the published version of the manuscript.

Funding: This research received no external funding.

Institutional Review Board Statement: The study was conducted in accordance with the Declaration of Helsinki and approved by the Ethics Committee of West Attica (3119/12 February 2024) for studies involving humans.

Informed Consent Statement: Informed consent was obtained from all subjects involved in the study.

Data Availability Statement: Data is available upon reasonable request from the corresponding author.

Conflicts of Interest: The authors declare no conflicts of interest.

References

1. Marsack-Topolewski, C.N.; Samuel, P.S.; Tarraf, W. Empirical evaluation of the association between daily living skills of adults with autism and parental caregiver burden. *PLoS ONE* **2021**, *16*, e0244844. [CrossRef] [PubMed]
2. Lecavalier, L.; Leone, S.; Wiltz, J. The impact of behavior problems on caregiver stress in young people with autism spectrum disorders. *J. Intellect. Disabil. Res.* **2006**, *50*, 172–183. [CrossRef] [PubMed]
3. Sánchez Amate, J.J.; Luque de la Rosa, A. The Effect of Autism Spectrum Disorder on Family Mental Health: Challenges, Emotional Impact, and Coping Strategies. *Brain Sci.* **2024**, *14*, 1116. [CrossRef]
4. Estes, A.; Olson, E.; Sullivan, K.; Greenson, J.; Winter, J.; Dawson, G.; Munson, J. Parenting-related stress and psychological distress in mothers of toddlers with autism spectrum disorders. *Brain Dev.* **2013**, *35*, 133–138. [CrossRef] [PubMed]
5. Papadopoulos, D. Mothers' experiences and challenges raising a child with autism spectrum disorder: A qualitative study. *Brain Sci.* **2021**, *11*, 309. [CrossRef]
6. Bögels, S.; Restifo, K. *Mindful Parenting: A Guide for Mental Health Practitioners*; Springer: New York, NY, USA, 2014.
7. van der Lubbe, A.; Swaab, H.; Vermeiren, R.; van Rossum, E.F.C.; van Balkom, I.D.C.; Ester, W.A. Chronic Parenting Stress in Parents of Children with Autism: Associations with Chronic Stress in Their Child and Parental Mental and Physical Health. *J. Autism Dev. Disord.* **2025**. [CrossRef]
8. Ekas, N.V.; Lickenbrock, D.M.; Whitman, T.L. Optimism, social support, and well-being in mothers of children with autism spectrum disorder. *J. Autism Dev. Disord.* **2010**, *40*, 1274–1284. [CrossRef]
9. Piro-Gambetti, B.; Greenlee, J.; Bolt, D.; Papp, L.M.; Hartley, S.L. Parent-couple satisfaction, parent depression, and child mental health in families with autistic children. *Front. Psychiatry* **2024**, *14*, 1306456. [CrossRef]
10. Davis, N.O.; Carter, A.S. Parenting stress in mothers and fathers of toddlers with autism spectrum disorders: Associations with child characteristics. *J. Autism Dev. Disord.* **2008**, *38*, 1278–1291. [CrossRef]
11. Carter, A.S.; Martínez-Pedraza, F.D.L.; Gray, S.A. Stability and individual change in depressive symptoms among mothers raising young children with ASD: Maternal and child correlates. *J. Clin. Psychol.* **2009**, *65*, 1270–1280. [CrossRef]
12. Lovejoy, M.C.; Graczyk, P.A.; O'Hare, E.; Neuman, G. Maternal depression and parenting behavior: A meta-analytic review. *Clin. Psychol. Rev.* **2000**, *20*, 561–592. [CrossRef] [PubMed]

13. Gladstone, T.R.G.; Beardslee, W.R.; Diehl, A. The impact of parental depression on children. In *Parental Psychiatric Disorder: Distressed Parents and Their Families*, 3rd ed.; Reupert, A., Maybery, D., Nicholson, J., Göpfert, M., Seeman, M.V., Eds.; Cambridge University Press: Cambridge, UK, 2015; pp. 117–126. [CrossRef]
14. Goodman, S.H.; Rouse, M.H.; Connell, A.M.; Broth, M.R.; Hall, C.M.; Heyward, D. Maternal depression and child psychopathology: A meta-analytic review. *Clin. Child Fam. Psychol. Rev.* **2011**, *14*, 1–27. [CrossRef] [PubMed]
15. Pan, B.; Gong, Y.; Wang, Y.; Miao, J.; Zhao, C.; Li, Y. The impact of maternal parenting stress on early childhood development: The mediating role of maternal depression and the moderating effect of family resilience. *BMC Psychol.* **2025**, *13*, 277. [CrossRef] [PubMed]
16. Chad-Friedman, S.; Zhang, I.; Donohue, K.; Chad-Friedman, E.; Rich, B.A. Reciprocal associations between parental depression and child cognition: Pathways to children's internalizing and externalizing symptoms. *Dev. Psychopathol.* **2025**, *37*, 29–39. [CrossRef]
17. Abbeduto, L.; Seltzer, M.M.; Shattuck, P.; Krauss, M.W.; Orsmond, G.; Murphy, M.M. Psychological well-being and coping in mothers of youths with autism, Down syndrome, or fragile X syndrome. *Am. J. Ment. Retard.* **2004**, *109*, 237–254. [CrossRef]
18. Dabrowska, A.; Pisula, E. Parenting stress and coping styles in mothers and fathers of preschool children with autism and Down syndrome. *J. Intellect. Disabil. Res.* **2010**, *54*, 266–280. [CrossRef]
19. Hayes, S.A.; Watson, S.L. The impact of parenting stress: A meta-analysis of studies comparing the experience of parenting stress in parents of children with and without autism spectrum disorder. *J. Autism Dev. Disord.* **2013**, *43*, 629–642. [CrossRef]
20. Yesilkaya, M.; Magallón-Neri, E. Parental Stress Related to Caring for a Child with Autism Spectrum Disorder and the Benefit of Mindfulness-Based Interventions for Parental Stress: A Systematic Review. *SAGE Open* **2024**, *14*, 21582440241235033. [CrossRef]
21. Dijkstra-de Neijs, L.; Swaab, H.; van Berckelaer-Onnes, I.A.; Ester, W.A. Resilience Within Families of Young Children with ASD. *J. Autism Dev. Disord.* **2025**. [CrossRef]
22. Chen, S.-Q.; Chen, S.-D.; Li, X.-K.; Ren, J. Mental health of parents of special needs children in China during the COVID-19 pandemic. *Int. J. Environ. Res. Public Health* **2020**, *17*, 9519. [CrossRef]
23. Papadopoulos, D. Impact of child and family factors on caregivers' mental health and psychological distress during the COVID-19 pandemic in Greece. *Children* **2023**, *11*, 7. [CrossRef]
24. Lovell, B.; Wetherell, M.A. Child behaviour problems mediate the association between coping and perceived stress in caregivers of children with autism. *Res. Autism Spectr. Disord.* **2015**, *20*, 17–23. [CrossRef]
25. Soke, G.N.; Rosenberg, S.A.; Rosenberg, C.R.; Vasa, R.A.; Lee, L.C.; DiGuiseppi, C. Brief Report: Self-injurious Behaviors in Preschool Children with Autism Spectrum Disorder Compared to Other Developmental Delays and Disorders. *J. Autism Dev. Disord.* **2018**, *48*, 2558–2566. [CrossRef] [PubMed]
26. Kim, I.; Ekas, N.V.; Hock, R. Associations between child behavior problems, family management, and depressive symptoms for mothers of children with autism spectrum disorder. *Res. Autism Spectr. Disord.* **2016**, *26*, 80–89. [CrossRef]
27. Postorino, V.; Sanges, V.; Giovagnoli, G.; Fatta, L.M.; De Peppo, L.; Armando, M.; Vicari, S.; Mazzone, L. Clinical differences in children with autism spectrum disorder with and without food selectivity. *Appetite* **2015**, *92*, 126–132. [CrossRef]
28. Karst, J.S.; Van Hecke, A.V. Parent and family impact of autism spectrum disorders: A review and proposed model for intervention evaluation. *Clin. Child Fam. Psychol. Rev.* **2012**, *15*, 247–277. [CrossRef]
29. Hartley, S.L.; Barker, E.T.; Seltzer, M.M.; Floyd, F.; Greenberg, J.; Orsmond, G.; Bolt, D. The relative risk and timing of divorce in families of children with an autism spectrum disorder. *J. Fam. Psychol.* **2010**, *24*, 449–457. [CrossRef]
30. Chan, K.K.S.; Leung, D.C.K. The Impact of Child Autistic Symptoms on Parental Marital Relationship: Parenting and Coparenting Processes as Mediating Mechanisms. *Autism Res.* **2020**, *13*, 1516–1526. [CrossRef]
31. Saini, M.; Stoddart, K.P.; Gibson, M.; Morris, R.; Barrett, D.; Muskat, B.; Nicholas, D.; Rampton, G.; Zwaigenbaum, L. Couple relationships among parents of children and adolescents with Autism Spectrum Disorder: Findings from a scoping review of the literature. *Res. Autism Spectr. Disord.* **2015**, *17*, 142–157. [CrossRef]
32. Weitlauf, A.S.; McPheeters, M.L.; Peters, B.; Sathe, N.; Travis, R.; Aiello, R.; Williamson, E.; Veenstra-VanderWeele, J.; Krishnaswami, S.; Jerome, R.; et al. *Therapies for Children with Autism Spectrum Disorder: Behavioral Interventions Update*; Agency for Healthcare Research and Quality: Rockville, MD, USA, 2014; Report No. 14-EHC036-EF. [PubMed]
33. Kersh, J.; Hedvat, T.T.; Hauser-Cram, P.; Warfield, M.E. The contribution of marital quality to the well-being of parents of children with developmental disabilities. *J. Intellect. Disabil. Res.* **2006**, *50*, 883–893. [CrossRef]
34. Brobst, J.B.; Clopton, J.R.; Hendrick, S.S. Parenting children with Autism Spectrum Disorders: The couple's relationship. *Focus Autism Other Dev. Disabil.* **2009**, *24*, 38–49. [CrossRef]
35. Sameroff, A.J. *The Transactional Model of Development: How Children and Contexts Shape Each Other*; American Psychological Association: Washington, DC, USA, 2009. [CrossRef]
36. Baker, B.L.; McIntyre, L.L.; Blacher, J.; Crnic, K.; Edelbrock, C.; Low, C. Pre-school children with and without developmental delay: Behaviour problems and parenting stress over time. *J. Intellect. Disabil. Res.* **2003**, *47*, 217–230. [CrossRef] [PubMed]

https://doi.org/10.3390/children13010053

37. Neece, C.L.; Green, S.A.; Baker, B.L. Parenting stress and child behavior problems: A transactional relationship across time. *Am. J. Intellect. Dev. Disabil.* **2012**, *117*, 48–66. [CrossRef] [PubMed]
38. Neece, C.L. Mindfulness-based stress reduction for parents of young children with developmental delays: Implications for parental mental health and child behavior problems. *J. Appl. Res. Intellect. Disabil.* **2014**, *27*, 174–186. [CrossRef]
39. Neece, C.L.; Baker, B. Predicting maternal parenting stress in middle childhood: The roles of child intellectual status, behavior problems, and social skills. *J. Intellect. Disabil. Res.* **2008**, *52*, 1114–1128. [CrossRef]
40. Baker, J.K.; Messinger, D.S.; Lyons, K.K.; Grantz, C.J. A pilot study of maternal sensitivity in the context of emergent autism. *J. Autism Dev. Disord.* **2010**, *40*, 988–999. [CrossRef]
41. Li, X.; Wang, Q.; Wu, Y.; Wang, S.; Huang, Y.; Li, T. Personality Characteristics and Neurocognitive Functions in Parents of Children with Autism Spectrum Disorder. *Shanghai Arch. Psychiatry* **2017**, *29*, 41–47. [CrossRef]
42. Wolff, S.; Narayan, S.; Moyes, B. Personality characteristics of parents of autistic children: A controlled study. *J. Child Psychol. Psychiatry* **1988**, *29*, 143–153. [CrossRef]
43. Pottie, C.G.; Ingram, K.M. Daily stress, coping, and wellbeing in parents of children with autism: A multilevel modeling approach. *J. Fam. Psychol.* **2008**, *22*, 855–864. [CrossRef]
44. Benson, P.R.; Karlof, K.L. Anger, stress proliferation, and depressed mood among parents of children with ASD: A longitudinal replication. *J. Autism Dev. Disord.* **2009**, *39*, 350–362. [CrossRef]
45. Smith, B.W.; Tooley, E.M.; Christopher, P.J.; Kay, V.S. Resilience as the ability to bounce back from stress: A neglected personal resource? *J. Posit. Psychol.* **2010**, *5*, 166–176. [CrossRef]
46. Phelps, K.W.; McCammon, S.L.; Wuensch, K.L.; Golden, J.A. Enrichment, stress, and growth from parenting an individual with an autism spectrum disorder. *J. Intellect. Dev. Disabil.* **2009**, *34*, 133–141. [CrossRef] [PubMed]
47. Haddock, L.R. Third-wave cognitive behavioral theories with mindfulness-based interventions. In *Counseling and Psychotherapy: Theories and Interventions*, 7th ed.; Capuzzi, D., Stauffer, M.D., Eds.; American Counseling Association: Alexandria, VA, USA, 2022; pp. 217–236.
48. Hayes, S.C.; Hofmann, S.G. "Third-wave" cognitive and behavioral therapies and the emergence of a process-based approach to intervention in psychiatry. *World Psychiatry* **2021**, *20*, 363–375. [CrossRef] [PubMed]
49. Whittingham, K. Parents of children with disabilities, mindfulness and acceptance: A review and a call for research. *Mindfulness* **2014**, *5*, 704–709. [CrossRef]
50. Kabat-Zinn, J. *Wherever You Go, There You Are: Mindfulness Meditation in Everyday Life*; Hyperion: New York, NY, USA, 1994.
51. Marlatt, G.A.; Kristeller, J.L. Mindfulness and meditation. In *Integrating Spirituality into Treatment: Resources for Practitioners*; Miller, W.R., Ed.; American Psychological Association: Washington, DC, USA, 1999; pp. 67–84. [CrossRef]
52. Davidson, R.J.; Kabat-Zinn, J.; Schumacher, J.; Rosenkranz, M.; Muller, D.; Santorelli, S.F.; Urbanowski, F.; Harrington, A.; Bonus, K.; Sheridan, J.F. Alterations in brain and immune function produced by mindfulness meditation. *Psychosom. Med.* **2003**, *65*, 564–570. [CrossRef]
53. Jha, A.P.; Stanley, E.A.; Kiyonaga, A.; Wong, L.; Gelfand, L. Examining the protective effects of mindfulness training on working memory capacity and affective experience. *Emotion* **2010**, *10*, 54–64. [CrossRef]
54. Bögels, S.M.; Lehtonen, A.; Restifo, K. Mindful parenting in mental health care. *Mindfulness* **2010**, *1*, 107–120. [CrossRef]
55. Singh, N.N.; Lancioni, G.E.; Winton, A.S.; Singh, J. Mindfulness training for parents and their children with ADHD increases the children's compliance. *J. Child Fam. Stud.* **2006**, *15*, 302–315. [CrossRef]
56. Segal, Z.V.; Williams, J.M.G.; Teasdale, J.D. *Mindfulness-Based Cognitive Therapy for Depression: A New Approach to Preventing Relapse*; Guilford Press: New York, NY, USA, 2002.
57. Segal, Z.V.; Williams, J.M.G.; Teasdale, J.D. *The Mindful Way Workbook: An 8-Week Program to Free Yourself from Depression and Emotional Distress*; Guilford Press: New York, NY, USA, 2014.
58. Bailie, C.; Smith, S.; Garbutt, J. Mindfulness-based cognitive therapy for parents of children with autism spectrum disorders: A qualitative evaluation. *J. Child Fam. Stud.* **2011**, *20*, 347–357.
59. Kabat-Zinn, J.; Kabat-Zinn, M. *Everyday Blessings: The Inner Work of Mindful Parenting*; Hachette Books: New York, NY, USA, 2014.
60. Bögels, S.; Hellemans, J.; van Deursen, S.; Römer, M.; van der Meulen, R. Mindful parenting in mental health care: Effects on parental and child psychopathology, parental stress, parenting, co-parenting, and marital functioning. *Mindfulness* **2010**, *1*, 107–120. [CrossRef]
61. Bögels, S.M.; Hoogstad, B.; van Dun, L.; de Schutter, S.; Restifo, K. Mindfulness training for adolescents with externalizing disorders, and their parents. *Behav. Cogn. Psychother.* **2008**, *36*, 1–17. [CrossRef]
62. van der Oord, S.; Bögels, S.M.; Peijnenburg, D. The effectiveness of mindfulness training for children with ADHD and mindful parenting for their parents. *J. Child Fam. Stud.* **2012**, *21*, 139–147. [CrossRef] [PubMed]
63. Beer, J.; Fernández, S.; Slusarchuk, C. Mindful parenting and maternal well-being in parents of children with autism spectrum disorder. *Mindfulness* **2013**, *4*, 220–233. [CrossRef]

https://doi.org/10.3390/children13010053

64. Conner, C.M.; White, S.W. Stress in mothers of children with autism: Trait mindfulness as a protective factor. *Res. Autism Spectr. Disord.* **2014**, *8*, 617–624. [CrossRef]
65. Faul, F.; Erdfelder, E.; Buchner, A.; Lang, A.-G. Statistical power analyses using G*Power 3.1: Tests for correlation and regression analyses. *Behav. Res. Methods* **2009**, *41*, 1149–1160. [CrossRef]
66. Lovibond, S.H.; Lovibond, P.F. *Manual for the Depression Anxiety Stress Scales*, 2nd ed.; Psychology Foundation of Australia: Sydney, Australia, 1995.
67. Rayan, A.; Ahmad, M. Mindfulness and parenting distress among parents of children with disabilities: The mediating role of parental self-efficacy. *Res. Dev. Disabil.* **2017**, *69*, 52–61.
68. Tellegen, C.L.; Sanders, M.R. A randomized controlled trial evaluating a brief parenting program with children with autism spectrum disorders. *J. Consult. Clin. Psychol.* **2014**, *82*, 1193–1200. [CrossRef]
69. Lyrakos, G.N.; Arvaniti, C.; Smyrnioti, M.; Kostopanagiotou, G. Translation and validation study of the Depression Anxiety Stress Scale in the Greek general population and in a psychiatric patient's sample. *Eur. Psychiatry* **2011**, *26*, 1731. [CrossRef]
70. Diener, E.; Emmons, R.A.; Larsen, R.J.; Griffin, S. The Satisfaction With Life Scale. *J. Pers. Assess.* **1985**, *49*, 71–75. [CrossRef]
71. Lyrakos, G.N.; Xatziagelaki, E.; Papazafiropoulou, A.K.; Batistaki, C.; Damigos, D.; Mathianakis, G.; Spinaris, V. Translation and validation study of the Satisfaction With Life Scale (SWLS) in the Greek general population, diabetes mellitus, and patients with emotional disorders. *Eur. Psychiatry* **2013**, *28*, 1. [CrossRef]
72. Watson, D.; Clark, L.A.; Tellegen, A. Development and validation of brief measures of positive and negative affect: The PANAS scales. *J. Pers. Soc. Psychol.* **1988**, *54*, 1063–1070. [CrossRef] [PubMed]
73. Benn, R.; Akiva, T.; Arel, S.; Roeser, R.W. Mindfulness training effects for parents and educators of children with special needs. *Dev. Psychol.* **2012**, *48*, 1476–1487. [CrossRef] [PubMed]
74. Daskalou, V.; Sigkollitou, E. Positive and Negative Affect Scale (PANAS). In *Psychometric Instruments in Greece*, 2nd ed.; Stalikas, A., Triliva, S., Roussi, P., Eds.; Pedio: Athens, Greece, 2012; p. 526.
75. Duncan, L.G.; Coatsworth, J.D.; Greenberg, M.T. A model of mindful parenting: Implications for parent–child relationships and prevention research. *Clin. Child Fam. Psychol. Rev.* **2009**, *12*, 255–270. [CrossRef] [PubMed]
76. George, D.; Mallery, P. *SPSS for Windows Step by Step: A Simple Guide and Reference*, 10th ed.; Pearson/Allyn & Bacon: Boston, MA, USA, 2010.
77. Hair, J.F.; Black, W.C.; Babin, B.J.; Anderson, R.E.; Tatham, R.L. *Multivariate Data Analysis*, 8th ed.; Cengage Learning: Andover, UK, 2019.
78. Cengiz, M.; Kılıç, D. The effects of mindfulness-based self-compassion training on stress, psychological resilience, and well-being in parents of autistic children: A randomized controlled study. *Curr. Psychol.* **2025**, *advance online publication*. [CrossRef]
79. Alibekova, R.; Chan, C.K.; Crape, B.; Kadyrzhanuly, K.; Gusmanov, A.; An, S.; Bulekbayeva, S.; Akhmetzhanova, Z.; Ainabekova, A.; Yerubayev, Z.; et al. Stress, anxiety and depression in parents of children with autism spectrum disorders in Kazakhstan: Prevalence and associated factors. *Global Ment. Health* **2022**, *9*, 472–482. [CrossRef]
80. Bazzano, A.; Wolfe, C.; Zylowska, L.; Wang, S.; Schuster, E.; Barrett, C. Mindfulness-based stress reduction (MBSR) for parents and caregivers of individuals with developmental disabilities: A community-based approach. *J. Child Fam. Stud.* **2015**, *24*, 298–308. [CrossRef]
81. Lunsky, Y.; Albaum, C.; Baskin, A.; Hastings, R.P.; Hutton, S.; Steel, L.; Wang, W.; Weiss, J. Group Virtual Mindfulness-Based Intervention for Parents of Autistic Adolescents and Adults. *J. Autism Dev. Disord.* **2021**, *51*, 3959–3969. [CrossRef]
82. Teasdale, J.D.; Segal, Z.V.; Williams, J.M.G.; Ridgeway, V.A.; Soulsby, J.M.; Lau, M.A. Prevention of relapse/recurrence in major depression by mindfulness-based cognitive therapy. *J. Consult. Clin. Psychol.* **2000**, *68*, 615–623. [CrossRef]
83. Ma, S.H.; Teasdale, J.D. Mindfulness-based cognitive therapy for depression: Replication and exploration of differential relapse prevention effects. *J. Consult. Clin. Psychol.* **2004**, *72*, 31–40. [CrossRef]
84. Greenberg, J.; Reiner, K.; Meiran, N. "Mind the trap": Mindfulness practice reduces cognitive rigidity. *PLoS ONE* **2012**, *7*, e36206. [CrossRef]
85. Azizi, M.; Sanaat, Z.; Jafarnejad, F.; Dadkhah, F. Increasing the tolerance of mothers with children with autism: The effectiveness of cognitive therapy based on mindfulness—Experimental research. *Ann. Med. Surg.* **2023**, *86*, 207–211. [CrossRef] [PubMed]
86. Sommerhoff, A.; Ehring, T.; Takano, K. Effects of induced mindfulness at night on repetitive negative thinking: Ecological momentary assessment study. *JMIR Ment. Health* **2023**, *10*, e44365. [CrossRef] [PubMed]
87. Hick, S.F.; Chan, L. Mindfulness-Based Cognitive Therapy for Depression: Effectiveness and Limitations. *Soc. Work Ment. Health* **2010**, *8*, 225–237. [CrossRef]
88. Cachia, R.L.; Anderson, A.; Moore, D.W. Mindfulness, stress and well-being in parents of children with autism spectrum disorder: A systematic review. *J. Child Fam. Stud.* **2016**, *25*, 1–14. [CrossRef]
89. Bluth, K.; Wahler, R.G. Does effort matter in mindful parenting? *Mindfulness* **2011**, *2*, 175–178. [CrossRef]
90. Lo, H.H.M.; Chan, S.K.C.; Szeto, M.P.; Chan, C.Y.H.; Choi, C.W. A feasibility study of a brief mindfulness-based program for parents of preschool children with developmental disabilities. *Mindfulness* **2017**, *8*, 1665–1673. [CrossRef]

https://doi.org/10.3390/children13010053

91. Burgdorf, W.; Szabó, M.; Abbott, M.J. Mindful parenting: A meta-analytic review of effects on parents, children, and parenting. *Clin. Psychol. Rev.* **2019**, *75*, 101799.
92. Singh, N.N.; Lancioni, G.E.; Karazsia, B.T.; Myers, R.E.; Hwang, Y.S.; Anālayo, B. Effects of mindfulness-based positive behavior support training are equally beneficial for mothers and their children with autism spectrum disorder or with intellectual disabilities. *Front. Psychol.* **2019**, *10*, 385. [CrossRef]
93. Weitlauf, A.S.; Vehorn, A.C.; Taylor, J.L.; Hampton, L.H. A pilot study of a remote parent-mediated early intervention for children with autism. *Autism* **2020**, *24*, 1288–1301. [CrossRef]
94. Cheung, R.Y.M.; Chan, S.K.C.; Chui, H.; Chan, W.M.; Ngai, S.Y.S. Enhancing parental well-being: Initial efficacy of a 21-day online self-help mindfulness-based intervention for parents. *Mindfulness* **2022**, *13*, 2812–2826. [CrossRef]
95. Garland, E.L.; Farb, N.A.; Goldin, P.R.; Fredrickson, B.L. The mindfulness-to-meaning theory: Extensions, applications, and challenges at the attention–appraisal–emotion interface. *Psychol. Inq.* **2015**, *26*, 377–387. [CrossRef]
96. Kunimatsu, M.M.; Marsee, M.A. Examining the presence of anxiety in aggressive individuals: The illuminating role of fight-or-flight mechanisms. *Child Youth Care Forum* **2012**, *41*, 247–258. [CrossRef]
97. Harnett, P.H.; Whittingham, K.; Puhakka, E.; Hodges, J.; Spry, C.; Dob, R. The short-term impact of a brief group-based mindfulness therapy program on depression and life satisfaction. *Mindfulness* **2010**, *1*, 183–188. [CrossRef]
98. Zhang, L. Mindfulness-based interventions and life satisfaction among parents of children with developmental disorders: A systematic review. *Int. J. Environ. Res. Public Health* **2023**, *20*, 2018. [CrossRef]
99. Alvarado-García, P.A.A.; Soto-Vásquez, M.R.; Infantes Gomez, F.M.; Guzman Rodriguez, N.M.; Castro-Paniagua, W.G. Effect of a mindfulness program on stress, anxiety, depression, sleep quality, social support, and life satisfaction: A quasi-experimental study in college students. *Front. Psychol.* **2025**, *16*, 1508934. [CrossRef]
100. Li, X.; Ma, L.; Li, Q. How mindfulness affects life satisfaction: Based on the mindfulness-to-meaning theory. *Front. Psychol.* **2022**, *13*, 887940. [CrossRef]
101. Extremera, N.; Rey, L. Ability emotional intelligence and life satisfaction: Positive and negative affect as mediators. *Pers. Individ. Dif.* **2016**, *102*, 98–101. [CrossRef]
102. Hölzel, B.K.; Carmody, J.; Vangel, M.; Congleton, C.; Yerramsetti, S.M.; Gard, T.; Lazar, S.W. Mindfulness practice leads to increases in regional brain gray matter density. *Psychiatry Res. Neuroimaging* **2011**, *191*, 36–43. [CrossRef]
103. Zheng, M.; Hong, T.; Zhou, H.; Garland, E.L.; Hu, Y. The acute effect of mindfulness-based regulation on neural indices of cue-induced craving in smokers. *Addict. Behav.* **2024**, *159*, 108134. [CrossRef]
104. Laurent, H.K.; Duncan, L.G.; Lightcap, A.; Khan, F. Mindful parenting predicts mothers' and infants' hypothalamic–pituitary–adrenal activity during a dyadic stressor. *Dev. Psychol.* **2017**, *53*, 417–424. [CrossRef]
105. Bergen-Cico, D.; Possemato, K.; Pigeon, W. Reductions in cortisol associated with primary care brief mindfulness program for veterans with PTSD. *Med. Care* **2014**, *52*, S25–S31. [CrossRef]
106. González-Martín, A.M.; Aibar-Almazán, A.; Rivas-Campo, Y.; Castellote-Caballero, Y.; Carcelén-Fraile, M.D.C. Mindfulness to improve the mental health of university students: A systematic review and meta-analysis. *Front. Public Health* **2023**, *11*, 1284632. [CrossRef] [PubMed]
107. Ruiz-Robledillo, N.; Moya-Albiol, L. Emotional intelligence modulates cortisol awakening response and self-reported health in caregivers of people with autism spectrum disorders. *Res. Autism Spectr. Disord.* **2014**, *8*, 1535–1543. [CrossRef]
108. Ahmed, A.N.; Raj, S.P. Self-compassion intervention for parents of children with developmental disabilities: A feasibility study. *Adv. Neurodev. Disord.* **2023**, *7*, 277–289. [CrossRef] [PubMed]
109. Ferraioli, S.; Harris, S.L. The impact of mindfulness-based interventions on the well-being of parents of children with autism spectrum disorders: A review. *Res. Autism Spectr. Disord.* **2013**, *7*, 1318–1331.
110. Chan, N.; Neece, C.L. Parenting stress and emotion dysregulation among children with developmental delays: The role of parenting behaviors. *J. Child Fam. Stud.* **2018**, *27*, 4071–4082. [CrossRef]
111. Button, K.S.; Ioannidis, J.P.; Mokrysz, C.; Nosek, B.A.; Flint, J.; Robinson, E.S.; Munafo, M.R. Power failure: Why small sample size undermines the reliability of neuroscience. *Nat. Rev. Neurosci.* **2013**, *14*, 365–376. [CrossRef]
112. Mo, Y.; Lei, Z.; Chen, M.; Deng, H.; Liang, R.; Yu, M.; Huang, H. Effects of self-help mindfulness-based cognitive therapy on mindfulness, symptom change, and suicidal ideation in patients with depression: A randomized controlled study. *Front. Psychol.* **2023**, *14*, 1287891. [CrossRef]
113. Meppelink, R.; de Bruin, E.I.; Wanders-Mulder, F.H.; Vennik, C.J.; Bögels, S.M. Mindful Parenting Training in Child Psychiatric Settings: Heightened Parental Mindfulness Reduces Parents' and Children's Psychopathology. *Mindfulness* **2016**, *7*, 680–689. [CrossRef]
114. Mann, J.; Kuyken, W.; O'Mahen, H.; Ukoumunne, O.C.; Evans, A.; Ford, T. Manual Development and Pilot Randomised Controlled Trial of Mindfulness-Based Cognitive Therapy Versus Usual Care for Parents with a History of Depression. *Mindfulness* **2016**, *7*, 1024–1033. [CrossRef]

115. De Los Reyes, A.; Kazdin, A.E. Informant discrepancies in the assessment of childhood psychopathology: A critical review, theoretical framework, and recommendations for further study. *Psychol. Bull.* **2005**, *131*, 483–509. [CrossRef]
116. Kuhlthau, K.; Payakachat, N.; Delahaye, J.; Hurson, J.; Pyne, J.M.; Kovacs, E.; Tilford, J.M. Quality of life for parents of children with autism spectrum disorders. *Res. Autism Spectr. Disord.* **2014**, *8*, 1339–1350. [CrossRef]
117. Kabat-Zinn, J.; Kabat-Zinn, M. *Mindful Parenting: Guide to Raising Compassionate Kids*; Piatkus: London, UK, 2021.

https://doi.org/10.3390/children13010053

children

MDPI

Article

Parental Burnout and Early-Childhood Behavioral Problems: Longitudinal Associations Beyond Maternal Depression

Anna Suarez [1,*] and Vera Yakupova [1,2]

[1] Faculty of Psychology, Lomonosov Moscow State University, 125009 Moscow, Russia; vera.yakupova@msupress.com
[2] Federal Science Center of Psychological and Interdisciplinary Research, 125009 Moscow, Russia
* Correspondence: anna.suarez.fig@msupress.com

Highlights

What are the main findings?

- This was a 3-year follow-up study investigating the distinct adverse effect of parental burnout on child development while controlling for maternal depression.
- Parental burnout was significantly associated with child internalizing and externalizing problems, independently of postpartum or present maternal depression at the dimensional level, even though associations with borderline/clinically significant outcomes were attenuated once overlapping maternal mental health factors were considered.

What are the implication of the main findings?

- Parental burnout presents a unique risk factor for child adverse outcomes in toddlerhood, distinct from maternal depression, which requires further research.
- It is crucial to recognize and support families where parents are experiencing significant burnout and caregiving-related exhaustion, particularly in contexts of limited social and institutional resources, regardless of the presence of a formal mental health diagnosis.

Abstract

Background: Parenting is increasingly recognized as a highly demanding and stressful role that, in the absence of sufficient resources, may lead to parental burnout (PB). This risk may be particularly pronounced in the Russian context, where limited access to childcare for children under three and reduced extended family support coincide with strong social expectations of intensive parenting. Although PB and maternal depression frequently co-occur, it remains unclear whether PB exerts a unique influence on child development, especially during toddlerhood. The present study examined the association between PB and behavioral problems in children aged 1.5 to 4 years while controlling for maternal depression assessed both during the first year postpartum and concurrently with PB. Methods: Using a longitudinal design, maternal mental health was assessed within the first 12 months postpartum (Stage 1) and again at follow-up (Stage 2), on average 2.24 years later, in 419 Russian mother–child dyads. Mothers completed measures of postpartum depression (PPD) (Edinburgh Postnatal Depression Scale), current depressive symptoms (Beck Depression Inventory-II), and PB (Parental Burnout Inventory). Child emotional and behavioral problems were assessed at Stage 2 using the Russian version of the Child Behavior Checklist (CBCL/1½–5). Results: Mothers of children with borderline/clinically significant internalizing, externalizing, and total problems had significantly higher PB, PPD, and present maternal depressive symptoms, although the effect sizes were small. PB

 https://doi.org/10.3390/children13020176

was strongly associated with all domains of child behavioral problems, also after correction for both postpartum and present depressive symptoms, as well as for other important covariates. Higher maternal PB symptoms further increased the odds of children having borderline/clinically significant internalizing and externalizing problems, although those effects were not independent of maternal depression. In turn, neither postpartum nor present maternal depressive symptoms were associated with any of the child behavioral problems domains. Conclusions: PB represents a distinct and clinically relevant risk factor for emotional and behavioral problems in toddlers, beyond the effects of maternal postpartum or present depression, in a context characterized by high caregiving demands and limited institutional support. These findings highlight an urgent need for programs aimed at identifying and supporting families in which parents experience high levels of exhaustion, regardless of whether they meet the criteria for other diagnosable mental health disorders. Addressing PB during toddlerhood may be critical for protecting both parental well-being and early child development.

Keywords: parental burnout; postpartum depression; maternal depression; child development; behavioral problems; internalizing problems; externalizing problems

1. Introduction

1.1. Background

Parenting is widely regarded as one of the most valuable human experiences, yet it is increasingly acknowledged as a demanding role accompanied by persistent stress. This phenomenon is often observed in Western cultures, where individualistic values foster heightened expectations of parents [1]. When these expectations exceed the resources available to parents, they may develop symptoms of parental burnout (PB). PB is characterized by physical and mental exhaustion, including somatic complaints and sleep disturbances, emotional distancing from children, and feelings of inadequacy in fulfilling parental responsibilities [2]. Preliminary investigations have identified various consequences of PB, such as escape ideations, suicidal thoughts, sleep disorders, addictions, marital conflicts, and instances of child abuse or neglect [3]. Factors contributing to PB include unrealistic expectations of parenting, insufficient support from partners or caregivers, and particular parental or child personality traits, such as high neuroticism [3,4].

The distinction between burnout and depression remains debated due to overlapping symptoms and diagnostic challenges, including sleep problems, substance use, somatic health issues, and relational conflicts [5–7]. However, several studies indicate that these constructs are related yet distinct. Specifically, low to moderate correlations have been reported between PB, work-related burnout, parental stress, and depressive mood [4,8]. Emerging evidence further suggests that the symptoms and consequences of PB and parental depression differ substantially [9,10]. Unlike depressive symptoms, PB is strongly associated with low parental satisfaction, neglect, and violence toward children [3] and appears to primarily affect family dynamics, whereas depression has broader impacts across multiple life domains [9]. These findings underscore the need for further research to clarify PB's unique implications for parental and child well-being.

Most PB studies have focused on mothers, who are often regarded as primary caregivers, particularly during the postpartum period [11,12]. Séjourné et al. identified a significant association between maternal burnout and a history of postpartum depression (PPD) [13]. Their findings also linked PB to anxiety, perceptions of a child as difficult, dissatisfaction with work–life balance, and parental stress. These results are consistent with

https://doi.org/10.3390/children13020176

cross-sectional studies conducted on 560 mothers in China and 1300 French-speaking mothers, both of which reported a positive association between PPD and PB [12,14]. However, longitudinal research examining depressive symptoms during both the postpartum period and later stages of parenthood in relation to PB remains limited.

PB affects not only parental well-being but also child development. Two studies from Russia found a positive association between PB and preschoolers' emotional and cognitive development, reporting improved executive functions and emotional comprehension skills in children of mothers with higher PB symptoms, independent of maternal depression [15,16]. Conversely, other studies have linked higher PB symptoms to increased internalizing and externalizing problems in Chilean preschoolers [17] and Chinese adolescents [11]. These discrepancies may reflect cultural differences in norms of intensive, child-centered parenting, as well as developmental stages, with PB potentially signaling overinvestment among Russian preschool mothers but reduced emotional availability and harsher parenting in other sociocultural contexts and at later ages. Therefore, further studies are warranted to explore the relationship between PB and child mental health problems during different stages of development and cultural contexts.

1.2. *Russia-Specific Context*

According to international consortium data, Russia is considered a country with high risks for PB exposure [1]. Consistent with the broader literature that has largely focused on parents of children aged four and older [17–19], Russian studies to date have been limited to parents of preschoolers [15,16] and primary school children [20]. Consequently, little is known about PB symptoms among Russian parents of toddlers.

The present study addresses this gap by focusing on the well-being of parents of toddlers, thereby extending knowledge on PB and its relation to child development in the earliest years. Russian parents may be particularly vulnerable to PB during toddlerhood, as this stage combines structural challenges—such as limited extended family support and the absence of free childcare for children under age three [21]—with increasing social pressures toward intensive parenting and high standards of "good parenting" [20,22].

1.3. *Aims of the Study*

Building on evidence that PB represents a parenting-specific form of distress with potential implications for early child development [23], the present study examines the association between maternal PB and socioemotional and behavioral problems in children aged 1.5 to 4 years, a sensitive developmental period. Using a longitudinal design, we aimed to assess whether PB is associated with child internalizing, externalizing, and total behavioral problems independently of maternal depressive symptoms assessed both during the first year postpartum and concurrently at follow-up. We hypothesized that higher levels of PB would be associated with greater child behavioral problems across all domains, beyond the effects of postpartum and current maternal depression.

2. Materials and Methods

2.1. *Procedure and Participants*

The present study employed a longitudinal design. At Stage 1, data collection occurred in two waves: February–March 2020 and February–March 2021. Participants were recruited through multiple channels, including childbirth education courses, maternity care providers (such as physicians and midwives), online forums and social media groups for expectant and new parents, and perinatal health professionals. Altogether, 2256 Russian women completed the online survey across these two time points.

https://doi.org/10.3390/children13020176

Eligibility criteria required that participants be at least 18 years old, literate in Russian, have given birth to a live infant within the past 12 months, and that the delivery occurred in Russia. The data was collected from different regions of Russia (Central region, Ural, Tatarstan, North and South regions), predominantly from big cities, i.e., Moscow, St. Petersburg, Ekaterinburg, Kazan, Novosibirsk, Ufa, Krasnodar.

Between August 2022 and July 2023, those who had previously participated and expressed interest in being contacted for continuous participation in the study were contacted via email and invited to join the follow-up phase (Stage 2). Respondents were mailed printed questionnaires. Stage 2 focused on assessing maternal mental health and child developmental outcomes 1.5–4 years after childbirth. Of the original cohort, 589 women returned the completed follow-up forms. Following data verification procedures—including matching Stage 1 and Stage 2 identifiers, removing duplicates, and excluding incomplete responses—419 mother–child dyads with complete datasets were retained for analysis. The retention rate was 18.5%. There were no statistically significant differences between women who chose to participate at Stage 2 of the study and those who did not in terms of EPDS scores, maternal age, marital status, mode of birth, and child gestational age at birth (p-values for all > 0.41). There were statistically significant differences in the levels of education (with slightly more women with higher education among the participants who answered at Stage 2 (90.8% vs. 95.5%, $p = 0.010$), child medical complications during pregnancy/childbirth (with mothers who participated at Stage 2 reporting their children having medical complications during pregnancy/childbirth more often (14.6% vs. 20.5%, $p = 0.023$), and parity (there were more first-time mothers among those who participated at Stage 2 (52.5% vs. 60.1%, $p = 0.020$).

The Ethical Committee of the Russian Psychological Society at Lomonosov Moscow State University approved the present study (No: 345/2019, 6 December 2021). All participants provided their informed consent using the online tool Testograph prior to filling in the survey. The study was conducted in accordance with the Declaration of Helsinki.

2.2. Measures

2.2.1. The Demographic Questionnaire

The online survey included questions regarding the participants' age at the time of testing, highest achieved level of education (primary/secondary or tertiary) and marital status (married/cohabiting with partner or single/divorced), gestational age at childbirth, the number of children in a family, mode of birth (vaginal (assisted vaginal)/cesarean (planned/emergency)), and perceived socioeconomic status in comparisons to other residents of their current region (low/middle/high). We also collected the data about the child's age at Stage 2 and the child's complications during pregnancy/childbirth (yes/no).

2.2.2. Parental Burnout

We used the Russian version of the Parental Burnout Inventory (PBI) [24,25] to analyze the level of maternal PB. The PBI is a 23-item questionnaire assessing four core symptoms of PB: emotional exhaustion (9 items; e.g., I feel completely run down by my role as a parent), contrast with previous parental self (6 items; e.g., I tell myself I'm no longer the parent I used to be), loss of pleasure in one's parental role (5 items; e.g., I do not enjoy being with my children), and emotional distancing from one's children (3 items; e.g., I am no longer able to show my children that I love them) [24]. The participants were asked to assess each statement using a seven-point frequency scale ranging from 0 to 6 (never, a few times a year, once a month or less, a few times a month, once a week, a few times a week, every day). The PB score is computed by summing the item scores: higher scores reflect higher parental burnout levels. The cut-off point for PB is 74 [26]. The internal consistency

https://doi.org/10.3390/children13020176

of the Russian version of the scale was Cronbach's alpha α = 0.97 [25], Cronbach's alpha for this sample was α = 0.98.

2.2.3. Edinburgh Postnatal Depression Scale

The Russian version (Cronbach's α = 0.84) of the Edinburgh Postnatal Depression Scale (EPDS) was used to estimate PPD symptoms [27,28]. It is a 10-item questionnaire scale rated on a 4-point Likert scale, ranging from 0 to 3, which indicates how the mother has felt during the previous week. A score of 10 and higher is considered to indicate clinically significant symptoms of depression [27]. Cronbach's alpha for the study sample was α = 0.88.

2.2.4. Beck Depression Inventory

The Russian version of the Beck Depression Inventory (BDI-II) was used to assess the levels of parental depression [29,30]. The BDI-II is a 21-item, self-report questionnaire measuring symptoms of depression [29]. Items are scored on a scale from 0 to 3, ranging from 0: "I do not feel guilty," 1: "I often feel guilty", and 2: "I feel guilty most of the time," to 3: "I feel guilty all the time". The depression score is obtained by summing the 21 item scores, with a score of 20 and higher indicating moderate and severe symptoms of depression [29]. For the Russian version, Cronbach's coefficient is α = 0.87 [30], with Cronbach's coefficient α = 0.89 in this sample.

2.2.5. Child Behavior Problems and Emotional Development

To study emotional and behavioral problems in children, the Russian version of the Child Behavior Checklist (CBCL/1½–5) was used [31,32]. It includes 99 statements describing various deviations in the behavior and emotional state of children. The child's parent marks each statement as incorrect (0), sometimes true or partially true (1), or very true (2). The raw scores were translated into T-scores, with $T \geq 65$ indicating a borderline level of severity of the problem and $T \geq 70$ corresponding to a clinical level of behavioral problems [31]. The CBCL/1½–5 behavior checklist evaluates three domains of behavioral problems: internalizing (emotional reactivity, anxiety/depression, somatic complaints, withdrawn symptoms), externalizing (attention problems, aggressive behavior), and total problems. Furthermore, there are five DSM-oriented scales (depressive problems, anxiety problems, autism spectrum problems, attention deficit/hyperactivity problems, oppositional defiant problems) that reflect psychological and behavioral syndromes aligned with diagnostic categories from the Diagnostic and Statistical Manual of Mental Disorders (DSM-V) [31]. The internal validity of the three domain scales in the Russian version is Cronbach's α = 0.91, α = 0.94, and α = 0.97 for internalizing, externalizing, and total problems, respectively [32]. In the present sample, Cronbach's α = 0.82 for internalizing, α = 0.87 for externalizing, and α = 0.90 for total problems.

2.3. Covariates

Statistical models were adjusted for maternal age at testing, level of education, family status, socioeconomic status, the number of children in a family, mode of birth, gestational age at childbirth, child's complications during pregnancy/childbirth, and child's age at Stage 2 as covariates.

2.4. Statistical Analysis

For all the analyses, maternal depressive symptom scores (both postpartum and present) were square root-transformed, and PB and CBCL scores were log-transformed to attain normality; the symptom scores were further standardized to a mean of 0 and an SD of 1 to facilitate interpretation.

https://doi.org/10.3390/children13020176

Spearman correlation analysis was used to examine the correlation between raw PB scores, postpartum and present depressive symptoms, and child behavioral problems and DSM-oriented scales. Although variables were transformed for parametric modeling, Spearman rank-order correlations were retained for bivariate analyses because the measures represent symptom severity scales and did not fully meet normality assumptions even after transformation. Spearman correlations were therefore used as a conservative, distribution-free descriptive approach, while transformed variables were applied in subsequent parametric analyses.

A one-way ANOVA was used to explore association of maternal PB, PPD, and present depressive symptoms with CBCL scores. After transformation, assumptions for parametric analyses were formally evaluated. Homogeneity of variance was assessed using Levene's test and was supported for the transformed variables ($p = 0.96$). Normality was examined using skewness indices and visual inspection of residual distributions.

Multiple linear regression analysis examined the association of PB scores with continuous child behavioral problem scores (internalizing, externalizing, and total problems as well as DSM-oriented scales), while binary logistic regression tested the association between maternal PB and borderline/clinical levels of child internalizing, externalizing, and total problems (yes/no).

For both groups of parametric analyses four models were tested: Model 1 was adjusted for the covariates listed above. Model 2 was further adjusted for PPD symptoms, while Model 3 included the covariates from Model 1 and present maternal depressive symptoms.

All statistical analyses were conducted using SPSS software, version 27 (IBM Corp, NY, USA, 2020) [33].

3. Results

The demographic characteristics of the mothers and their children are presented in Table 1. The data indicate that the majority of mothers originate from middle-income families (58.9%), are married or have a partner (95.2%), have higher education (95.5%), and have one child (60.1%). Our sample further consisted of young children with a mean age of 2.24 years, most of whom had no reported complications during pregnancy or childbirth, although approximately one fifth experienced at least one complication (Table 1).

Table 1 shows that, among the participants, 10.3% of mothers reported clinically significant current depressive symptoms, while 35% showed clinically significant symptoms of PPD and 16.2% of mothers reported PBI scores above the cut-off point. PB scores were highly correlated with present depressive symptoms and moderately correlated with PPD (Spearman correlation coefficient = 0.65 and 0.36, respectively, $p < 0.001$ for both) (Supplemental Table S1).

Spearman correlation analysis further showed that all the CBCL scales correlated strongly with PB scores and with postpartum and present depressive symptoms ($p < 0.01$), with two exceptions: there was only a modest correlation between the DSM-oriented autism problems scale and present maternal depression (rho = 0.11, $p = 0.03$), while there was no significant correlation between the same CBCL scale and PPD symptoms (rho = 0.08, $p = 0.095$) (Supplemental Table S1).

One-way ANOVAs revealed statistically significant associations between PB, PPD, and current maternal depressive symptoms and all three domains of child behavioral problems. Specifically, PB scores were significantly higher among mothers of children with borderline/clinically significant internalizing ($F(1418) = 5.03$, $p = 0.025$), externalizing ($F(1418) = 7.35$, $p < 0.01$), but not total behavioral problems ($F(1418) = 3.22$, $p = 0.074$). Similarly, maternal PPD symptoms were significantly elevated in cases of child internalizing ($F(1418) = 8.18$, $p < 0.01$), externalizing ($F(1418) = 9.38$, $p < 0.01$), and total problems

https://doi.org/10.3390/children13020176

(F(1418) = 7.76, $p < 0.01$). Current maternal depressive symptoms were also significantly higher among mothers of children with borderline/clinically significant internalizing (F(1418) = 9.91, $p < 0.01$), externalizing (F(1418) = 8.12, $p < 0.01$), and total behavioral problems (F(1418) = 8.74, $p < 0.01$). Figure 1 illustrates these group differences. Importantly, the figure reflects untransformed scores of PBI, EPDS, and BDI-II scores for ease of clinical interpretation.

Table 1. Characteristics of the sample (N = 419).

Characteristics		Mean/N	SD/%	Range
	Parental characteristics			
Age (years)		33.34	4.29	23–49
Education	primary/secondary	19	4.5%	
	tertiary	400	95.5%	
Family status	married/cohabiting with a partner	399	95.2%	
	single/divorced	20	4.8%	
Gestational age at childbirth		39.36	1.92	27–42
The number of children in a family	1	252	60.1%	
	2	92	22.0%	
	3	49	11.7%	
	4	18	4.3%	
	5	4	1.0%	
	6	2	0.5%	
	7	2	0.5%	
Mode of birth	Vaginal (including medical interventions	300	71.6%	
	Cesarean (planned/emergency)	119	28.4%	
EPDS total score		9.23	6.01	0–29
Had clinically significant PPD symptoms (score ≥ 10)		148	35%	
BDI total score		8.99	7.66	0–39
Had clinically significant present maternal depressive symptoms (score ≥ 20)		43	10.3%	
PBI total score		39.82	33.51	0–138
PBI score above the cut-off point		68	16.2%	
	Child characteristics			
Age (years)		2.24	0.63	1.5–4
Child's complications during pregnancy/childbirth	No	329	78.5%	
	Yes	90	21.5%	
	CBCL checklist			
Internalizing problems		48.15	9.78	29–78
Had borderline/clinically significant internalizing problems (score ≥ 65)		23	5.5%	
Externalizing problems		48.92	8.96	28–80
Had borderline/clinically significant externalizing problems (score ≥ 65)		26	6.2%	
CBCL total score		49.35	9.24	28–76
Had borderline/clinically significant total behavioral problems (score ≥ 65)		22	5.3%	
	DSM-oriented scales			
Depressive problems		1.28	1.34	0–9
Anxiety problems		3.21	2.25	0–13
Autism spectrum problems		1.53	1.83	0–11
Attention deficit/Hyperactivity problems		4.57	2.52	0–12
Oppositional defiant problems		2.61	2.05	0–11

EPDS—Edinburgh Postnatal Depression Scale; PPD—postpartum depression; BDI—Beck Depression Inventory; PBI—Parental Burnout Inventory; CBCL—Child Behavior Checklist; DSM—Diagnostic and Statistical Manual of Mental Disorders.

Table 2 shows that PB is strongly associated with all the scales of child behavioral problems. Importantly, the association remains significant in the models additionally adjusted for both postpartum and present maternal depressive symptoms. In turn, neither PPD nor present maternal depression were significantly associated with any of the outcomes (Table 2).

https://doi.org/10.3390/children13020176

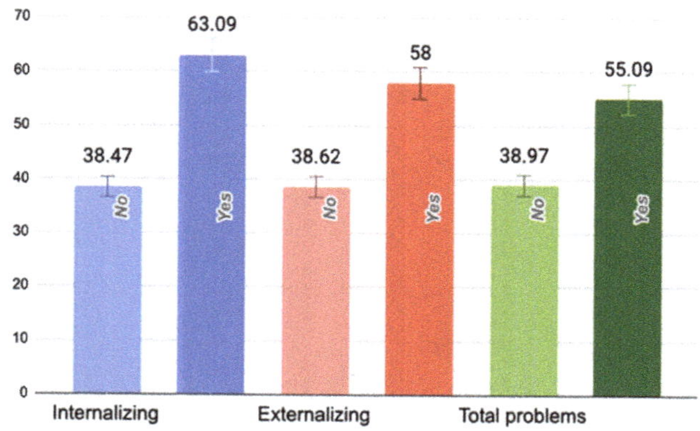

(**A**)

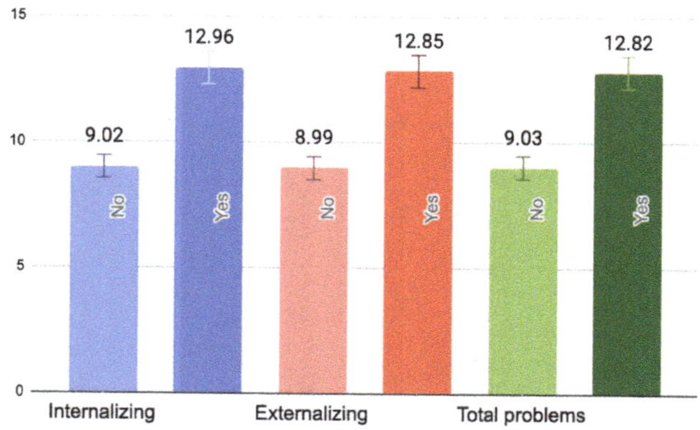

(**B**)

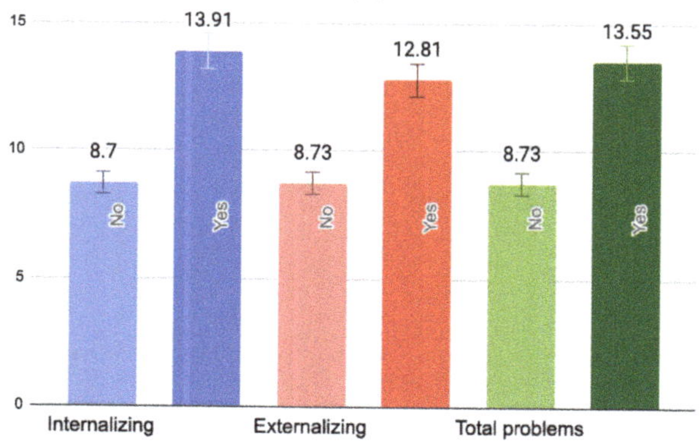

(**C**)

Figure 1. Mean levels of maternal parental burnout (**A**), postpartum depressive symptoms (**B**), and present maternal depressive symptoms (**C**) by child behavioral problem status. (**A**) Mean differences between parental burnout symptoms (raw PBI scores) in mothers of children with and without borderline/clinically significant behavioral problems. (**B**) Mean differences between postpartum depression symptoms (raw EPDS scores) in mothers of children with and without borderline/clinically significant

https://doi.org/10.3390/children13020176

behavioral problems. (**C**) Mean differences between present maternal depressive symptoms (raw BDI-II scores) in mothers of children with and without borderline/clinically significant behavioral problems.

Table 2. Multiple linear regression models: association between PB scores at Stage 2 and CBCL scores (Stage 2), excluding and including PPD (Stage 1) and present maternal depression (Stage 2).

Regression Models/Outcomes	β (95%CI)	β (95%CI)	Adjusted R^2
Model 1. Parental Burnout			
Internalizing problems	0.202 (0.109, 0.295) **		0.10
Externalizing problems	0.309 (0.219, 0.400) **		0.15
Total problems	0.294 (0.204, 0.384) **		0.15
DSM Depressive problems	0.211 (0.116, 0.305) **		0.07
DSM Anxiety problems	0.667 (0.457, 0.877) **		0.10
DSM Autism spectrum problems	0.147 (0.051, 0.242) **		0.05
DSM Attention deficit/hyperactivity problems	0.264 (0.172, 0.356) **		0.12
DSM Oppositional defiant problems	0.208 (0.117, 0.300) **		0.13
Model 2. Parental Burnout (PB) and Postpartum Depression (PPD)			
	PB	PPD	
Internalizing problems	0.181 (0.083, 0.279) **	0.067 (−0.033, 0.168)	0.10
Externalizing problems	0.301 (0.206, 0.397) **	0.025 (−0.073, 0.124)	0.14
Total problems	0.282 (0.187, 0.377) **	0.038 (−0.059, 0.136)	0.15
DSM Depressive problems	0.201 (0.101, 0.301) **	0.031 (−0.071, 0.134)	0.07
DSM Anxiety problems	0.619 (0.397, 0.840) **	0.153 (−0.074, 0.380)	0.10
DSM Autism spectrum problems	0.166 (0.065, 0.266) **	−0.060 (−0.163, 0.044)	0.05
DSM Attention deficit/hyperactivity problems	0.263 (0.165, 0.360) **	0.004 (−0.096, 0.104)	0.11
DSM Oppositional defiant problems	0.213 (0.116, 0.309) **	−0.015 (−0.114, 0.085)	0.13
Model 3. Parental Burnout (PB) and Present Maternal Depression			
	PB	Present Maternal Depression	
Internalizing problems	0.142 (0.030, 0.254) *	0.109 (−0.005, 0.223)	0.10
Externalizing problems	0.292 (0.183, 0.402) **	0.031 (−0.080, 0.143)	0.14
Total problems	0.243 (0.135, 0.352) **	0.092 (−0.019, 0.202)	0.16
DSM Depressive problems	0.150 (0.036, 0.264) **	0.110 (−0.006, 0.225)	0.08
DSM Anxiety problems	0.665 (0.411, 0.919) **	0.003 (−0.255, 0.262)	0.09
DSM Autism spectrum problems	0.149 (0.034, 0.265) *	-0.004 (−0.122, 0.113)	0.05
DSM Attention deficit/hyperactivity problems	0.283 (0.171, 0.394) **	−0.034 (−0.147, 0.079)	0.11
DSM Oppositional defiant problems	0.246 (0.135, 0.356) **	−0.068 (−0.18, 0.045)	0.13

Note. β—standardized regression coefficients from a multiple linear regression model; 95% CI—95% Confidence Interval; PB—parental burnout; PPD—postpartum depression. DSM—The Diagnostic and Statistical Manual of Mental Disorders. All models are adjusted for maternal age at testing, level of education, family status, socioeconomic status, the number of children in a family, mode of birth, gestational age at childbirth, child's complications during pregnancy/childbirth, and child age at Stage 2. * $p < 0.05$, ** $p < 0.001$.

Table 3 demonstrates statistically significant associations between PB and child borderline/clinically significant internalizing and externalizing behavioral problems. Specifically, higher levels of PB were associated with a 70% increase in the odds of internalizing problems (OR = 1.70, 95% CI [1.03, 2.82]) and a 74% increase in the odds of externalizing problems (OR = 1.74, 95% CI [1.05, 2.87]). These effect sizes indicate small-to-moderate associations. However, these associations were attenuated after adjustment for postpartum or current maternal depressive symptoms. In turn, neither postpartum nor present maternal depressive symptoms were associated with any of the child behavioral problems domains (Table 3).

https://doi.org/10.3390/children13020176

Table 3. Binary logistic regression models: association between PB scores at Stage 2 and child borderline/clinically significant child behavioral problems (Stage 2), excluding and including PPD (Stage 1) and present maternal depression (Stage 2).

Regression Models/Outcomes	OR (95% CI)	OR (95% CI)
Model 1. Parental Burnout		
Internalizing problems	1.70 (1.03, 2.82) *	
Externalizing problems	1.74 (1.05, 2.87) *	
Total problems	1.44 (0.87, 2.37)	
Model 2. Parental Burnout (PB) and Postpartum Depression (PPD)		
	PB	PPD
Internalizing problems	1.54 (0.92, 2.61)	1.36 (0.80, 2.34)
Externalizing problems	1.59 (0.94, 2.67)	1.32 (0.79, 2.23)
Total problems	1.32 (0.79, 2.21)	1.37 (0.79, 2.37)
Model 3. Parental Burnout (PB) and Present Maternal Depression		
	PB	Present Maternal Depression
Internalizing problems	1.42 (0.78, 2.56)	1.36 (0.77, 2.39)
Externalizing problems	1.69 (0.92, 3.14)	1.04 (0.60, 1.79)
Total problems	1.21 (0.67, 2.20)	1.33 (0.75, 2.38)

Note. OR—odds ratio coefficient from the binary logistic regression model; 95% CI—95% Confidence Interval; PB—parental burnout; PPD—postpartum depression. All models are adjusted for maternal age at testing, level of education, family status, socioeconomic status, the number of children in a family, mode of birth, gestational age at childbirth, child's complications during pregnancy/childbirth, and child age at Stage 2. * $p < 0.05$

4. Discussion

The present study examined the associations between maternal psychological distress, namely, PB, PPD, and present depression, and child behavioral and emotional problems, as measured by the CBCL/1½–5, in children aged 1.5 to 3.5 years. The longitudinal design allowed us to control for PPD measured during the first year postpartum while simultaneously assessing PB and present depressive symptoms at 2.24 years later. This constitutes an important methodological advancement, as previous research linking PB to child internalizing and externalizing problems rarely adjusted for either postpartum or concurrent maternal depression [17,34]. Overall, our findings underscore significant associations between maternal mental health and child outcomes and provide novel evidence for the distinct contribution of PB to early childhood behavioral problems.

In our sample, PB was prevalent in 16.2% of mothers, substantially higher than the 2.3% previously reported among Russian parents of preschoolers [16]. This suggests that toddlerhood, like adolescence, may represent a particularly vulnerable developmental period for parental exhaustion in Russia.

This heightened vulnerability likely stems from structural and cultural pressures that are especially pronounced during the toddler years. Unlike parents of preschoolers, parents of toddlers in Russia typically lack access to free public childcare for children under three, and private options are often financially inaccessible. At the same time, extended family support has become less accessible due to urbanization and geographic mobility, reducing opportunities for shared caregiving. These constraints coincide with intensified societal expectations of "good parenting", which emphasize constant engagement, developmental stimulation, and high emotional availability [34]. Together, these factors place substantial and sustained demands on parents of toddlers, potentially explaining why burnout appears more common in this group than among parents of older children [35].

Despite a comparable or even higher prevalence than maternal depression, however, PB remains unrecognized in Russian clinical guidelines. The absence of systematic screening, professional training, or specialized support services likely contributes to underdiagnosis and leaves many mothers without necessary psychological assistance.

This lack of structured support systems may amplify the impact of PB on both maternal well-being and child outcomes, highlighting the pressing need for policy and clinical frameworks targeting parental exhaustion. In line with our hypothesis, the regression

https://doi.org/10.3390/children13020176

models revealed significant associations between PB and all domains of child behavioral problems, even after controlling for both postpartum and present maternal depressive symptoms. This pattern reinforces prior evidence that PB uniquely contributes to child maladjustment [17,36]. Interestingly, findings from Russian samples of preschool-aged children have shown a different pattern, with higher maternal PB being associated with better emotional and cognitive outcomes in children, independently of maternal depression [15,16]. The heterogeneity of findings across studies examining PB and child outcomes may, therefore, reflect important moderating factors. In particular, child developmental stages may shape how parental exhaustion affects children: during toddlerhood, children are highly dependent on primary caregivers and possess limited self-regulatory capacities, which may render them more vulnerable to reduced parental emotional availability. In contrast, among preschool-aged children, greater autonomy and engagement with broader social environments may alter the ways in which parental exhaustion is expressed and experienced, giving rise to different interactional pathways. In the Russian context, higher parental burnout in mothers of preschoolers may reflect sustained overinvestment in children's development rather than reduced caregiving quality, consistent with strong cultural norms encouraging intensive, child-centered parenting [15,16]. It is also plausible that specific parenting behaviors, such as positive involvement or psychologically intrusive control, mediate or moderate these associations; however, such mechanisms were not assessed in the present study and warrant dedicated investigation in future work.

When examining borderline or clinically significant child behavioral problems, we found that mothers of children with difficulties above the cut-off reported higher levels of PB, PPD, and present depressive symptoms across the board. As a result, the associations between PB and clinically significant/borderline internalizing and externalizing problems in binary regression analyses were attenuated once overlapping maternal mental health factors were considered. This might suggest that in cases of more severe child difficulties, multiple maternal mental health challenges co-occur, making it harder to isolate the unique contribution of PB [37]. Furthermore, it is possible that PB may be particularly relevant for explaining subthreshold and mild-to-moderate child behavioral problems, whereas more severe psychopathology likely reflects a broader constellation of maternal mental health difficulties. In other words, PB may capture parenting-specific strain that is closely tied to everyday child behavior, while depression and other comorbid conditions may become more salient as predictors when child behavior reaches clinical levels of impairment. PB may influence child outcomes primarily through changes in parenting behavior, such as reduced emotional availability, harsher or more inconsistent discipline, and increased psychological intrusion or control, which have been linked to higher internalizing and externalizing symptoms in children. While emerging longitudinal work suggests that such parenting strategies can partly mediate the association between PB and child adjustment, these mechanisms remain preliminarily tested only in parent–adolescent dyads [38].

Crucially, these relationships are likely bi-directional [39,40]. Children exhibiting emotional or behavioral difficulties may place additional demands on parents, increasing parental exhaustion and PB. Conversely, parents experiencing burnout may be less responsive or emotionally available, which can further exacerbate children's vulnerability to internalizing and externalizing symptoms [17]. While these effects are particularly pronounced for parents of children with more severe problems, evidence indicates that all parents benefit from support, regardless of the severity of child difficulties [41].

Contrarily, neither postpartum nor current maternal depressive symptoms were significantly associated with child behavioral outcomes once PB was accounted for. While this may appear counter to prior research [42–44], including findings from the same longitudinal cohort in which children of mothers with persistently high depressive symptoms exhibited pronounced behavioral problems [45], several explanations are possible. Current depressive symptoms were highly correlated with PB (rho = 0.65), indicating substantial overlap. It is therefore plausible that maternal depression influences child behavior indirectly via PB, with regression models isolating the variance specifically attributable to parental exhaustion, the aspect most proximally linked to child outcomes. PB is uniquely characterized by fatigue, emotional depletion, and reduced emotional availability in the parent–child relationship. These symptoms can lead to less responsive and more punitive parenting, which, in turn, may increase child internalizing and externalizing problems [34,46,47]. Prior research further demonstrates that PB predicts child maltreatment, including verbal aggression and neglect [3,36], both strong risk factors for child behavioral difficulties [48–50]. Unlike depressive symptoms, which may arise from diverse life stressors, PB is specific to parenting demands and captures the unique burden of parental responsibilities. Importantly, research on PB remains limited; while maternal depression and child development have been extensively studied for decades, few studies have explicitly examined PB or accounted for its influence independently. Consequently, the current findings highlight PB as a key proximal mechanism linking maternal mental health and child outcomes and the need for further studies in this field.

Thus, it is crucial to recognize PB as a distinct and clinically significant risk factor, implement systematic screening in pediatric and maternal healthcare settings, and develop targeted interventions aimed at reducing parental exhaustion to safeguard both maternal well-being and child developmental outcomes.

4.1. Strengths and Limitations

The strengths of our study include the longitudinal study design, which allows us to uniquely estimate the association of maternal PB and child behavioral problems while controlling for PPD symptoms measured within 12 months after childbirth, thus allowing us to evaluate the effects of PB, PPD, and present maternal depression independent of each other. The use of validated questionnaires and controlling for a number of significant covariates (such as child's gestational age at birth, child health complications during pregnancy/postpartum, maternal education, and socioeconomic status) can also be considered as strengths. Particularly, the use of the CBCL/1½–5, a well-validated and internationally standardized instrument, allowed for comprehensive assessment of both internalizing and externalizing behavioral problems in early childhood and facilitated comparison of our findings with existing international research [31].

Nonetheless, certain limitations must be acknowledged.

First, child behavioral data were obtained exclusively through maternal reports, which introduces the possibility of reporter bias, particularly in studies involving parental mental health. Although the CBCL/1½–5 is a reliable and widely used instrument designed to minimize subjective interpretation, maternal perceptions may still be influenced by emotional states such as burnout or depressive symptoms. This risk is inherent to research conducted in early childhood contexts where mothers are typically the primary, and often the sole, caregivers, which is the case in Russia, where alternative informants are rarely available for children under three years old. While our analyses did not identify significant associations between maternal depression and child behavioral problems after accounting for PB, reliance on a single informant nevertheless limits the interpretability of the directionality of the effects.

Second, we observed a high attrition rate: only 18.5% of participants from Stage 1 returned the completed surveys at Stage 2. Although substantial dropout is common in longitudinal research, in our study, it may have been exacerbated by the use of printed CBCL/1½–5 questionnaires mailed to parents. This shift from an online format was necessary because the researchers who validated the CBCL/1½–5 in Russia had obtained distribution rights only for the printed version. As a result, the change in administration mode may have contributed to lower response rates.

Furthermore, sample attrition may also have been influenced by the high level of stigma surrounding maternal mental health in the context of child development in Russia. Sociological research shows that Russian society is predominantly child-centered, with strong social expectations that parents, particularly mothers, prioritize their children's needs above their own [51,52]. Consequently, when women were invited to participate in a study that included questions about both child behavioral difficulties and their own mental health, many may have been reluctant to disclose personal struggles. Future research would benefit from improved access to more vulnerable groups, alongside broader public awareness and psychoeducational efforts aimed at reducing the stigma around parental mental health.

Importantly, the follow-up sample did not differ in PPD scores from the baseline sample, allowing us to examine groups with comparable levels of vulnerability. Notably, a higher proportion of first-time mothers (52.5% vs. 60.1%) and mothers of children with medical complications during pregnancy/childbirth (14.6% vs. 20.5%) participated at Stage 2. This may reflect heightened concern about their children's development, as well as possible increased caregiving challenges and associated fatigue.

Finally, our findings are limited by the absence of objective medical data on maternal mental health at both stages of the study, as well as obstetric and child medical information. Instead, the study relies solely on self-reported data—a common limitation in contexts such as Russia, where registry-based medical records are either unavailable or not publicly accessible [49].

4.2. Further Directions

Future research should aim to build on the present findings by addressing several methodological and conceptual limitations. First, expanding the sample size and enhancing representativeness is essential to improve external validity. Studies including fathers, families from diverse socioeconomic backgrounds, and participants from different cultural and regional contexts would allow for a more comprehensive understanding of PB and its role in child development.

Second, future studies would benefit from incorporating additional informants and methodologies to reduce the shared method bias inherent in self-report designs. Collecting data from fathers, other caregivers, teachers, or healthcare professionals, as well as using observational assessments of parent–child interactions or clinician-rated measures of child behavior, would strengthen the objectivity and robustness of findings. Although such approaches are currently challenging in early childhood contexts in Russia, their inclusion represents an important goal for future research efforts.

Third, to clarify the directionality and causal mechanisms linking PB and child behavioral outcomes, future longitudinal studies should include additional measurement waves and apply cross-lagged panel or other dynamic modeling approaches. This would allow for examination of reciprocal effects between parental exhaustion and child behavior over time.

Finally, future research should consider a broader range of contextual and individual confounders, such as parenting styles, marital satisfaction, social support, child temperament, and parental coping strategies. Examining protective factors alongside risk mechanisms may help identify pathways through which PB affects child development and inform the design of targeted preventive and intervention programs.

https://doi.org/10.3390/children13020176

5. Conclusions

The present work contributes to understanding the unique role of PB in early childhood development, showing that PB is associated with all domains of child behavioral problems independently of postpartum or present maternal depression at the dimensional level, even though associations with borderline/clinical outcomes were attenuated once overlapping maternal mental health factors were considered. Unlike much previous research, our longitudinal design allowed us to account for both postpartum and concurrent depressive symptoms, providing clearer evidence that exhaustion from parental responsibilities alone can negatively affect children. These findings underscore the importance of recognizing and addressing PB, even in the absence of depression, and point to a high need for emotional and practical support for parents, particularly during the toddler years, when parenting demands are especially intense and designated help (e.g., accessible childcare, extended family support) is often lacking, as in the Russian context. There is an urgent need for clinical guidelines and institutional programs that identify and support families where parents experience high levels of PB, regardless of whether they also meet the criteria for other mental health disorders, to promote parental well-being, healthier parent–child interactions, and optimal child development.

Supplementary Materials: The following supporting information can be downloaded at https://www.mdpi.com/article/10.3390/children13020176/s1, Table S1: Spearman correlations between parental burnout, postpartum depressive symptoms, present maternal depressive symptoms, and Child Behavior Checklist scales.

Author Contributions: A.S. and V.Y. contributed to conception and design of the study. V.Y. organized the database and wrote sections of the manuscript. A.S. performed the statistical analysis, wrote sections of the manuscript and edited the manuscript. All authors have read and agreed to the published version of the manuscript.

Funding: This research received no external funding.

Institutional Review Board Statement: The Ethical Committee of the Russian Psychological Society at Lomonosov Moscow State University approved the present study (No: 345/2019) on 6 December 2021. The study was conducted in accordance with the Declaration of Helsinki.

Informed Consent Statement: Informed consent was obtained from all subjects involved in the study.

Data Availability Statement: We are ready to provide an anonymized dataset, syntaxes and the survey form (in Russian) by request.

Acknowledgments: The authors are grateful to all the women who took part in this study and to Evgenia Vasilyeva for her help with the research administration.

Conflicts of Interest: The authors declare no conflicts of interest.

References

1. Roskam, I.; Aguiar, J.; Akgun, E.; Arikan, G.; Artavia, M.; Avalosse, H.; Aunola, K.; Bader, M.; Bahati, C.; Barham, E.J.; et al. Parental Burnout Around the Globe: A 42-Country Study. *Affect. Sci.* **2021**, *2*, 58–79. [CrossRef]
2. Roskam, I.; Brianda, M.E.; Mikolajczak, M. A step forward in the conceptualization and measurement of parental burnout: The parental burnout assessment (PBA). *Front. Psychol.* **2018**, *9*, 758. [CrossRef]
3. Mikolajczak, M.; Brianda, M.E.; Avalosse, H.; Roskam, I. Consequences of parental burnout: A preliminary investigation of escape and suicidal ideations, sleep disorders, addictions, marital conflicts, child abuse and neglect. *Child Abuse Negl.* **2018**, *80*, 134–145. [CrossRef]
4. Furutani, K.; Kawamoto, T.; Alimardani, M.; Nakashima, K. Exhausted parents in Japan: Preliminary validation of the Japanese version of the Parental Burnout Assessment. *New Dir. Child Adolesc. Dev.* **2020**, *174*, 33–49. [CrossRef]
5. Lai, J.; Cleary, M.; Sitharthan, T.; Hunt, G.E. Prevalence of comorbid substance use, anxiety and mood disorders in epidemiological surveys, 1990–2014: A systematic review and meta-analysis. *Drug Alcohol Depend.* **2015**, *151*, 1–13. [CrossRef]

https://doi.org/10.3390/children13020176

6. Moussavi, S.; Chatterji, S.; Verdes, E.; Tandon, A.; Patel, V.; Ustun, B. Depression, chronic diseases, and decrements in health: Results from the World Health Surveys. *Lancet* **2007**, *370*, 851–858. [CrossRef]
7. Shelton, K.H.; Harold, G.T. Interparental conflict, negative parenting, and children's adjustment: Bridging links between parents' depression and children's psychological problems. In *Rutter's Child and Adolescent Psychiatry*; Rutter, M.J.H., Bishop, D.V.M., Pine, D.S., Scott, S., Stevenson, J., Taylor, E., Thapar, A., Eds.; Blackwell Publishing: Oxford, UK, 2008; pp. 330–350.
8. Van Bakel, H.J.A.; Van Engen, M.L.; Peters, P. Validity of the Parental Burnout Inventory Among Dutch Employees. *Front. Psychol.* **2018**, *9*, 697. [CrossRef] [PubMed]
9. Mikolajczak, M.; Gross, J.J.; Stinglhamber, F.; Lindahl Norberg, A.; Roskam, I. Is parental burnout distinct from job burnout and depressive symptoms? *Clin. Psychol. Sci.* **2020**, *8*, 673–689. [CrossRef]
10. Sánchez-Rodríguez, R.; Orsini, É.; Laflaquière, E.; Callahan, S.; Séjourné, N. Depression, anxiety, and guilt in mothers with burnout of preschool and school-aged children: Insight from a cluster analysis. *J. Affect. Disord.* **2019**, *259*, 244–250. [CrossRef] [PubMed]
11. Chen, B.-B.; Qu, Y.; Yang, B.; Chen, X. Chinese mothers' parental burnout and adolescents' internalizing and externalizing problems: The mediating role of maternal hostility. *Dev. Psychol.* **2022**, *58*, 58–69. [CrossRef]
12. Lebert-Charron, A.; Dorard, G.; Wendland, J.; Boujut, E. Who are and are not the burnout moms? A cluster analysis study of French-speaking mothers. *J. Affect. Disord. Rep.* **2021**, *5*, 100173. [CrossRef]
13. Séjourné, N.; Sanchez-Rodriguez, R.; Leboullenger, A.; Callahan, S. Maternal burn-out: An exploratory study. *J. Reprod. Infant Psychol.* **2018**, *36*, 276–288. [CrossRef] [PubMed]
14. Huang, Y.; Mao, F.; Zhang, X.; Wang, J.; Xu, Z.; Cao, F. Exploring the relationship between postnatal depressive symptoms and parental burnout from the perspective of the population and individual level. *BMC Psychiatry* **2023**, *23*, 409. [CrossRef]
15. Yakupova, V.A.; Suarez, A. Parental burnout, depression and emotional development of the preschoolers. *Front. Psychol.* **2023**, *14*, 1123456. [CrossRef]
16. Yakupova, V.A.; Suarez, A. Maternal depression and burnout and preschoolers' executive function development. *Panam. J. Neuropsychol.* **2024**, *18*, 203.
17. Woine, A.; Escobar, M.J.; Panesso, C.; Szczygieł, D.; Mikolajczak, M.; Roskam, I. Parental Burnout and Child Behavior: A Preliminary Analysis of Mediating and Moderating Effects of Positive Parenting. *Children* **2024**, *11*, 353. [CrossRef] [PubMed]
18. Paula, A.J.; Condeles, P.C.; Moreno, A.L.; Ferreira, M.B.G.; Fonseca, L.M.M.; Ruiz, M.T. Parental burnout: A scoping review. *Rev. Bras. Enferm.* **2021**, *74*, e20210203. [CrossRef]
19. He, Q.; Zhao, B.; Wei, H.; Huang, F. The relationship between parental phubbing and learning burnout of elementary and secondary school students: The mediating roles of parent-child attachment and ego depletion. *Front. Psychol.* **2022**, *13*, 963492. [CrossRef]
20. Apanovich, T.M.; Serykh, A.B. Emotional Burnout Symptoms in Mothers of Primary School Children: Role of Intensive Parenting Attitudes and Parenting Styles. *Russ. Psychol. J.* **2024**, *21*, 22–34.
21. Kalabikhina, I.; Kyznetsova, P. Who needs (or doesn't) three years of parental leave? *Demogr. Rev.* **2022**, *9*, 24–43. [CrossRef]
22. Avdeeva, A.; Isupova, O.; Kuleshova, A.; Chernova, Z.H.; Shpakovskaya, L. *Parenting 2.0: Why Modern Parents Need to Know Everything*; Alpina Publisher: Moscow, Russia, 2021.
23. Woodard, K.; Pollak, S.D. Is there evidence for sensitive periods in emotional development? *Curr. Opin. Behav. Sci.* **2020**, *36*, 1–6. [CrossRef]
24. Roskam, I.; Raes, M.E.; Mikolajczak, M. Exhausted parents: Development and preliminary validation of the parental burnout inventory. *Front. Psychol.* **2017**, *8*, 163. [CrossRef] [PubMed]
25. Starchenkova, E. Social-psychological factors of parental burnout. In *Psychology of Stress and Coping Behavior: Challenges, Resources, Well-Being*; Kostroma State University: Kostroma, Russia, 2019; pp. 109–113.
26. Brianda, M.E.; Mikolajczak, M.; Bader, M.; Bon, S.; Déprez, A.; Favez, N.; Holstein, L.; Le Vigouroux, S.; Lebert-Charron, A.; Sánchez-Rodríguez, R.; et al. Optimizing the Assessment of Parental Burnout: A Multi-informant and Multimethod Approach to Determine Cutoffs for the Parental Burnout Inventory and the Parental Burnout Assessment. *Assessment* **2023**, *30*, 2234–2246. [CrossRef]
27. Cox, J.L.; Holden, J.M.; Sagovsky, R. Detection of postnatal depression: Development of the 10-item Edinburgh Postnatal Depression Scale. *Br. J. Psychiatry* **1987**, *150*, 782–786. [CrossRef]
28. Yakupova, V.A. The impact of psychological and physiological conditions of motherhood on postnatal depression. *Russ. Psychol. J.* **2018**, *15*, 8–23. [CrossRef]
29. Beck, A.T.; Ward, C.H.; Mendelson, M.; Mock, J.; Erbaugh, J. An inventory for measuring depression. *Arch. Gen. Psychiatry* **1961**, *4*, 561–571. [CrossRef]
30. Zlobina, M.V.; Pervushina, O.N. Analysis of Two Depression Questionnaires PHQ-9 and BDI-II. *Reflexio* **2018**, *11*, 83–98. [CrossRef]
31. Achenbach, T.M.; Rescorla, L.A. *Manual for the ASEBA Preschool Forms & Profiles: An Integrated System of Multi-Informant Assessment*; Department of Psychiatry, University of Vermont: Cardiff, UK, 2000.

https://doi.org/10.3390/children13020176

32. Kolmagorova, A.V.; Slobodskaya, E.R.; Kinsht, I.A. Assessment of mental health in early age. *Bull. Sib. Branch Russ. Acad. Med. Sci.* **2007**, *125*, 45–52.
33. IBM Corp. *IBM SPSS Statistics for Macintosh*; mIBM Corp: New York, NY, USA, 2020.
34. Thériault, R.L.; Bernier, A.; Deneault, A.A. Maternal and paternal parenting stress: Direct and interactive associations with child externalizing and internalizing behavior problems. *Early Child. Res. Q.* **2025**, *71*, 114–122. [CrossRef]
35. Nisskaya, A.K.; Tsyganova, E.M. Parental Practices of Controlling and Supporting the Autonomy of Elementary School Children and Early Adolescents in Russia: A Qualitative Study. *Psychol. Russ. State Art* **2024**, *17*, 3–22. [CrossRef] [PubMed]
36. Schittek, A.; Roskam, I.; Mikolajczak, M. Parental burnout and borderline personality stand out to predict child maltreatment. *Sci. Rep.* **2023**, *13*, 12153. [CrossRef]
37. Lowthian, E.; Bedston, S.; Kristensen, S.M.; Akbari, A.; Fry, R.; Huxley, K.; Johnson, R.; Kim, H.S.; Owen, R.K.; Taylor, C.; et al. Maternal Mental Health and Children's Problem Behaviours: A Bi-Directional Relationship? *Res. Child Adolesc. Psychopathol.* **2023**, *51*, 1611–1626. [CrossRef]
38. Zhou, Y.B.; Ruan, S.J.; Bu, Y.R.; Zhong, C.; Bao, Q. Effects of parental burnout and psychological intrusion on adolescent resilience. *Sci. Rep.* **2025**, *15*, 38441. [CrossRef]
39. Curci, S.G.; Somers, J.A.; Winstone, L.K.; Luecken, L.J. Within-dyad bidirectional relations among maternal depressive symptoms and child behavior problems from infancy through preschool. *Dev. Psychopathol.* **2023**, *35*, 547–557. [CrossRef]
40. Gawlik, K.S.; Melnyk, B.M.; Tan, A. Burnout and Mental Health in Working Parents: Risk Factors and Practice Implications. *J. Pediatr. Health Care.* **2025**, *39*, 41–50. [CrossRef] [PubMed]
41. Roskam, I.; Aguiar, J.; Akgun, E.; Arena, A.F.; Arikan, G.; Aunola, K.; Besson, E.; Beyers, W.; Boujut, E.; Brianda, M.E.; et al. Three reasons why parental burnout is more prevalent in individualistic countries: A mediation study in 36 countries. *Soc. Psychiatry Psychiatr. Epidemiol.* **2024**, *59*, 681–694. [CrossRef] [PubMed]
42. Closa-Monasterolo, R.; Gispert-Llaurado, M.; Canals, J.; Luque, V.; Zaragoza-Jordana, M.; Koletzko, B.; Grote, V.; Weber, M.; Gruszfeld, D.; Szott, K.; et al. The Effect of Postpartum Depression and Current Mental Health Problems of the Mother on Child Behaviour at Eight Years. *Matern. Child Health J.* **2017**, *21*, 1563–1572. [CrossRef]
43. Kingston, D.; Kehler, H.; Austin, M.P.; Mughal, M.K.; Wajid, A.; Vermeyden, L.; Benzies, K.; Brown, S.; Stuart, S.; Giallo, R. Trajectories of maternal depressive symptoms during pregnancy and the first 12 months postpartum and child externalizing and internalizing behavior at three years. *PLoS ONE* **2018**, *13*, e0195365. [CrossRef] [PubMed]
44. Netsi, E.; Pearson, R.M.; Murray, L.; Cooper, P.; Craske, M.G.; Stein, A. Association of Persistent and Severe Postnatal Depression with Child Outcomes. *JAMA Psychiatry* **2018**, *75*, 247–253. [CrossRef]
45. Suarez, A.; Shraibman, L.; Yakupova, V. Long-Term Effects of Maternal Depression during Postpartum and Early Parenthood Period on Child Socioemotional Development. *Children* **2023**, *10*, 1718. [CrossRef]
46. Ren, X.; Cai, Y.; Wang, J.; Chen, O. A systematic review of parental burnout and related factors among parents. *BMC Public Health* **2024**, *24*, 376. [CrossRef]
47. Guseva, U. Features of emotions understanding development in Russian children. *Natl. Psychol. J.* **2025**, *20*, 100–114. [CrossRef]
48. Tsunga, L.; Heron, J.; Lake, M.T.; Halligan, S.L.; Malcolm-Smith, S.; Hoffman, N.; Zar, H.J.; Fraser, A.; Stein, D.J.; Donald, K.A. Exposure to Violence and Mental Health Outcomes Among Pre-schoolers in a South African Birth Cohort. *Res. Child Adolesc. Psychopathol.* **2024**, *52*, 1635–1646. [CrossRef] [PubMed]
49. Ivanov, M.V.; Boksha, I.S.; Balakireva, E.E.; Klyushnik, T.P. Epidemiological Study on the Early Detection of Mental Disorders in Young Children in Russia. *Consort. Psychiatr.* **2022**, *3*, 18–26. [CrossRef] [PubMed]
50. Rean, A.; Egorova, A.; Konovalov, И. The Relationship Between Screen Time Use and Various Types of Aggression in Late Adolescence. *Moscow Univ. Bull. Ser. 14 Psychol.* **2025**, *48*, 60–83. [CrossRef]
51. Tikhonova, I.V.; Misiyk, Y.V.; Khazova, S.A. About some factors of stress generation of parental role in "intensive" parents. *Vestn. Kostroma State Univ. Ser. Pedagogy Psychol. Sociokinetics* **2023**, *29*, 99–108.
52. Misiyk, Y.; Khazova, S. Study of the expression of attitudes on intensive parenting in Russian women. *Vestn. Kostroma State Univ. Ser. Pedagogy Psychol. Sociokinetics* **2021**, *27*, 91–98. [CrossRef]

https://doi.org/10.3390/children13020176

children

MDPI

Article

Using Co-Design to Adapt a Digital Parenting Program for Parents Seeking Mental Health Support

Meg Louise Bennett [1], Ling Wu [2], Joshua Paolo Seguin [2], Patrick Olivier [2], Andrea Reupert [3], Anthony F. Jorm [4], Sylvia Grant [5], Helen Vaxevanis [5], Mingye Li [2], Jue Xie [2] and Marie Bee Hui Yap [1,*]

1 Turner Institute for Brain and Mental Health, School of Psychological Sciences, Monash University, Clayton, VIC 3800, Australia; meg.bennett1@monash.edu
2 Action Lab, Faculty of Information Technology, Monash University, Clayton, VIC 3800, Australia
3 School of Educational Psychology and Counselling, Faculty of Education, Monash University, Clayton, VIC 3800, Australia
4 Melbourne School of Population and Global Health, The University of Melbourne, Parkville, VIC 3010, Australia
5 IPC Health, P.O. Box 171, Deer Park, VIC 3023, Australia
* Correspondence: marie.yap@monash.edu

Abstract

Background/Objectives: Parental mental health challenges are associated with parenting difficulties and child mental health issues. Parenting interventions can support families; however, parents with mental health challenges face barriers to accessing parenting support, which is not consistently offered within adult mental health settings. Embedding technology-assisted parenting programs into these settings could provide accessible, holistic support. Partners in Parenting Kids (PiP Kids) is a digital parenting program designed to prevent child anxiety and depression, yet its suitability for parents with mental health challenges and fit within mental health services remains unclear. This study aimed to co-design and adapt PiP Kids for future implementation in an Australian adult mental health service. **Methods**: Parents who recently sought mental health support (n = 8) and service providers (n = 7) participated in co-design workshops to explore needs and preferences for a technology-assisted parenting program and iteratively develop a prototype. Parents (n = 3) trialled the online component of the prototype and participated in qualitative interviews to assess acceptability. **Results**: The adapted clinician-supported program was designed to facilitate (1) parent and clinician readiness for parenting support; (2) emotional and social support for parents and clinicians; (3) practical, personalised parenting knowledge; (4) parent-led empowerment; and (5) accessible, integrated support. Prototype clinician training was developed to strengthen the clinician-support component. Parents indicated initial acceptability of the online prototype while reiterating the value of including face-to-face support. **Conclusions**: This study co-designed an online, clinician-supported parenting program for future embedding within adult mental health settings. The findings highlight key considerations for developing and implementing technology-assisted interventions that promote family-focused care for parents seeking mental health support.

Keywords: co-design; parenting; parental mental health; service design; parenting intervention; digital health; mental health services; clinician; acceptability

1. Introduction

Children of parents experiencing mental health challenges, such as anxiety and depression, are up to twice as likely to experience their own mental health difficulties, especially if families do not have adequate support [1,2]. Parental mental health challenges are linked with an increased likelihood of parenting difficulties, including reduced warmth and increased overcontrolling, harsh, or inconsistent parenting [3–7]. These parenting difficulties have been identified as a key mechanism in the intergenerational transmission of mental health issues [8–10] and can worsen parents' mental health, creating a vicious cycle of distress within families [11,12]. Fortunately, parenting is a modifiable factor, with evidence-based parenting interventions shown to improve parenting and child outcomes for parents with and without mental health challenges [13–15]. However, access to parenting intervention for these parents can be limited, and they are not consistently offered parenting support within mental health treatment pathways [16]. This is a missed opportunity given the well-established interrelationships between parenting, parental mental health, and child outcomes [17,18].

Integrating parenting support into parent mental health care can offer holistic, family-focused care for families, while enhancing the recovery of parents [11,19]. Research shows that for parents with mental health issues, interventions targeting both parental mental health and parenting yield more wide-ranging benefits across parent symptoms, parenting, and child outcomes compared to those targeting either issue alone [19,20]. Adult mental health services are well placed to provide a combined approach, as they can extend their support of parent mental health to address parenting as one aspect of the parent's identity, functioning, and wellbeing [21,22]. There are several face-to-face interventions and initiatives that integrate parenting support within adult mental health services [21,23–25], for example, Let's Talk about Children [26,27] and the ParentingWell practice approach [28,29]. These have been found to be acceptable among parents and clinicians and to be effective in improving parent mental health, parenting, and child outcomes, as well as clinician confidence and skills in supporting parenting [27,30]. Despite this, implementation of family-focused support into mental health settings can be hindered by service barriers, including a lack of resources, training, time, and clinician confidence to deliver parenting intervention alongside mental health care [31,32]. Additionally, parents experiencing mental health challenges often face barriers to accessing in-person support, such as stigma, competing priorities, fluctuating mood, low energy, childcare demands, and transportation difficulties [33–35].

One promising approach is implementing technology-assisted parenting programs in existing mental health services, where parenting support is provided partially or entirely via technology [36]. Technology has the potential to provide parents with accessible, flexible parenting support alongside mental health treatment, by minimising barriers such as stigma, lack of time, and scheduling demands [37,38]. By reducing reliance on clinicians, this approach can also decrease service burden and costs and support feasible long-term implementation in resource-limited adult mental health services [39,40]. Importantly, evidence is emerging that technology-assisted parenting programs are acceptable and effective in improving parenting and child outcomes among parents with mental health challenges [41–43]. However, to our knowledge these programs have not yet been embedded within adult mental health settings.

Partners in Parenting Kids (PiP Kids; formerly known as Parenting Resilient Kids or PaRK) is a digital parenting program that may be well-suited for integration. PiP Kids is a fully online program that provides parents with evidence-based parenting strategies to reduce the risk of anxiety and depression in their primary school-aged children [44,45]. The original program comprises a self-assessment of parenting practices, a tailored feedback report, and self-guided online modules [44]. In a randomised controlled trial, parents who received PiP Kids showed greater improvements in parenting behaviours compared to those receiving a factsheet intervention [46]. This evidence of efficacy, together with the

https://doi.org/10.3390/children13010129

successful adaptation of PiP Kids to family services for parents of children experiencing adversity [47], suggests its potential for integration within adult mental health treatment.

Yet, it remains unclear how well a digital parenting program such as PiP Kids will fit into the existing clinician and service practices at adult mental health services. Additionally, parents with mental health challenges have unique parenting needs, including talking with children about parental mental health, managing their mental health symptoms alongside parenting, and navigating increased parenting stress [48–50]. These parents may also face unique barriers to engaging with parenting programs, such as debilitating symptoms, low literacy, socioeconomic disadvantage, and social isolation [34,35]. Generic or fully digital parenting programs such as PiP Kids may therefore not adequately address the specific needs or preferences of these parents [21,51]. This highlights the importance of adapting PiP Kids to ensure its acceptability and compatibility with existing service practices and family circumstances.

Co-design or collaboration with relevant stakeholders and end-users is an ideal approach for ensuring a thorough understanding of and tailoring to the needs of parents and existing health services [52]. Actively engaging parents in designing programs is needed to develop an intervention that meets their needs and preferences [53,54]. Similarly, service provider perspectives are crucial as they possess specialised knowledge of service practices, are instrumental in advocating for families, and may also be key end users involved in program delivery [47]. Research suggests that adapting programs to fit the context, procedures, and workload of the existing health service, while retaining evidence-based content, helps ensure the program is relevant and successfully integrated [29,35].

The aim of this study was therefore to co-design and adapt an evidence-based digital parenting program (PiP Kids) for future integrative implementation in an existing adult mental health service, to support parents seeking mental health care. Specifically, this study used co-design methods to (1) identify design considerations for integrating technology-assisted parenting programs by exploring the needs and preferences of parents with lived experience of seeking mental health support and service providers who support these parents. This study then aimed to (2) design, develop, and refine an adapted prototype parenting program, and (3) deliver the online component of the prototype program to parents, to understand its initial acceptability and identify what further adaptations are needed.

2. Materials and Methods

2.1. Study Setting

This study was conducted as part of a larger research program, in partnership with a major provider of community health services in Victoria, Australia. As this study specifically focuses on parents seeking mental health support, the mental health services within this community health organisation (including therapeutic counselling for individuals experiencing mild-to-severe mental health challenges, gambling, and alcohol and other drug use) were selected as the most appropriate setting for the study.

2.2. Recruitment

We aimed to recruit a small number of participants in this initial study to gain detailed insights into parent and service needs. Small sample sizes are generally considered acceptable in in-depth qualitative studies [55]. Co-developing and piloting an initial prototype on a small scale is considered a feasible and cost-effective way of designing and refining new interventions during the development stages [56]. Findings from these initial iterations can then be used to guide larger-scale iterations and eventual implementation.

https://doi.org/10.3390/children13010129

2.2.1. Service Providers

Service providers were clinicians and clinical leads employed at the collaborating mental health service, who spoke English and had experience providing mental health support to parents of children aged 5–11 years. All eligible service providers within the collaborating mental health service were invited to participate via an emailed flyer.

2.2.2. Parents

All parent participants were parents or primary caregivers of children aged 5–11 years who spoke English and lived in Australia. Parents were either (1) currently seeking mental health support at the collaborating community health service or (2) had received psychological support for their mental health in the community within the past year. Recruitment occurred via two methods. First, clinicians at the collaborating mental health service distributed flyers to potentially eligible parent clients. Second, flyers were distributed via websites, social media, waiting rooms, and mailing lists of community organisations across Australia that support parents with mental health challenges. Although the study aimed to recruit across parents experiencing general mental health challenges, gambling, and alcohol and other drug use, the recruited parents all self-reported general mental health challenges such as anxiety, depression, or stress.

2.3. Study Design and Procedure

The Double Diamond design process guided the co-design methods in this study [57]. Each diamond represents a process of examining an issue broadly followed by taking focused action. As shown in Figure 1, this study was conducted in three phases that align with the Double Diamond stages. Phase 1 involved workshops with parents and service providers to 'discover' needs and preferences and 'define' design considerations for integrating technology-assisted parenting programs into a mental health service. Phase 2 involved workshops with parents and service providers to 'develop' an initial prototype and validate and refine this design and the design considerations. Phase 3 involved 'delivering' the online component of the refined prototype to parents and conducting one-on-one interviews to explore initial acceptability and identify further adaptations for the next iteration. See Supplementary Table S1 for a summary of the aims and methods. Due to the iterative nature of the study, further methodological details for each phase are provided within their respective Methods Sections below, with each phase informed by findings from the previous one.

2.4. Ethical Considerations

All procedures were approved by the Monash University Human Research Ethics Committee (approval numbers #35059 and #44564). Participants were provided with a plain-language explanatory statement and the opportunity to ask questions prior to consenting. Parent participants were reimbursed with a $35 gift card for each hour spent engaging in a workshop or interview. Service provider participants were not financially compensated, as research activities were conducted during their working hours. For parents currently seeking support at the collaborating service, clinicians initially provided parent contact details to the research team. Once parents were recruited, all individual parent data were collected and stored securely by the research team and were not shared with the partner service, regardless of whether parents were currently seeking support from the collaborating service.

Co-design workshops were conducted separately for each participant group to create a safe environment for open discussion and minimise the influence of power imbalances. To ensure parent participant wellbeing, all workshops and interviews were facilitated by

https://doi.org/10.3390/children13010129

a provisional psychologist (the first author) with formal training in mental health, under the supervision of a registered psychologist. Regardless of whether parent participants demonstrated distress, the first author contacted them within 24 h of their workshop or interview to assess for distress and offer support and crisis resources.

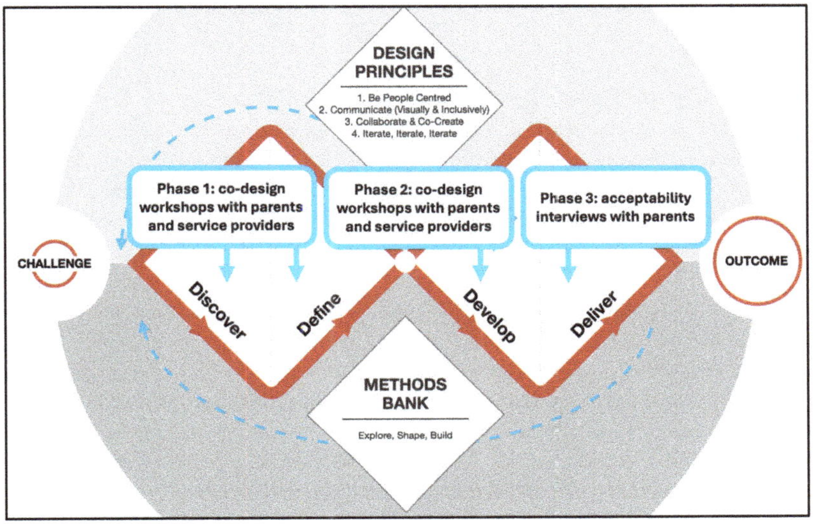

Figure 1. The Double Diamond design process, illustrating how the discover, define, develop, and deliver stages align with the phases of the current study, as indicated by the blue arrows.

2.5. Researcher Positionality and Reflexivity

The first author is a female clinical psychology PhD candidate and provisional psychologist with interests in mental health, parenting, and evidence-based intervention. Other co-authors involved in data interpretation included two academics with expertise in co-design and qualitative research and one professor who is a parent and psychologist with 14 years' experience working with parents, young people, and service providers in co-designing and developing parenting interventions. The remaining co-authors who reviewed the findings and manuscript included professors with expertise in parental mental health, prevention and intervention in mental health, co-design and human–computer interaction, as well as service providers with expertise in clinical service delivery and management, several of whom have lived experience of parenting themselves. The first author facilitated all workshops and interviews. While the prompts used during these activities were designed to be open-ended, the first author's choice of prompts and management of group dynamics may have influenced participant responses. Group workshops may have encouraged sharing of perspectives, whereas individual sessions may have encouraged more personal reflection. The first author kept a reflexive journal following each activity, documenting her reflections, including how facilitator choices may have influenced data. During analysis, a conscious effort was also made to ensure a balanced integration of perspectives across all three participant groups (parents, clinician, and clinical leads) when triangulating findings and identifying themes.

https://doi.org/10.3390/children13010129

3. Phase 1 Methods and Results: Discover and Define Design Considerations

3.1. Phase 1 Methods

3.1.1. Participants

Parent participants (n = 8) were all mothers aged 39–46 years (M = 41.1). One was currently seeking mental health support at the collaborating health service, and seven had recent lived experience of seeking mental health support in the community. Parents' self-reported mental health challenges included high stress (n = 7), anxiety (n = 5), depression (n = 4), trauma (n = 3), and one each with psychosis, bipolar disorder, and grief. Parents' reported cultural backgrounds included Australian/New Zealand (n = 4), European (n = 2), Pacific Islander (n = 2), and one each of East Asian, Middle Eastern, and South Asian.

Service provider participants included clinicians (n = 5) and clinical leads (n = 2), all of whom were women. Clinicians were aged 25–50 years (M = 37.8) and included counsellors (n = 2) and social workers (n = 3) who primarily worked with mild-to-severe mental health challenges (n = 4) or gambling concerns (n = 1). Clinicians' reported cultural backgrounds included one each of Australian/New Zealand, European, Middle Eastern, Pacific Islander, South Asian, and Māori. Clinical leads were aged 52–59 years (M = 55.5) and included one team leader who was a psychologist and one service manager who was a social worker. Clinical leads reported their cultural backgrounds as one each of Australian/New Zealand and European. Three clinicians were also mothers with lived experience of depression and/or anxiety, with many of their responses combining their personal and professional perspectives. Several of these instances are highlighted in the results. Supplementary Table S2 details further demographic characteristics of the Phase 1 participants.

3.1.2. Data Collection

Phase 1 workshops explored parent and service provider needs and preferences for any technology-assisted parenting program integrated into mental health care. Participants completed a brief demographic questionnaire using REDCap (Research Electronic Data Capture) [58,59] before taking part in workshops. Workshop focus and format were informed by relevant literature on co-design, parenting in the context of parental mental health challenges, parenting programs, program adaptation, real-world implementation, and clinician experiences and training. All workshops were conducted via Zoom, with audio and video recording. Each workshop lasted 2 h, including a 5–10 min break.

3.1.3. Parent Workshops

Each parent participated in one individual or group workshop during this phase. As parents with mental health challenges often describe feeling guilt, shame, and helplessness [60,61], this workshop used case-vignettes to create psychological distance where parents could draw on their lived experience reflectively and empathetically without being overwhelmed [62,63]. In the vignettes, parent participants role-played as helpline workers providing advice to the vignette parents. Activities explored challenges faced by parents in parenting, engaging with parenting programs, and applying parenting knowledge, as well as strategies to support parents in these areas. Figure 2 provides examples of activities from the parent workshop.

3.1.4. Service Provider Workshops

Service providers attended two rounds of workshops in this phase. The first round examined the service context, focusing on day-to-day service delivery for clinicians and on broader program integration and organisational resources for clinical leads. This round also explored general challenges faced by parents in applying parenting knowledge and

https://doi.org/10.3390/children13010129

opportunities and barriers within the service to support them. The second round of workshops built on findings from prior workshops by first exploring service provider feedback on emerging themes. Findings from the first round of workshops with parents and clinicians indicated a clear need for clinicians to support parents in engaging with any digital parenting program. Consequently, this round of workshops focused on how to enable clinicians to provide this support. For clinicians, this involved identifying the resources and support they would need, while for clinical leads the focus was on determining what organisational resources could be provided to address these needs. Figure 3 presents example activities from these workshops.

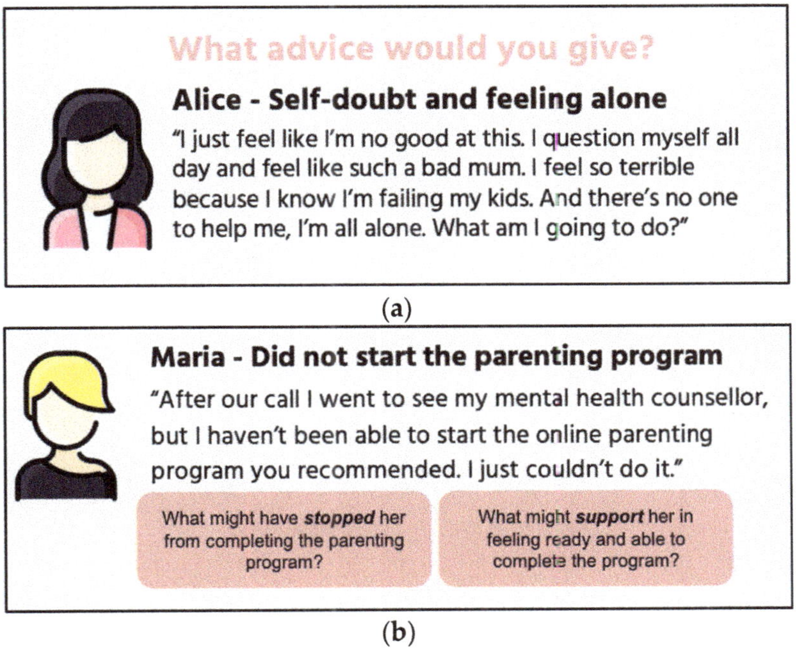

Figure 2. Examples of activities from the Phase 1 parent workshop demonstrating (**a**) an activity exploring strategies for supporting parents with parenting challenges; (**b**) an activity exploring barriers to engaging with parenting programs and strategies for support.

3.1.5. Data Analysis

Recordings were transcribed verbatim by an automatic artificial intelligence transcription service (Descript version 2.10.0) and corrected by the research team. Transcripts were analysed with the support of NVivo qualitative software version 15.3.0, using Braun and Clarke's reflexive thematic analysis approach [64,65]. Data were coded inductively as the purpose of this phase was to broadly explore the needs and preferences of parents and service providers. We followed the six-phase process of reflexive thematic analysis: (1) data familiarisation; (2) iterative data coding; (3) initial theme generation; (4) theme development and review; (5) refining, defining, and naming themes; and (6) writing up the findings [65,66]. The development and refinement of themes was carried out by the first author in collaboration with the broader research team.

https://doi.org/10.3390/children13010129

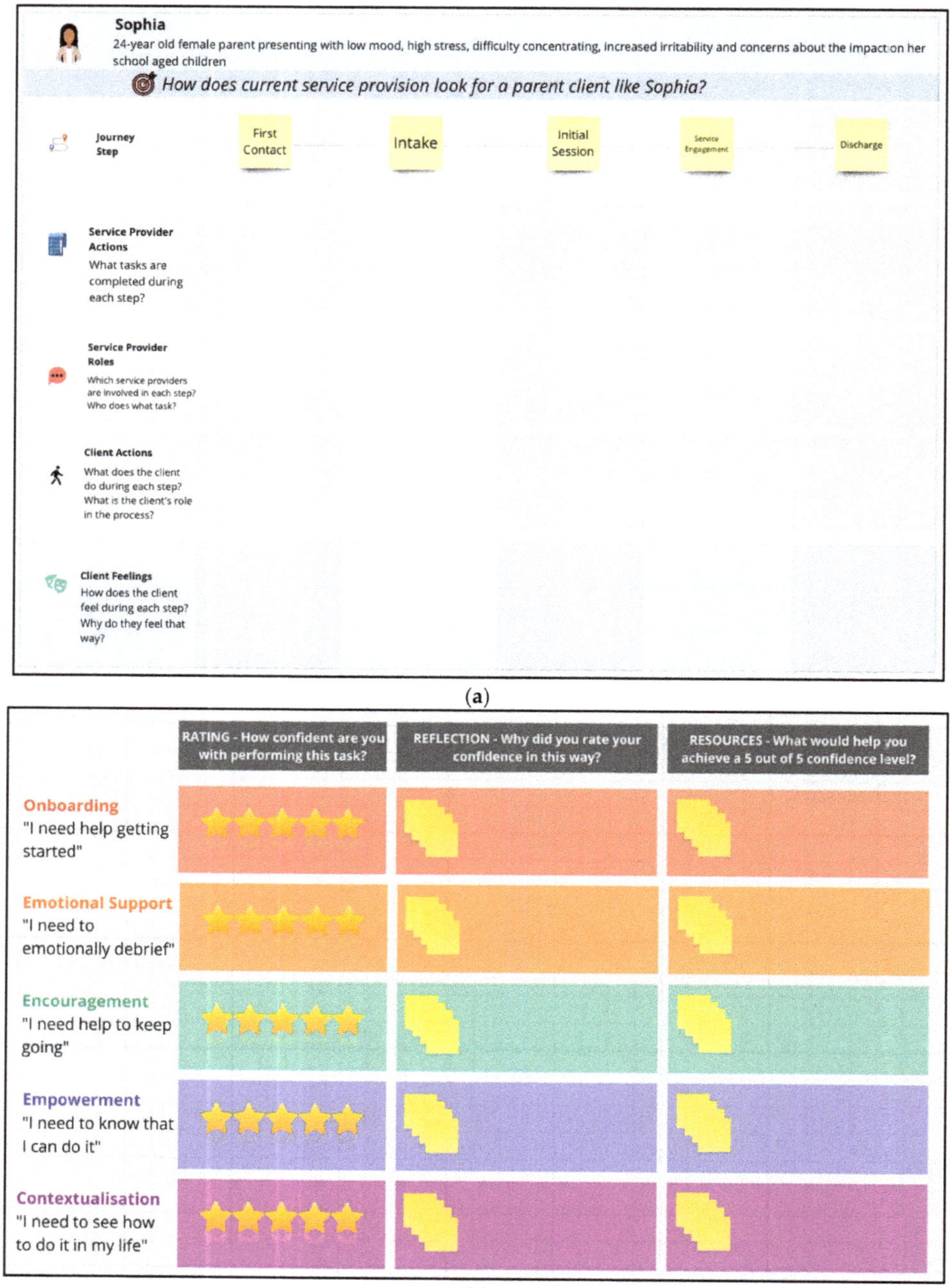

(a)

(b)

Figure 3. Examples of activities from Phase 1 service provider workshops demonstrating (**a**) an activity from the round-one workshops that mapped service provision and clinician roles within the collaborating mental health service; (**b**) an activity from the round-two workshops that explored clinician confidence in undertaking parenting support tasks and identified supports to strengthen this confidence. Yellow stars and sticky notes were used to record participant responses during the activities.

https://doi.org/10.3390/children13010129

3.2. Phase 1 Results

Participants described five design considerations for adapting the parenting program to address parent and service provider needs and preferences, as identified in the following themes: (1) building parent and clinician readiness for parenting support, (2) emotional and social support for parents and clinicians, (3) practical and personalised parenting knowledge, (4) parent-led empowerment, and (5) accessible and integrated support. Supplementary Table S3 presents each theme and subtheme with additional indicative quotes.

3.2.1. Theme 1: Building Readiness for Parenting Support

Participants described foundational factors influencing parent and clinician readiness to engage in parenting-focused support. Readiness was seen to depend on the wellbeing and safety of parents and their family, clinician training, and both groups' understanding of the purpose and value of the program.

Parental wellbeing foundations

All participants emphasised that parents' mental health, safety, and physical wellbeing are prerequisites for their capacity to parent effectively and engage with parenting support. Parent self-care, breaks from parenting, and attention to physical health were highlighted as particularly important. Declining mental health, or risk concerns such as family conflict, suicide risk, or child protection, were seen as needing stabilisation prior to parenting support. Service providers similarly emphasised the service's primary focus on parental mental health, with parenting considered a secondary focus when relevant to parent wellbeing.

> "They would talk about the difficulties they have with their young kids... but the main focus... the reason they came to me was because of their own mental health. That was the primary issue." [Clinician 4]

Program understanding and confidence

Participants identified understanding the program and feeling confident about its value and use as essential prerequisites among parents and service providers. All groups highlighted their need for a detailed program introduction, including its purpose, content, benefits, and technology. Parents suggested a clinician could support their introduction and help overcome barriers such as program uncertainty, fear of change, and difficulty starting. Some clinicians expressed low confidence in parenting issues and requested refresher training on child development, parenting, and supporting parents.

> "Not training on just the program but training on just working specifically with mums... low self-esteem, feelings of guilt, shame, all that stuff that comes along with being a mum." [Clinician 5]

Clinical leads proposed that clinicians already possess this knowledge and that training should primarily focus on the program and building clinicians' confidence in applying their clinical skills to providing support on parenting.

3.2.2. Theme 2: Emotional and Social Support

Emotional support and social and peer connection were seen as crucial for both parents and clinicians.

Emotional support and validation

Participants (including clinicians with lived experience) highlighted the need to provide parents with non-judgmental emotional support that avoids criticising them for their mental health difficulties. Normalisation and validation of parent experiences were emphasised to remind parents they are not alone, acknowledge struggles as common, and foster

https://doi.org/10.3390/children13010129

hope. Participants stressed the need for parents to emotionally debrief with support people who listened with empathy and understanding. Strong therapeutic relationships with counsellors or psychologists built on trust, continuity, and rapport were seen as essential for parents to safely engage in support.

> "You don't often share what's in your mind for fear of judgment... and that is the independent source that is hopefully listening and not judging and giving empathy... Just someone to listen to you is extremely powerful." [Parent 6]

Social and peer connection

Social support was seen as vital for parents and clinicians. Participants noted that connecting parents to family experiences or peers with lived experience of mental health challenges fostered support, belonging, and joy, and reduced isolation and self-blame.

> "It would be good for her to meet other mums... so you get to share experiences and... gets to hear that she's not alone... everyone goes through that same feeling that she's going through... just getting connected and being able to hear other mums, I think that would be good for her." [Parent 3]

These connections were seen to provide practical support, such as sharing strategies or help with housework and childcare, which was described as particularly crucial when parental mental health was poor. However, participants expressed how social connection, such as support groups, could have downsides, including parents feeling shame or anxiety. Clinicians stressed their need for working in specialised, collaborative teams of peers to enhance confidence, shared learning, and work quality.

> "As a clinician and working in this particular area if it was kind of specific... working within a team where we're all on the same page and we're able to kind of help and support one another... that's how I'd build on my confidence." [Clinician 1]

3.2.3. Theme 3: Practical and Personalised Knowledge

Participants expressed that parents need program content that extends beyond information to provide practical and personalised guidance.

Practical knowledge

Participants, including clinicians drawing on personal experience, emphasised that parents would benefit from concrete examples of how to use strategies and plans, reminders, and goal setting to translate knowledge into action. Practicing skills through role-playing with others and trying strategies with children was seen as essential. Participants highlighted that parents need practical steps and support for problem-solving barriers. Parents and clinical leads suggested that this be supported by a clinician who could follow up on issues, answer questions, and help parents consolidate and implement strategies.

> "They might have read something and they were like, 'I'm not really understanding how to put this into practice... I've read it, but I'm not sure how to implement it'. So maybe the clinician can assist with that." [Clinical Lead 2]

Personalised knowledge

Participants clarified that knowledge is effective only when tailored and contextualised to each parent, as every family is different. All participants described personalisation as requiring understanding of each parent's unique context, mental health challenges, and barriers, then adapting strategies to be relevant and useful. Parents suggested that clinicians could support this through recommending modules and customising strategies based on each parent's changing needs.

https://doi.org/10.3390/children13010129

> "That kind of personalised process... to understand what a parenting program means to her... Or maybe... she doesn't have the time, so maybe the counsellor can help her prioritise... that would be hard for [parent] to do on her own, and it's probably not a component of the parenting program itself." [Parent 5]

Parents and service providers also highlighted the need for content that is culturally inclusive and specific to parenting with mental health challenges, to ensure parents can see their family context in the program.

3.2.4. Theme 4: Parent-Led Empowerment

All participants emphasised the importance of supporting parent empowerment and autonomy through helping parents feel more capable, confident, and in control.

Guided autonomy

Participants identified autonomy as central to empowering parents in their mental health and parenting, whilst acknowledging that parents would need professionals to support this autonomy through guidance and encouragement. It was seen as essential that this support was collaborative to help parents feel in control and guided rather than directed. Online and clinician support was viewed as most powerful when it respected parents' ideas and helped them reflect, build on existing knowledge, and generate their own solutions. Participants stressed the need for clinicians to adopt a parent-centred approach led by parent preferences and priorities, consistent with the service's client-led model.

> "Sometimes people, they know what's the best to do, but... don't have the capacity. So I definitely agree with... not to tell her what to do. I would like to ask her... what do you think we can do in this situation... what's your suggestion?" [Parent 4]

Parent self-efficacy and self-worth

All participants, including clinicians with lived experience, emphasised the need to support parent self-efficacy and self-esteem to counter feelings of guilt, shame, inadequacy, and self-blame. Encouraging parents to embrace 'good enough' parenting, set realistic goals, and approach tasks one step at a time were viewed as crucial for building self-worth and a sense of achievement. Participants described the value of reinforcing parents' existing strengths and acknowledging incremental progress to boost parent confidence and motivation to keep going. Clinicians were identified as playing a key role in this.

> "Helping the parents to look... at the positives first... working within the strength-based model. And helping parents to identify their own character strengths so they can use that to... build on their parenting." [Clinician 3]

3.2.5. Theme 5: Accessible and Integrated Support

Parents and service providers emphasised that program delivery must be accessible, flexible, and seamlessly embedded into everyday life and clinical practice

Low-burden accessibility

All participants valued a simple, engaging, and adaptable program to maximise usability. A mix of written, visual, and interactive delivery was perceived as important for maintaining parent engagement across learning styles. Participants asked for easy-to-follow, plain-language content to accommodate parents with diverse literacy levels or reduced cognitive functioning. They also recommended minimising the burden for parents with limited time and fluctuating symptoms by dividing the program into short sections with breaks, providing reminders, and ensuring flexibility to access the program at any time of day and to pause and re-engage as needed.

https://doi.org/10.3390/children13010129

"It can't be too long... parents might have things they need to organise for the kids... Breaking it down into smaller portions so that it's achievable... because they could be tired and they may not be able to concentrate for too long." [Parent 8]

Participants highlighted the importance of the program being low-cost and offering user-friendly technology accessible across devices, to suit parents with different incomes and technology resources, as well as parents and clinicians with varying digital skills.

Seamless integration

Participants highlighted that effective program delivery depends on seamless integration into routine clinical practice, reflecting their view that mental health and parenting are closely intertwined. A self-directed program complemented by clinician check-ins during existing sessions was suggested to minimise clinician burden, leverage existing clinician skills, and extend support beyond limited clinician contact.

"Can kind of check in with people during that session... if it's within... that timeframe, yes. But outside of that, it might be a challenge because of the other demands of clients." [Clinician 1]

Service providers emphasised the need to use case-coordination, secondary consultation, or referrals to specialists when parents' needs exceed expertise or service scope, which parents also valued. Clinician training was recommended to be brief and flexible, including ensuring staff can learn at their own pace, revisit content, and access optional extra resources to accommodate diverse needs and schedules. While clinicians suggested supervision from parenting specialists, clinical leads considered this infeasible and proposed that this support be provided by existing supervisors instead.

3.2.6. Intervention Design

The research team synthesised the above findings and translated the design considerations into relevant design features for the intended adapted parenting program. Features were designed and refined iteratively, drawing on relevant literature, features from the original PiP Kids program, and multidisciplinary meetings with psychology and human–computer interaction researchers from the team. For example, the subtheme 'Parent self-efficacy and self-worth' was conceptualised as including strengths-based and encouraging language, achievable strategies, and progress indicators within each online module, among other features. All concretised features are presented in Supplementary Table S4, mapped to the theme and subtheme they were designed to address and the program component where they would be embedded. Broadly, the adapted parenting program, named 'Partners in Parenting Kids Parental Mental Health (PiP Kids PMH; herein 'the program'), is intended to include four key components and a clinician training package. See Table 1 for a description of the main components of the program.

Table 1. Key components of the intended adapted parenting program and the clinician training package, developed through the translation of design considerations into program components.

Program Component	Description
Self-directed online modules	- Short 10–15 min, interactive online modules providing parents with evidence-based parenting knowledge and practical strategies in easy-to-understand, validating language.
End-of-module reflection questions	- Reflection questions at the end of each module to help parents set individualised goals, reflect on implementing goals, and identify areas where they may benefit from further support from clinicians or their broader support network.

https://doi.org/10.3390/children13010129

Table 1. *Cont.*

Program Component	Description
Clinician-support component	- Clinician-support component integrated into parents' existing mental health counselling sessions to supplement module content. Conversations are scaffolded by parents' goals and reflection responses, which clinicians access via their own dashboard. Clinicians provide tailored guidance, support implementation of strategies, highlight parent strengths, and offer non-judgmental encouragement and emotional support.
Written summary of each counselling session	- A written summary of the key takeaways, goals, and plans from each counselling session, co-created between clinician and parent to help parents remember and implement learnings at home.
Clinician training package	- To support clinicians in delivering the clinician-support component. It includes (a) Self-paced online training modules introducing the program, the clinicians' role, and each parenting topic (b) Access to the parent modules so they can explore the program content and delivery; (c) A one-off group workshop to discuss the training and practise skills with peers; (d) Ongoing supervision delivered by existing clinical supervisors within clinician's regular supervision sessions.

4. Phase 2 Methods and Results: Develop and Validate the Initial Prototype Design

4.1. Phase 2 Methods

4.1.1. Participants

Participants included the same parents (n = 8) and all service providers from Phase 1, except one social worker clinician who had left the collaborating service (n = 2 clinical leads; n = 4 clinicians).

4.1.2. Data Collection

Based on Phase 1 findings, the research team developed an initial prototype of the adapted parenting program and associated clinician training, each demonstrating the dashboard and two example modules. Figure 4 shows the online dashboard pages from the initial parenting program prototype and the accompanying clinician training modules. Phase 2 workshops aimed to validate and refine the program design with parents and service providers. Each parent and service provider participated in one workshop during this phase. All parents attended individual workshops due to difficulties scheduling group workshops, and service providers participated in either individual or group sessions. Workshops were conducted via Zoom with audio and video recording and lasted 2 h (with a 5–10 min break).

Workshops explored parent and service provider feedback on the preliminary Phase 1 design considerations to sense-check whether these reflected their needs and preferences. Feedback was then sought on the broad program design, including its four main components. Parents and service providers were then given access to the online component of the initial program prototype and encouraged to share their feedback aloud. Service providers were also provided with access to a prototype of the online component of the clinician training in this way. Follow-up questions explored participant preferences (e.g., what they liked, what they would change, and how design features should be structured and delivered) and how well the program addressed the design considerations.

https://doi.org/10.3390/children13010129

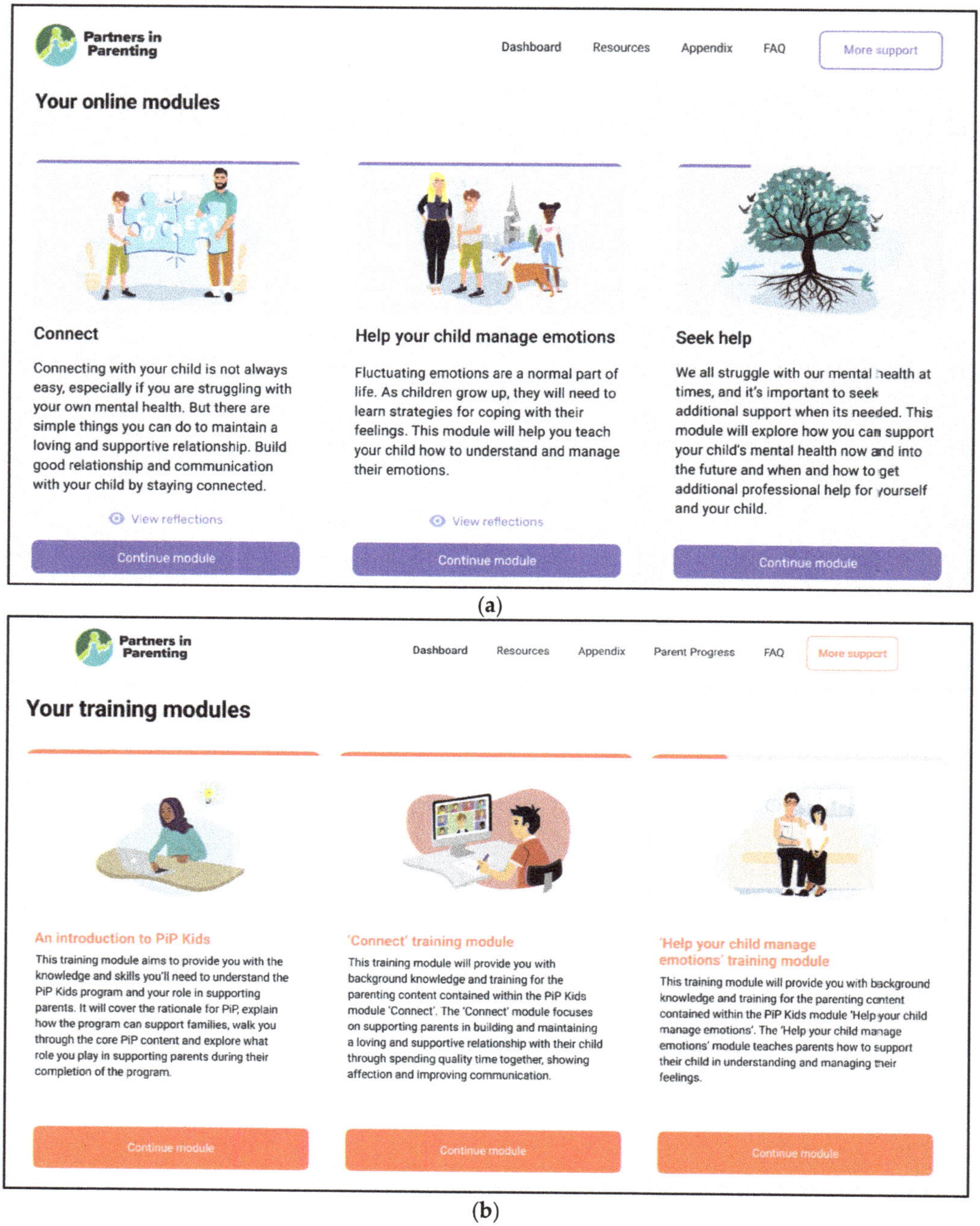

Figure 4. Dashboard pages including example modules from the online components of the initial prototype of the (**a**) parenting program and (**b**) associated clinician training modules, demonstrating the layout, wording, example topics, and functionality of the prototype.

4.1.3. Data Analysis

Interviews were transcribed automatically via Zoom or by a third-party transcription service and checked by the first author for accuracy. Transcribed data were coded with the

https://doi.org/10.3390/children13010129

support of NVivo software, using Braun and Clarke's six-phase reflexive thematic-analysis approach [64,65]. Data were analysed deductively using the five design considerations from Phase 1, as the purpose of this phase was to sense-check these themes and validate if and how the initial prototype met these needs. Additional themes were identified inductively to capture novel insights beyond these pre-defined themes. To avoid confirmation bias and ensure any novel insights would be captured, each transcript was initially coded openly before being coded to the Phase 1 themes. Throughout the analysis process, the research team also actively sought findings that may contradict the Phase 1 themes or suggest that the prototype did not meet these design considerations.

4.2. Phase 2 Results

Participants frequently reiterated findings from Phase 1, confirming the relevance of these for the program. For this reason, a summary of how well the initial prototype met the design considerations is provided in Supplementary File S1, with illustrative quotes. A novel theme was also developed, highlighting the program's role in facilitating communication between parents and clinicians, and considerations for how this could occur. The results below outline this new theme as well as suggestions for improvement according to each design consideration.

4.2.1. Building Readiness for Parenting Support

Suggestions for the next program iteration included a quick-exit button and extra mental health resources within module pages. Participants also suggested more clearly specifying for parents the program's purpose, better highlighting the benefits of parent and clinician reflection questions, and introducing the program in terms of its potential benefits to parental mental health.

4.2.2. Emotional and Social Support

Suggestions for the next program iteration included more explicitly acknowledging that parenting is difficult, additional 24/7 support options, more lived-experience examples, and additional prompts or opportunities to reach out to support networks or peers. Clinicians suggested that training should include ongoing group supervision and specify that clinician reflections are designed to be shared with other clinicians.

4.2.3. Practical and Personalised Knowledge

Suggestions for the next program iteration included pictures of real people, space for parents to note personalised goals and strategies and answer goal prompts, and more example strategies within modules. Participants also recommended more goal options, a search function, and a personalised dashboard picture. Other suggestions included more contextualising of content to parenting with mental health challenges, more examples for fathers, and ensuring images include a balanced representation of different cultures.

4.2.4. Parent-Led Empowerment

Suggestions for the next program iteration included space for parents to note extra comments or record their existing skills, while also ensuring parents have control over whether they share goals and reflections with clinicians. Participants recommended increasing and bolding encouraging language, removing language that may be deficit- or pressure-focused, and providing more obvious progress indicators.

4.2.5. Accessible and Integrated Support

Suggestions for the next program iteration included improving the readability of content; minimising open text responses; more audio, including the option for text to be read aloud; versions in other languages; and encouraging parents to download content. They also suggested including videos and more images, colours, and activities. Parents recommended providing estimates of how long activities might take and acknowledging financial concerns as a potential challenge. Clinical leads recommended that parents be given a timeframe for program completion. Clinicians asked for a supervisor with parenting expertise and the option to contact parents to check in on progress between sessions.

4.2.6. Emergent Theme: Bridge for Communication

Participants described how the program was able to facilitate communication between parents and clinicians. The end-of-module reflection questions were seen as helpful for starting and guiding sessions by communicating parent needs to clinicians. This feature was seen as an efficient way for parents to express priorities or sensitive issues that might be difficult to say aloud, though it was noted that these should not replace therapeutic conversation. Participants described the benefit of parents completing reflections while they were in the mindset of the program to help them record points to discuss later. Parents and clinicians appreciated clinicians having direct dashboard access to parent progress and reflections to facilitate easy communication, and clinicians' ability to review these in advance for session preparation.

> "Some people still find it hard to talk face-to-face... so I feel like this is really good because you're getting this information to them. It's like, when you fill out a questionnaire, and you almost feel anonymous... cause you're not saying it. It's another way of communicating without having to speak." [Parent 7]

Suggestions for the next iteration of the program included having more frequent reminders within the content to speak with clinicians and extra space for parents to note comments or questions to share. Clinical leads raised issues with clinicians having dashboard access to parent progress and reflections, including concerns about confidentiality, data security if a clinician or parent leaves the service, and added administrative burden. They concluded that parents should instead share their progress and reflections with clinicians directly unless logistical issues with the clinician dashboard can be resolved.

4.2.7. Intervention Refinements

The research team refined the design of the initial prototype based on the Phase 2 findings. For example, sharing each module's goals and reflection responses was made optional to give parents control over if and when they share this information with their clinician or other support people. Supplementary Table S5 provides a full outline of all prototype refinements as well as additional considerations for future iterations of the program beyond the scope of the current study.

As only a limited number of modules could be developed for this first iteration, topics were prioritised based on Phase 1 and 2 findings, our systematic review comparing parental factors between parents with and without anxiety and/or depression [48], and a broader literature review of parenting domains linked to parental mental health and child outcomes [5,45,67–69]. Particularly salient parenting domains identified from this search included talking with children about parental mental health, seeking help, self-care, parenting stress, effective discipline, aversiveness, withdrawal, warmth, parental self-efficacy, and parent–child relationship quality. The topics 'Talking with children about parental mental health' and 'Showing affection and acceptance' were chosen, with information on self-care and help-seeking integrated throughout these modules. These topics were selected to cover as many of the key domains as possible, while including content specific to parenting in the

https://doi.org/10.3390/children13010129

context of parental mental health challenges and prioritising warmth as a factor repeatedly linked to parent–child relationship quality and child outcomes [45,68].

Evidence-based content for the 'Showing affection and acceptance' module was retained from the original PiP Kids program, with features and wording adapted for contextualisation to parenting with mental health challenges. Content for the 'Talking with children about parental mental health' topic was divided into two modules, (1) 'Getting ready for conversations' and (2) 'Having conversations', to keep each module manageable for parents. This new content was developed by reviewing existing resources on the topic [69–76]. The content and its presentation were comprehensively reviewed by research team members with expertise in psychology, parenting, and parental mental health. Modules were initially designed to take 10–15 min to complete; however, incorporating all design considerations while including evidence-based content required extending the duration of modules to approximately 15–25 min. Supplementary File S2 provides images of the refined parenting program prototype, including the dashboard and selected module pages.

5. Phase 3 Methods and Results: Deliver the Refined Prototype

5.1. Phase 3 Methods

5.1.1. Participants

Recruitment followed the same methods as Phase 1, and parents from earlier phases were also invited to participate. Six parents expressed interest, including four from Phases 1 and 2. Five parents consented, including one newly recruited parent and the four returning participants. One of the returning participants withdrew due to competing life circumstances, and another was lost to follow-up after partially completing the prototype.

In total, three parents completed all three prototype modules and the interview, and their data were included for analysis. The parents were mothers (n = 2) and a grandmother (n = 1) aged 41–56 years (M = 47). The newly recruited parent was seeking mental health support at the collaborating health service, while the other two parents had lived experience of accessing support in the broader community within the past six months. Parents' self-reported mental health challenges included high stress (n = 3), anxiety (n = 2), trauma (n = 2), and depression (n = 1). Parents' reported cultural backgrounds included Australian/New Zealand (n = 2), East Asian (n = 1), and Middle Eastern (n = 1). Their highest education levels were one each of technical qualifications, a bachelor's degree, and a postgraduate degree. All three were single parents and concession card holders. Supplementary Table S6 presents further demographic characteristics of the Phase 3 parent participants.

5.1.2. Data Collection

Phase 3 focused on piloting the refined prototype with parents to explore its initial acceptability and identify areas for improvement. For this study, only the online module component of the refined prototype was piloted, not the clinician-support component or clinician training. A staged approach was considered valuable given the newly co-designed content and program features. This online-only trial served as a logical first step in evaluating the modules before integrating them with clinician support.

Parents completed a demographic questionnaire via REDCap before commencing the refined prototype. Parents were encouraged to complete one module per week, with the first author monitoring progress and sending weekly, personalised reminder emails based on each parent's goals and progress. Approximately one month after commencing the prototype, parents completed a 1 hour semi-structured feedback interview. Interviews were conducted using a guide adapted from prior related research [47,77,78] to explore prototype acceptability and adaptations for the next iteration of the program. The interview schedule (Supplementary File S3) was adapted from the Theoretical Framework of Acceptability (TFA) questionnaire, a theory-informed approach to evaluating the acceptability of healthcare interventions [79,80]. Open questions asking parents for their perspectives on a clinician-support component were also included. Interviews were conducted one-on-one via Zoom with audio recording. Parents were reimbursed with a $35 gift card for the interview and an additional $10 for each online parenting module completed.

5.1.3. Data Analysis

Interview recordings were automatically transcribed by Zoom and manually cleaned by the research team. Parents were invited to review their transcripts for alignment with their experience of the interview [81]; however, no parent chose to review their transcript. The transcripts were analysed with the support of NVivo using a reflexive thematic-analysis approach [64,65]. Themes were identified deductively using the seven constructs of the TFA [79,80], with subthemes developed inductively, including those not covered by the TFA but still relevant to acceptability.

5.2. Phase 3 Results

Themes reflecting the acceptability of the refined prototype were developed using the seven TFA constructs, with subthemes capturing specific contributors to acceptability and suggestions for improvement. Table 2 defines the TFA constructs and presents the subthemes with illustrative quotes.

Table 2. Acceptability themes, subthemes, and illustrative quotes for Phase 3.

TFA [a] Construct: Definition	Subtheme of TFA [a] Construct	Illustrative Quotes
Affective attitude: How an individual feels about the intervention.	Positive overall experience	- "All this online resources are self-guided evidence base. It's really really good. And you always give the link to us where it's from... so I think if people really interested, they... can go to do their own research." [Parent 2]
	Accessible and user-friendly	- "There's no difficulties... even though English is my second language, so... the language is really good. The content is easy to follow, easy to remember." [Parent 2]
	Engaging and interactive	- "It was interactive, it was easy to interact with. It was different stuff... audio, text... big, small, different size... it just keeps you like, it's not boring." [Parent 3]
	Supportive and encouraging	- "Not in a way that I feel like they're judging me they're telling me what to do... It's just some extra information... it was like easy to go ahead and friendly." [Parent 3]
Intervention coherence: The extent to which the individual understands the intervention and how it works.	Some uncertainty about program instructions	- "Sometimes...English being my second language, I was not sure what I need to do when I read them, so it was not clear enough, like the instruction... Is it a question? Is this just information?... What do I need to do?" [Parent 3]
	Unclear program scope and users	- "Another thing was not clear to me is that at the end, who is going to use these resources... and is it self-referral, is it like advice by GP?" [Parent 3] - "I thought there were more [modules] coming." [Parent 1]

Table 2. *Cont.*

TFA [a] Construct: Definition	Subtheme of TFA [a] Construct	Illustrative Quotes
Perceived effectiveness: The extent to which the intervention achieved its intended purpose.	Reinforced parent self-efficacy	- "It increased the knowledge of my strength... my belief in myself, and that, I do have the strength to do this... it just reaffirmed to me... That in the eyes of what people would recommend, I'm doing it." [Parent 1]
	Encouraged some reflection and practice	- "It definitely give me a stop point to rethink what I have done, what I can improve, because there's always room to improve. So not huge changes, but definitely helping to make small changes, adjustments." [Parent 2]
	Content was familiar but helpful	- "I think it's really really helpful for all parents across the board, no matter how much the parents already know the knowledge itself." [Parent 2]
Ethicality: The extent to which the intervention has a good fit with an individual's value system.	Ability to tailor to individual parents	- "I was able to choose my own goal, they didn't choose it for me... If it was not reasonable or doable, I wouldn't choose them." [Parent 3]
	Inclusivity valued but could be improved	- "From the picture... it was inclusive... it was not just from one gender, one nationality it was kind of like inclusive." [Parent 3] - "Four people family has been showing so many different pages, and I haven't seen... families in other shapes... single parents, grandparents, same-sex parents, or just a traditional core mum and dad children." [Parent 2]
Burden: The amount of effort required to participate in the intervention.	Time and cognitive effort required	- "It was so text based... it did take me a long time... I had to really concentrate... It's not something that I could do while I had [child] around." [Parent 1] - "It's not too difficult. If I sit down for one hour, I can finish a module." [Parent 2]
	Balancing competing life demands	- "I had set myself aside time to do it but life got in the way" [Parent 1] - "I'm working, I'm single mother I have a lot to do... sometimes those goals will be on top of my priority list sometimes there's other things happening that they can't wait so... to fit that in my busy schedule was difficult." [Parent 3]
Opportunity costs: The benefits, profits, or values that were given up to engage in the intervention.	No sacrifices other than time and internet	- "Time, internet, some people they don't have money to... like you need computer, internet and time." [Parent 3] - "I didn't have to sacrifice anything other than time." [Parent 1]

https://doi.org/10.3390/children13010129

Table 2. *Cont.*

TFA [a] Construct: Definition	Subtheme of TFA [a] Construct	Illustrative Quotes
Self-efficacy in completing program: The individual's confidence that they can perform the behaviour(s) required to participate in the intervention.	Confidence in eventual completion	- "I was confident I'd finish it. But I wasn't confident of when." [Parent 1]
	Difficulty completing some program activities	- "The goal setting and the making it happen page, I didn't really like them personally, because I hated school... I don't like to have to write down all this stuff... and it's like... How do I put that into words?" [Parent 1]
	Goals helpful but challenging to implement	- "I had to work out how to do it and it was just like, with the way [child]'s been lately. Concentrating on stuff... problem solving, and that sometimes there's not, so clear for me how to do it." [Parent 1] - "It was good that I have a goal... and it will benefit me... but on a negative side there was no manual ... how to achieve this goal." [Parent 3]
Additional acceptability subthemes:	Normalising challenges	- "The clear message is... No parents are perfect. You don't have to be perfect. It's okay to take a take a moment... we're all humans" [Parent 2] - "It does normalise it because I wasn't thinking mental health the whole time... I just viewed it as this is for parents." [Parent 1]
	Desire for human support and connection	- "Ifwe have a live person behind this website... is it just got something for people to read?... Follow up outside this website would be very beneficial." [Parent 3] - "If there is sort of like an in-person opportunity, or possibly even a group... know that they can get together and talk about things." [Parent 1]
	Opportunity for child feedback	- "Will that be a possible, children friendly versions like the little questionnaire or something?... So actually, I can get some feedback from my kids." [Parent 2]

[a] TFA = Theoretical Framework of Acceptability.

5.2.1. Affective Attitude

Parents expressed a positive experience with the program, including its self-directed, evidence-based content and optional further reading. They found it accessible and user-friendly with clear language, summaries, audio, and images to support understanding. The simple technology was appreciated, but parents recommended adding the ability to enlarge text and easily return to previous pages. Parents found the program engaging and interactive due to its varied text, visuals, and activities; however, they mentioned that interactive boxes could be more clearly indicated. The program was described as being supportive through non-judgmental and non-directive language, calming colours, and progress indicators, but parents suggested adding encouraging music when completing activities.

5.2.2. Intervention Coherence

While parents generally had a good understanding of the program, they were occasionally uncertain about program instructions, such as whether some sections were informational or required a response. They suggested including a video to introduce the program, as written instructions may not be accessible for everyone. There was also some

https://doi.org/10.3390/children13010129

uncertainty about the program's scope and users, as some parents expected extra modules and were unsure about who the program was for and how it would be accessed.

5.2.3. Perceived Effectiveness

Parents reported that they felt the program helped strengthen their self-efficacy and self-belief by reinforcing their existing strengths. Parents said that reflective activities and practical suggestions prompted them to think about their parenting and make small adjustments. However, they stated that the end-of-module reflection questions did not encourage them to seek additional support as intended. Parents described the content as familiar, noting that while it included some new information, its main value was in reminding them of what they already knew. Parents suggested this may be most beneficial for new parents or those less familiar with the content. To further support reflection and practice, parents suggested including more topics, space for open reflection, and quizzes.

5.2.4. Ethicality

Parents appreciated that the modules could be tailored to the needs of individual parents, such as being able to select strategies that were relevant and achievable for them. Parents also valued that the program was inclusive and represented diverse cultures in images, but they recommended depicting a broader range of family types and incorporating parenting examples from other cultures. They also mentioned that the content was not always catered to individual circumstances, such as low literacy, neurodivergence, or unique family contexts. Parents suggested ways to further tailor the program, such as uploading their own avatar and including space to note reflections specific to their situation.

5.2.5. Burden

Parents had different experiences with the time and cognitive effort required for the program. They mentioned that it took around an hour to finish a module, which was longer than intended. Some found this manageable, but others found reading the text-heavy content demanding of their limited time and energy. Parents recommended shorter modules, less information displayed at once, faster page transitions, and more audio and video options. Although the self-directed modules allowed parents to fit the program flexibly around competing demands, they said that busy schedules still interrupted progress. Parents appreciated that all modules were available at once, and they found email reminders helpful, but suggested adding optional text message reminders.

5.2.6. Opportunity Costs

All parents reported that participating in the program was worthwhile and required no sacrifices beyond time and internet access. However, one parent noted that internet access might be a challenge for some families.

5.2.7. Self-Efficacy in Completing Program

Parents reported feeling confident they would complete the program, although uncertain how long it might take. Some open activities were perceived as difficult due to the need to put responses into words, and parents suggested more multiple-choice activities. Goals were seen as helpful and achievable, but applying them in daily life could be challenging given the need to problem-solve. Parents appreciated the goal reminders but suggested extra reminders and the ability to track goals on the dashboard.

5.2.8. Additional Acceptability Subthemes

Parents valued that the program normalised parenting and mental health challenges and emphasised that no parent is perfect. They reinforced the importance of incorporating

https://doi.org/10.3390/children13010129

human support and connection, noting the benefit of flexible access to a clinician and peer-based social opportunities. One parent suggested incorporating opportunities for parents to receive feedback from their children on their parenting.

6. Discussion

This co-design study aimed to adapt an evidence-based digital parenting program (PiP Kids) for future implementation in an existing adult mental health service, to support parents seeking mental health care. Triangulation of findings across parents, clinicians, and clinical leads provided a multifaceted understanding of end-user needs, strengthened by the lived experience of several clinicians. The main findings identified from Phase 1 and reinforced in Phase 2 underpinned design considerations regarding the needs and preferences of parents and service providers. These design considerations are discussed in detail below, with reference to the existing literature and future research directions. Initial acceptability findings and suggestions for improvement from Phase 3 are integrated into the themes where relevant.

6.1. Building Parent and Clinician Readiness for Parenting Support

The first design consideration identified several factors impacting parent and clinician readiness for parenting support, including parent wellbeing and safety, clinician training, and both groups' understanding of the purpose and value of the program. The Phase 1 and 2 findings regarding building parents' readiness align with prior research emphasising that the immediate wellbeing of families should be addressed before they can engage in parenting support, particularly in contexts involving risk, safety concerns, or family violence [34]. Managing parental mental and physical health and engaging in self-care have also been identified as foundational for parenting capacity [17,82]. Participants from Phase 2 appreciated that the prototype helped support parent and family wellbeing through content that encouraged self-care and help-seeking, in addition to clinicians directly supporting parent mental health. Consistent with prior research, participants from Phase 1 viewed mental health treatment as the main role of the adult mental health service, with clinicians extending to parenting when it helped support the parent's mental health goals or after acute concerns were addressed [24,29]. This suggests that parenting programs integrated within adult mental health services should prioritise parental mental health first, either by allowing treatment before the program begins or by supporting the parent's mental health goals directly. Our adapted version of PiP Kids aims to address this by utilising a flexible, largely self-directed format that can be introduced at any stage of treatment, allowing clinicians to prioritise parental mental health goals while integrating parenting support as appropriate.

Additionally, our results suggest that a thorough introduction to the program may be particularly valuable for parents with mental health challenges, as this was expressed across all three phases. In the intended program design, this is supported through an introductory email sent to parents as well as clinicians introducing the program's purpose, its intended benefits, and how to access and use it. We found that parents in Phase 2 particularly appreciated the clinicians' role in supporting this introduction, similar to prior research [34]. However, it was repeatedly suggested that an initial video may also be beneficial. The importance of a clear introduction has also been found in previous research, with suggestions that setting clear expectations and describing the benefits of programs can help ease parent anxiety, support engagement, create stability, and minimise the uncertainty that has occurred across this and other programs for parents with mental health challenges [23,34].

https://doi.org/10.3390/children13010129

Findings regarding clinician readiness also suggested the importance of clinicians understanding the program and feeling confident about its value and use. Clinicians from Phase 2 appreciated that the program would provide them with not just program training but also brief refreshers on parenting content and how their existing skills translate to parenting support. Since practitioner confidence and skills related to parenting are key factors in the likelihood of family-focused practice [83], this approach may support successful implementation into a range of settings, since it does not require extensive parenting-specific training [29]. Together, these findings suggest that integration of parenting support into adult mental health care should begin with a period of building readiness and addressing foundational factors with both parents and clinicians.

6.2. Facilitating Emotional, Social, and Peer Support for Parents and Clinicians

The second design consideration suggested that for parents, normalising non-judgmental emotional support and social connection is crucial, whereas for clinicians, professional peer support is required. In particular, initial acceptability feedback from parents in Phase 3 indicated that they found the supportive, non-judgmental language of the online modules helpful. Consistent with existing literature, parenting was described as a potentially sensitive topic, especially for parents with mental health challenges who often fear being judged as incompetent, which can act as a barrier to help-seeking [82,84]. This highlighted the importance of validating module content and empathetic emotional support from clinicians [85]. Specifically, across Phases 1 and 2, participants emphasised that parenting-related emotional support provided in an existing parent–clinician relationship would be particularly beneficial. This aligns with research suggesting the importance of establishing a trusting relationship prior to introducing parenting programs, to create a safe, non-critical, reflective environment for parents [34].

Across Phases 2 and 3, parents also valued that the module content encouraged social support from family and friends beyond the therapeutic alliance. This finding aligns with prior studies suggesting that parents benefit from social connection as it provides emotional support, shared parenting strategies, and support with practical parenting tasks [17,86]. Participants across all phases consistently reiterated the potential benefits of adding peer support from other parents with mental health challenges, which has been described by parents and clinicians previously [21,34,50]. Likely benefits include reduced social isolation as well as normalisation, reassurance, and learning from others in similar situations [23,84]. However, consistent with earlier findings [84,86], some participants in Phase 1 described the potential negative effects of peer groups, such as anxiety, shame, or reluctance to share personal information. It may be beneficial for future studies to investigate how to leverage existing technology to design peer support communities that enable the benefits of peer support while minimising the concerns articulated by participants.

Peer support was also valued by clinicians in Phases 1 and 2, as they highlighted the importance of connection with other clinicians delivering the program, similar to previous work [34]. Clinicians suggested that ongoing group supervision would be more valuable than a one-off workshop; however, clinical leads indicated this may be challenging in their busy health service. Future studies could explore implementation options for feasible group supervision, such as having a brief dedicated peer supervision or an embedded approach where parenting-related discussions are integrated within existing group supervision to reduce time demands on clinicians and services.

6.3. Providing Parents with Practical and Personalised Parenting Knowledge

The third design consideration highlighted the importance of providing parenting knowledge that is practical, relevant, and tailored to each parent's unique family, context,

https://doi.org/10.3390/children13010129

and mental health challenges to help them implement strategies that work for them. This aligns with previous findings emphasising the benefit of practical strategies [82], clinician modelling [34], clinicians adapting content for each family [17,21], and support for problem-solving implementation of strategies [51,87]. Goals within the module content were also valued for helping parents action changes, consistent with research identifying goal setting as a key process in both parenting and mental health recovery [22]. During Phase 2, the written summaries of each counselling session were highlighted as a particularly helpful aspect for supporting implementation of learned strategies, but the usefulness of this in practice will need to be trialled in the future when piloting the clinician-support component. In Phase 3, parents suggested the helpfulness of the module's practical tips, but noted that much of the content felt familiar, suggesting we may have reached parents with relatively high parenting literacy. This initial acceptability data suggested that for parents in this study, their main challenges were less about gaining parenting information, but more in relation to applying the content to their unique circumstances and putting strategies into action in their lives. Together, these findings suggest that even when module content is easy to understand, making changes in parenting may be the difficult part, especially for parents with mental health challenges [21]. This indicates a need for applied and personalised support beyond what a fully self-directed program can provide. Findings echo the potential benefit of clinician-support provided by the parent's mental health clinician who already has the context of the parent's family and mental health challenges for tailoring strategies [18].

Additionally, participants across Phases 2 and 3 liked the program's consistent focus specifically on parenting in the context of mental health issues, which has been shown to be crucial to program engagement and acceptability for these parents [21,49]. For example, we and other studies have found the need for parenting programs to support parents in talking with their children about parental mental health [49,88], given children's desire to receive this information from their parents and parents' uncertainty about how to have these conversations [54,89]. These findings are consistent with past research, which suggests that generic parenting programs that fail to address parental mental health may be insufficient for parents with mental health concerns [21,43]. Finally, participants across all phases highlighted the importance of ensuring that module content reflects diverse family types and cultures, consistent with prior calls for inclusive and culturally sensitive design [29,51].

6.4. Encouraging Parent-Led Empowerment for Parents

The fourth design consideration demonstrated the importance of parents having autonomy and control while receiving the strengths-based support they need. Parents and service providers in Phase 2 described the value of the program's self-directed module content for encouraging parent autonomy and independence, similar to prior work [34]; but they also reinforced the need for adjunct clinician support of such autonomy. Specifically, our initial acceptability data from Phase 3 indicated that fully self-directed programs may be less suitable for parents with mental health issues unless some degree of human support and encouragement is provided. These findings are consistent with emerging evidence suggesting that self-directed parenting programs may be acceptable for parents with mental health issues, but guidance is needed due to the potential impact of mental health symptoms on parents' capacity to engage [34,51]. Incorporating clinician support to scaffold parents' completion of an autonomous, self-directed program may not only enhance program engagement but also outcomes for parents and families [90]. Additionally, consistent with previous findings [29,82], we found the need for this clinician support to take a collaborative, parent-led approach to promote parent autonomy and empowerment.

https://doi.org/10.3390/children13010129

Parents have reported positive experiences when given the opportunity to participate in decisions about their care [91], reinforcing the importance of this finding.

Participants across all phases also emphasised the value of strengths-based support that acknowledges parents' existing parenting strengths and fosters confidence in their parenting abilities. This aligns with previous evidence suggesting the importance of working with parents to promote a positive identity related to parenting [17,49]. To do this, findings echoed the need for interventions and clinicians to promote self-compassion and acceptance of imperfection, to help parents feel competent as parents and people [17,23]. Participants in Phases 2 and 3 appreciated the role of clinicians in promoting parent confidence and encouraging them to make progress with the program, consistent with prior work [34,82]. This focus on empowerment seems especially important given that feelings of inadequacy are common among parents with mental health challenges [86]. Initial acceptability data from Phase 3 suggested that parents felt the online modules supported their self-efficacy in parenting, similar to another study of a guided self-help parenting intervention [51]. Importantly, promoting parents' self-efficacy, positive sense of self, agency, and independent problem-solving capacity have been identified as key influences on parenting changes [92] and mental health recovery [93], highlighting the value of interventions that target these aspects.

6.5. Embedding Accessible and Integrated Support into Existing Practices

The final design consideration highlighted that program delivery must be accessible and integrated into the everyday life of parents and clinicians. Across all phases, flexibility for parents to disengage and re-engage was valued to accommodate fluctuating symptoms and competing life demands, similar to prior suggestions for parents with mental health challenges [94]. Parents in Phases 2 and 3 found module features that reduced cognitive burden to be helpful, such as reminders, summaries, and multiple-choice questions. This is not surprising, given the barriers parents with mental health challenges face when engaging with parenting programs, including fluctuating mood, competing priorities, and memory difficulties [34]. Initial acceptability data from Phase 3 suggested that parents generally found the online modules to be clear, engaging, user-friendly, and interactive. However, our findings and those of others suggest that the accessibility of module content could be improved by minimising text, presenting content visually or in videos, and making the program available in other languages [34,40,51].

Parents in Phase 3 suggested making the modules shorter, similar to findings that brief interventions are particularly beneficial for parents facing social disadvantage [36]. Notably, attempts were made to break the 'Talking with children' module into two parts to make it more cognitively manageable; however, parents suggested that further breaking down modules into even smaller chunks would be ideal. Furthermore, parents stated that modules took them approximately one hour to complete, despite an intended design of 15–25 min, based on the original PiP Kids program. This discrepancy could suggest that parents with mental health challenges may require additional time for module completion due to factors such as difficulties with mental health symptoms, reading comprehension, engagement, or digital literacy. Parents from Phase 3 reported confidence in their ability to complete modules eventually; however, parents across all phases said that the largely self-directed program may not be appropriate for parents with low English proficiency, limited technology literacy, or reading difficulties, unless extra support is available to help with completing modules. Future iterations of the adapted program should explore ways to balance evidence-based PiP Kids content with parent preferences for brevity, such as by implementing suggestions including videos or bite-sized modules that were not feasible in the current project. To further guide the development of future iterations,

https://doi.org/10.3390/children13010129

we suggest prioritising core features to maintain program accessibility while minimising burden on parents. Features that are likely essential to retain, due to their reiteration across all study phases, include a clear program introduction, inclusivity of diverse family types and cultures, content specific to parenting in the context of parental mental health, strengths-based language, clinician and social support, flexibility to engage and re-engage, and features that reduce cognitive burden. The remaining features may offer added value, but whether they are essential remains to be tested in the future.

The need to embed the program into existing mental health practice was also emphasised across Phases 1 and 2, to ensure the program becomes a feasible and sustainable part of routine care. Our findings align with existing literature suggesting that parenting is closely intertwined with parent mental health recovery, providing challenging and positive experiences, hope, and motivation [91]. Parenting is a central factor in the lives of many parents, suggesting the need for parenting support to be integrated within individual mental health care, not isolated in a separate service [29,82]. This is supported by evidence that parents experience positive outcomes when parenting is included in mental health treatment [32,91] and that interventions that integrate parenting with mental health support may best serve parents with mental health issues [20]. Notably, parental mental health and parenting support are often delivered separately, with parents experiencing frustration when their parenting is not addressed by psychologists and they have to repeat themselves to multiple clinicians [91,95]. Our technology-assisted adaptation of PiP Kids aims to address this gap with the intention of embedding digital parenting support within existing mental health service provision. This approach has the potential to not only reduce the need for parents to engage with multiple providers but also allow clinicians to provide parenting support without delivering parenting content, unlike face-to-face parenting programs that often rely on clinician delivery [21,23]. A technology-assisted program such as this is thus likely to be beneficial in community mental health settings where clinicians often manage large caseloads, limited numbers of sessions, and competing demands [30,35].

Importantly, clinicians from Phase 2 indicated that the intended embedded program seems to align with existing service practices, including using existing clinician skills and clinicians referring parents to other services when support needs fall outside the scope. These referrals are likely to be especially important for parents with mental health issues who often present with complex needs, including child mental health problems and socioeconomic disadvantage [96,97]. Additionally, clinicians differed in their confidence levels regarding parenting, suggesting the need for clinician training that is flexible in not only timing but also content. Our self-directed clinician training with optional additional resources seemed to be well-regarded for addressing these needs once implemented. Overall, these findings suggest the need for there to be clear compatibility between parenting programs and service needs for successful integration of programs into routine practice.

6.6. Creating a Bridge for Communication Between Parents and Clinicians

A novel finding in Phase 2 of this study was the potential role of the program in facilitating communication between parents and clinicians. Previous research has shown that vignettes, written resources, or other program components can be useful for starting difficult parenting conversations [24,30]. Our findings extend this by suggesting that a technology-assisted parenting program has the potential to serve as a structured communication mechanism embedded within the service model, allowing parents to regularly articulate their parenting needs and experiences. However, preliminary acceptability findings from Phase 3 suggest that without integrated clinician support, the end-of-module reflection questions may not encourage parents to communicate their support needs to

https://doi.org/10.3390/children13010129

others. Future research might examine whether the program serves this communication function when clinician support is incorporated.

Moreover, the clinician dashboard, which would allow clinicians to view parent progress and end-of-module reflections, was seen by parents and clinicians in Phase 2 to have potential value for streamlining communication. However, clinical leads identified practical challenges for implementation, including confidentiality concerns and logistical issues when clinicians or parents leave the service. While identifying design considerations and assessing initial acceptability is a critical early step in this research, only these two clinical leads discussed the real-world feasibility of implementing the integrated program design. Thus, future work is needed to further explore how suggestions such as the clinician dashboard could be integrated and to identify facilitators and barriers to implementation of the program in everyday practice.

6.7. Limitations

This study has several limitations that should be considered when interpreting the findings. First, although parents had recent lived experience of seeking mental health care, several were not currently in treatment. This may have limited the study sample to parents with stable levels of mental health challenges, but not necessarily parents with current mental health challenges. Additionally, the recruited parents self-reported general mental health challenges such as anxiety and depression, and not all presentations seen at adult mental health services were represented (e.g., alcohol and other drug use, gambling, eating disorders). It may therefore be helpful for future evaluations to trial the program with parents who are all currently accessing mental health support and for a broader range of presentations.

Second, recruitment difficulties and dropout affected sample size, consistent with prior research noting problems engaging parents with mental health issues, potentially due to stigma or low energy [21,49]. Due to recruitment difficulties, we engaged parents from all over Australia, which may not reflect the demographics of the collaborating health service, potentially impacting the external validity of the findings. Third, all parent participants spoke English, were female, and were primarily mothers, as we were unable to recruit any fathers. All clinicians were also female, employed at a single organisation, and no clinicians from the alcohol and other drug (AOD) service could be recruited. This sample homogeneity further limits the generalisability of findings to other populations or service settings. Although the inclusion of only mothers is common in parenting research [51], it is important to repeat this research with fathers, linguistically diverse families, and clinicians from multiple service contexts to increase transferability. Additionally, although the participants had diverse cultural backgrounds, the socioeconomic background of participants was only assessed in Phase 3, and it is therefore unclear how socioeconomic diversity may have influenced Phase 1 and 2 findings.

Fourth, the collaborating health service already emphasises parenting within its model of care, consistent with the shift in Australia towards family-focused practice [98]. However, this may not be reflective of other services; for example, less than half of adult-mental health clinicians in a study in the United Kingdom worked on parenting with their parent clients [16]. Future research should explore whether findings differ in countries or services with less family-oriented care.

Fifth, for feasibility reasons, Phase 3 piloted only the online component of the adapted program. Although this precluded exploration of the implementation of the whole program, Phase 3 nonetheless provided valuable preliminary insights into areas for improvement in the online modules. Delivering the full intervention, including the clinician-support component, on a small-scale to assess implementation and clinical outcomes is thus a

https://doi.org/10.3390/children13010129

priority for the next phase of this research. Lastly, due to feasibility, only a limited number of content topics were included in this first iteration of the adapted program. Other important topics such as effective discipline, aversive parenting, and withdrawal should be a priority for inclusion in future iterations of the program.

7. Conclusions

To our knowledge, this is the first study to adapt a digital parenting program with the intention of embedding it within routine adult mental health care. It provides an in-depth exploration of the needs and preferences of parents seeking mental health support and the service providers who support them when it comes to technology-assisted parenting programs. The identified design considerations indicate the importance of readiness, support, personalisation, practical knowledge, empowerment, accessibility, and integration for designing helpful technology-assisted parenting programs for this population. Based on these findings, this study develops a unique model of care in which parents would access digital parenting content and adjunct clinician support from their existing mental health clinician, whilst minimising burden on clinicians. Such an approach advances the literature on family-focused practice by moving beyond siloed parent and child services to address the parent's caregiving role within their mental health care, with the aim of better supporting parents and reducing the intergenerational risk of mental health issues. While the integrated, clinician-supported program is yet to be trialled, preliminary findings suggest the potential value of adopting this holistic, family-focused approach that integrates technology-assisted parenting support within adult mental health settings.

Although this study focused specifically on the PiP Kids program within one adult mental health service, the insights and design considerations may have broader implications for any technology-assisted parenting program aimed at supporting parents with mental health challenges. The results highlight the importance of co-designing these interventions with end users to ensure they are acceptable and accommodate parent and service needs. Collectively, findings contribute to implementation science in this field of research by exploring considerations for the future tailoring and implementation of digital parenting programs into real-world mental health services. Researchers, clinicians, and service developers seeking to design technology-assisted parenting programs for this population or implement interventions within existing mental health settings can consider our findings in their work.

Supplementary Materials: The following supporting information can be downloaded at: https://www.mdpi.com/article/10.3390/children13010129/s1, Table S1: Co-design methods and aims; Table S2: Demographics of Phase 1 parent and service provider participants; Table S3: Themes, subthemes and additional illustrative quotes for Phase 1; Table S4: Concrete features of the initial adapted parenting program alongside Phase 1 themes and subthemes; Table S5: Refinements made to the initial prototype and considerations for future iterations alongside Phase 2 themes; Table S6: Demographics of Phase 3 parent participants; File S1: Summary of Phase 2 findings regarding how well the initial prototype met the design considerations; File S2: Selected images of the refined parenting program prototype incorporating features from Phase 1 and 2 findings; File S3: Phase 3 parent interview schedule.

Author Contributions: Conceptualization, M.L.B., L.W., J.P.S., P.O., A.R., A.F.J. and M.B.H.Y.; methodology, M.L.B., L.W., J.P.S., P.O., A.R., A.F.J. and M.B.H.Y.; software, J.P.S., M.L. and J.X.; formal analysis, M.L.B., L.W. and J.P.S.; investigation, M.L.B.; resources, S.G. and H.V.; data curation, M.L.B.; writing—original draft preparation, M.L.B.; writing—review and editing, L.W., J.P.S., P.O., A.R., A.F.J., S.G., H.V., M.L., J.X. and M.B.H.Y.; visualisation, M.L.B.; supervision, L.W., P.O., A.R., A.F.J. and M.B.H.Y.; project administration, M.L.B. All authors have read and agreed to the published version of the manuscript.

Funding: This project is affiliated with the Centre of Research Excellence (CRE) in Childhood Adversity and Mental Health, a five-year research program (2019–2023) co-funded by the National Health and Medical Research Council (NHMRC) and Beyond Blue. The first author is funded by a Research Training Program Scholarship (Monash University) and was awarded a top-up scholarship from the NHMRC Centres of Research Excellence Grant APP1153419 titled 'Centre of Research Excellence in Childhood Adversity and Associated Depression and Anxiety'. This research was funded by these scholarships.

Institutional Review Board Statement: The study was conducted in accordance with the Declaration of Helsinki and approved by the Monash University Human Research Ethics Committee (ID #35059 approved 19 August 2022 and ID #44564 approved 20 September 2024).

Informed Consent Statement: Informed consent was obtained from all participants in the study.

Data Availability Statement: The data from this study are not publicly available to protect participant privacy and anonymity. Deidentified summaries of the data are available on request from the corresponding author.

Acknowledgments: The research team extends sincere thanks to the parents and service providers involved for generously contributing their time and lived experience. The team also gratefully acknowledges the community health service for supporting and promoting the study. The first author extends gratitude to Olivia Bruce and Sunita Bayyavarapu for co-facilitating workshops, and to the research interns on the team for their contribution to refining artificial intelligence (AI)-generated transcripts.

Conflicts of Interest: M.B.H.Y. and A.F.J. are co-authors of the Partners in Parenting Kids (PiP Kids) program, which forms the basis of the program examined in this research. They receive no financial benefits from the program or the current study. The authors declare no other conflict of interest.

Abbreviations

The following abbreviations are used in this manuscript:

PaRK	Parenting Resilient Kids
PiP	Partners in Parenting
PTSD	Post-Traumatic Stress Disorder
TFA	Theoretical Framework of Acceptability

References

1. Wolicki, S.B.; Bitsko, R.H.; Cree, R.A.; Danielson, M.L.; Ko, J.Y.; Warner, L.; Robinson, L.R. Mental Health of Parents and Primary Caregivers by Sex and Associated Child Health Indicators. *Adv. Res. Sci.* **2021**, *2*, 125–139. [CrossRef]
2. Johnson, S.E.; Lawrence, D.; Perales, F.; Baxter, J.; Zubrick, S.R. Prevalence of Mental Disorders Among Children and Adolescents of Parents with Self-Reported Mental Health Problems. *Community Ment. Health J.* **2018**, *54*, 884–897. [CrossRef] [PubMed]
3. Friedman, H.P.; Bilsky, S.A.; Luber, M.J. Parent Anxiety, Child Anxiety, Parental Beliefs about Anxiety, and Parenting Behaviors: Examining Direct and Indirect Associations. *J. Child Fam. Stud.* **2023**, *32*, 3419–3429. [CrossRef]
4. Vreeland, A.; Gruhn, M.A.; Watson, K.H.; Bettis, A.H.; Compas, B.E.; Forehand, R.; Sullivan, A.D. Parenting in Context: Associations of Parental Depression and Socioeconomic Factors with Parenting Behaviors. *J. Child Fam. Stud.* **2019**, *28*, 1124–1133. [CrossRef]
5. Christie, H.; Hamilton-Giachritsis, C.; Alves-Costa, F.; Tomlinson, M.; Halligan, S.L. The Impact of Parental Posttraumatic Stress Disorder on Parenting: A Systematic Review. *Eur. J. Psychotraumatol.* **2019**, *10*, 1550345. [CrossRef]
6. Engur, B. Parents with Psychosis: Impact on Parenting & Parent-Child Relationship- A Systematic Review. *Glob. J. Addict. Rehabil. Med.* **2017**, *1*, 36–40. [CrossRef]
7. Campbell, L.; Poon, A.W.C. Parenting Challenges for Persons with a Serious Mental Illness. In *Mental Health and Social Work*; Ow, R., Poon, A.W.C., Eds.; Springer: Singapore, 2020; pp. 457–474.
8. Goodman, S.H.; Simon, H.F.M.; Shamblaw, A.L.; Kim, C.Y. Parenting as a Mediator of Associations between Depression in Mothers and Children's Functioning: A Systematic Review and Meta-Analysis. *Clin. Child Fam. Psychol. Rev.* **2020**, *23*, 427–460. [CrossRef]

https://doi.org/10.3390/children13010129

9. Xu, F.; Cui, W.; Lawrence, P.J. The Intergenerational Transmission of Anxiety in a Chinese Population: The Mediating Effect of Parental Control. *J. Child Fam. Stud.* **2020**, *29*, 1669–1678. [CrossRef]
10. Kluczniok, D.; Boedeker, K.; Hindi Attar, C.; Jaite, C.; Bierbaum, A.-L.; Fuehrer, D.; Paetz, L.; Dittrich, K.; Herpertz, S.C.; Brunner, R.; et al. Emotional Availability in Mothers with Borderline Personality Disorder and Mothers with Remitted Major Depression Is Differently Associated with Psychopathology among School-Aged Children. *J. Affect. Disord.* **2018**, *231*, 63–73. [CrossRef]
11. Hine, R.H.; Maybery, D.J.; Goodyear, M.J. Identity in Recovery for Mothers with a Mental Illness: A Literature Review. *Psychiatr. Rehabil. J.* **2018**, *41*, 16–28. [CrossRef]
12. Löchner, J.; Ulrich, S.M.; Lux, U. The Impact of Parents' Stress on Parents' and Young Childrens' Mental Health—Short- and Long-Term Effects of Risk and Resilience Factors in Families with Children Aged 0–3 in a Representative Sample. *Stress Health* **2024**, *40*, e3400. [CrossRef]
13. Phelan, R.F.; Howe, D.J.; Cashman, E.L.; Batchelor, S.H. Enhancing Parenting Skills for Parents with Mental Illness: The Mental Health Positive Parenting Program. *Med. J. Aust.* **2013**, *199*, S30–S33. [CrossRef]
14. Giannakopoulos, G.; Solantaus, T.; Tzavara, C.; Kolaitis, G. Mental Health Promotion and Prevention Interventions in Families with Parental Depression: A Randomized Controlled Trial. *J. Affect. Disord.* **2021**, *278*, 114–121. [CrossRef] [PubMed]
15. Sandler, I.; Ingram, A.; Wolchik, S.; Tein, J.-Y.; Winslow, E. Long-Term Effects of Parenting-Focused Preventive Interventions to Promote Resilience of Children and Adolescents. *Child Dev. Perspect.* **2015**, *9*, 164–171. [CrossRef] [PubMed]
16. Dunn, A.; Startup, H.; Cartwright-Hatton, S. Adult Mental Health Service Engagement with Patients Who Are Parents: Evidence from 15 English Mental Health Trusts. *Br. J. Clin. Psychol.* **2022**, *61*, 335–348. [CrossRef]
17. Awram, R.; Hancock, N.; Honey, A. Balancing Mothering and Mental Health Recovery: The Voices of Mothers Living with Mental Illness. *Adv. Ment. Health* **2017**, *15*, 147–160. [CrossRef]
18. Solantaus, T.; Reupert, A.; Maybery, D. Working with Parents Who Have a Psychiatric Disorder. In *Parental Psychiatric Disorder: Distressed Parents and Their Families*, 3rd ed.; Reupert, A., Maybery, D., Nicholson, J., Göpfert, M., Seeman, M.V., Eds.; Cambridge University Press: New York, NY, USA, 2015; pp. 238–247.
19. Everett, Y.; Martin, C.G.; Zalewski, M. A Systematic Review Focusing on Psychotherapeutic Interventions That Impact Parental Psychopathology, Child Psychopathology and Parenting Behavior. *Clin. Child Fam. Psychol. Rev.* **2021**, *24*, 579–598. [CrossRef] [PubMed]
20. Barrett, S.; Muir, C.; Burns, S.; Adjei, N.; Forman, J.; Hackett, S.; Hirve, R.; Kaner, E.; Lynch, R.; Taylor-Robinson, D.; et al. Interventions to Reduce Parental Substance Use, Domestic Violence and Mental Health Problems, and Their Impacts Upon Children's Well-Being: A Systematic Review of Reviews and Evidence Mapping. *Trauma Violence Abus.* **2024**, *25*, 393–412. [CrossRef]
21. Isobel, S.; Meehan, F.; Pretty, D. An Emotional Awareness Based Parenting Group for Parents with Mental Illness: A Mixed Methods Feasibility Study of Community Mental Health Nurse Facilitation. *Arch. Psychiatr. Nurs.* **2016**, *30*, 35–40. [CrossRef]
22. Maybery, D.; Reupert, A.; Goodyear, M. Goal Setting in Recovery: Families Where a Parent Has a Mental Illness or a Dual Diagnosis. *Child Fam. Soc. Work* **2015**, *20*, 354–363. [CrossRef]
23. Hestbaek, E.; Mikkelsen, P.A.; Thomas, R.E.; Sleed, M.; Holm, C.; Corlin, A.B.; Sørensen, P.; Væver, M.S.; Simonsen, S. A Mentalization-Based Parenting Intervention (Lighthouse Parenting Programme) for Parents with Various Mental Disorders in Adult Mental Health Service: A Feasibility Study. *Ment. Health Prev.* **2025**, *38*, 200415. [CrossRef]
24. McCarthy, K.L.; Lewis, K.L.; Bourke, M.E.; Grenyer, B.F.S. A New Intervention for People with Borderline Personality Disorder Who Are Also Parents: A Pilot Study of Clinician Acceptability. *Bord. Pers. Disord. Emot. Dysregul.* **2016**, *3*, 10. [CrossRef] [PubMed]
25. Falkov, A.; Grant, A.; Hoadley, B.; Donaghy, M.; Weimand, B.M. The Family Model: A Brief Intervention for Clinicians in Adult Mental Health Services Working with Parents Experiencing Mental Health Problems. *Aust. N. Z. J. Psychiatry* **2020**, *54*, 449–452. [CrossRef] [PubMed]
26. Solantaus, T.; Toikka, S. The Effective Family Programme: Preventative Services for the Children of Mentally Ill Parents in Finland. *Int. J. Ment. Health Promot.* **2006**, *8*, 37–44. [CrossRef]
27. Allchin, B.; Solantaus, T. An Evidence-Based Practice Developed in-Situ: Let's Talk About Children and a Consolidation of Its Evidence Base. *Front. Psychiatry* **2022**, *13*, 824241. [CrossRef]
28. Heyman, M.; Nicholson, J.; English, K. The ParentingWell Practice Approach: Facilitating Implementation in U.S. Adult Mental Health Services. *Front. Psychiatry* **2024**, *15*, 1377088. [CrossRef]
29. Nicholson, J.; Heyman, M.; English, K.; Biebel, K. The ParentingWell Practice Approach: Adaptation of Let's Talk About Children for Parents with Mental Illness in Adult Mental Health Services in the United States. *Front. Psychiatry* **2022**, *13*, 801065. [CrossRef]
30. Gray, A.S.; Townsend, M.L.; Bourke, M.E.; Grenyer, B.F.S. Effectiveness of a Brief Parenting Intervention for People with Borderline Personality Disorder: A 12-Month Follow-up Study of Clinician Implementation in Practice. *Adv. Ment. Health* **2019**, *17*, 33–43. [CrossRef]

https://doi.org/10.3390/children13010129

31. Sherman, M.D.; Hooker, S.A. Supporting Families Managing Parental Mental Illness: Challenges and Resources. *Int. J. Psychiatry Med.* **2018**, *53*, 361–370. [CrossRef]
32. Gregg, L.; Adderley, H.; Calam, R.; Wittkowski, A. The Implementation of Family-focused Practice in Adult Mental Health Services: A Systematic Review Exploring the Influence of Practitioner and Workplace Factors. *Int. J. Ment. Health Nurs.* **2021**, *30*, 885–906. [CrossRef]
33. Riemersma, I.; Van Santvoort, F.; Van Doesum, K.; Hosman, C.; Janssens, J.; Van Der Zanden, R.; Otten, R. 'You Are Okay': Effects of a Support and Educational Program for Children with Mild Intellectual Disability and Their Parents with Mental Health Concerns. *J. Intellect. Disabil.* **2022**, *26*, 70–89. [CrossRef]
34. Butler, J.; Gregg, L.; Calam, R.; Wittkowski, A. Exploring Staff Implementation of a Self-Directed Parenting Intervention for Parents with Mental Health Difficulties. *Community Ment. Health J.* **2021**, *57*, 247–261. [CrossRef] [PubMed]
35. Ordway, M.R.; McMahon, T.J.; De Las Heras Kuhn, L.; Suchman, N.E. Implementation of an Evidenced-Based Parenting Program in a Community Mental Health Setting. *Infant Ment. Health J.* **2018**, *39*, 92–105. [CrossRef] [PubMed]
36. Harris, M.; Andrews, K.; Gonzalez, A.; Prime, H.; Atkinson, L. Technology-Assisted Parenting Interventions for Families Experiencing Social Disadvantage: A Meta-Analysis. *Prev. Sci.* **2020**, *21*, 714–727. [CrossRef] [PubMed]
37. Opie, J.E.; Esler, T.B.; Clancy, E.M.; Wright, B.; Painter, F.; Vuong, A.; Booth, A.T.; Newman, L.; Johns-Hayden, A.; Hameed, M.; et al. Universal Digital Programs for Promoting Mental and Relational Health for Parents of Young Children: A Systematic Review and Meta-Analysis. *Clin. Child Fam. Psychol. Rev.* **2024**, *27*, 23–52. [CrossRef]
38. Hall, C.M.; Bierman, K.L. Technology-Assisted Interventions for Parents of Young Children: Emerging Practices, Current Research, and Future Directions. *Early Child. Res. Q.* **2015**, *33*, 21–32. [CrossRef]
39. Breitenstein, S.M.; Gross, D.; Christophersen, R. Digital Delivery Methods of Parenting Training Interventions: A Systematic Review: Digital Delivery of Parent Training. *Worldviews Evid. Based Nurs.* **2014**, *11*, 168–176. [CrossRef]
40. Ramos, G.; Chavira, D.A. Use of Technology to Provide Mental Health Care for Racial and Ethnic Minorities: Evidence, Promise, and Challenges. *Cogn. Behav. Pract.* **2022**, *29*, 15–40. [CrossRef]
41. van der Zanden, R.A.; Speetjens, P.A.; Arntz, K.S.; Onrust, S.A. Online Group Course for Parents with Mental Illness: Development and Pilot Study. *J. Med. Internet Res.* **2010**, *12*, e1394. [CrossRef]
42. Jones, S.; Calam, R.; Sanders, M.; Diggle, P.J.; Dempsey, R.; Sadhnani, V. A Pilot Web Based Positive Parenting Intervention to Help Bipolar Parents to Improve Perceived Parenting Skills and Child Outcomes. *Behav. Cogn. Psychother.* **2014**, *42*, 283–296. [CrossRef]
43. Kaplan, K.; Solomon, P.; Salzer, M.S.; Brusilovskiy, E. Assessing an Internet-Based Parenting Intervention for Mothers with a Serious Mental Illness: A Randomized Controlled Trial. *Psychiatr. Rehabil. J.* **2014**, *37*, 222–231. [CrossRef] [PubMed]
44. Fernando, L.M.N.; Sim, W.H.; Jorm, A.F.; Rapee, R.; Lawrence, K.A.; Yap, M.B.H. Parenting Resilient Kids (PaRK), an Online Parenting Program to Prevent Anxiety and Depression Problems in Primary School-Aged Children: Study Protocol for a Randomised Controlled Trial. *Trials* **2018**, *19*, 236. [CrossRef] [PubMed]
45. Yap, M.B.H.; Jorm, A.F. Parental Factors Associated with Childhood Anxiety, Depression, and Internalizing Problems: A Systematic Review and Meta-Analysis. *J. Affect. Disord.* **2015**, *175*, 424–440. [CrossRef] [PubMed]
46. Sim, W.H.; Fernando, L.M.N.; Jorm, A.F.; Rapee, R.M.; Lawrence, K.A.; Mackinnon, A.J.; Yap, M.B.H. A Tailored Online Intervention to Improve Parenting Risk and Protective Factors for Child Anxiety and Depression: Medium-Term Findings from a Randomized Controlled Trial. *J. Affect. Disord.* **2020**, *277*, 814–824. [CrossRef]
47. Aldridge, G.; Wu, L.; Seguin, J.P.; Robinson, J.; Battaglia, E.; Olivier, P.; Yap, M.B.H. Embedding Technology-Assisted Parenting Interventions in Real-World Settings to Empower Parents of Children with Adverse Childhood Experiences: Co-Design Study. *JMIR Form. Res.* **2024**, *8*, e55639. [CrossRef]
48. Bennett, M.; McClure, A.; Khalesi, H.; Vu, M.T.N.; Feng, J.; Reupert, A.; Yap, M.B.H. Differences in Parental Factors between Parents with and Without Depression or Anxiety Issues: A Systematic Review and Meta-Analysis. *J. Affect. Disord.* **2026**, *392*, 120085. [CrossRef]
49. McFarland, L.; Fenton, A. Unfogging the Future: Investigating a Strengths-Based Program to Build Capacity and Resilience in Parents with Mental Illness. *Adv. Ment. Health* **2019**, *17*, 21–32. [CrossRef]
50. Coates, D.; Phelan, R.; Heap, J.; Howe, D. "Being in a Group with Others Who Have Mental Illness Makes All the Difference": The Views and Experiences of Parents Who Attended a Mental Health Parenting Program. *Child. Youth Serv. Rev.* **2017**, *78*, 104–111. [CrossRef]
51. Wolfenden, L.; Calam, R.; Drake, R.J.; Gregg, L. The Triple P Positive Parenting Program for Parents with Psychosis: A Case Series with Qualitative Evaluation. *Front. Psychiatry* **2022**, *13*, 791294. [CrossRef]
52. Slattery, P.; Saeri, A.K.; Bragge, P. Research Co-Design in Health: A Rapid Overview of Reviews. *Health Res. Policy Syst.* **2020**, *18*, 17. [CrossRef]

https://doi.org/10.3390/children13010129

53. Morris, H.; O'Connor, A.; Cummins, J.; Valentine, C.; Dwyer, A.; Goodyear, M.; Skouteris, H. A Pilot Efficacy Study of Parents Building Solutions: A Universal Parenting Program Using Co-Design and Strength-Based Approaches. *Child. Youth Serv. Rev.* **2019**, *105*, 104447. [CrossRef]
54. Goodyear, M.; Zechmeister-Koss, I.; Bauer, A.; Christiansen, H.; Glatz-Grugger, M.; Paul, J.L. Development of an Evidence-Informed and Codesigned Model of Support for Children of Parents with a Mental Illness—"It Takes a Village" Approach. *Front. Psychiatry* **2022**, *12*, 806884. [CrossRef] [PubMed]
55. Boddy, C.R. Sample Size for Qualitative Research. *Qual. Mark. Res. Int. J.* **2016**, *19*, 426–432. [CrossRef]
56. Hawkins, J.; Madden, K.; Fletcher, A.; Midgley, L.; Grant, A.; Cox, G.; Moore, L.; Campbell, R.; Murphy, S.; Bonell, C.; et al. Development of a Framework for the Co-Production and Prototyping of Public Health Interventions. *BMC Public Health* **2017**, *17*, 689. [CrossRef]
57. Framework for Innovation—Design Council. Available online: https://www.designcouncil.org.uk/our-resources/framework-for-innovation/ (accessed on 4 September 2025).
58. Harris, P.A.; Taylor, R.; Thielke, R.; Payne, J.; Gonzalez, N.; Conde, J.G. Research Electronic Data Capture (REDCap)—A Metadata-Driven Methodology and Workflow Process for Providing Translational Research Informatics Support. *J. Biomed. Inform.* **2009**, *42*, 377–381. [CrossRef]
59. Harris, P.A.; Taylor, R.; Minor, B.L.; Elliott, V.; Fernandez, M.; O'Neal, L.; McLeod, L.; Delacqua, G.; Delacqua, F.; Kirby, J.; et al. The REDCap Consortium: Building an International Community of Software Platform Partners. *J. Biomed. Inform.* **2019**, *95*, 103208. [CrossRef]
60. Yates, S.; Gatsou, L. Idealisation and Stigmatisation of Parenting in Families with Parental Mental Illness. *SSM Qual. Res. Health* **2021**, *1*, 100020. [CrossRef]
61. Chan, S.Y.Y.; Ho, G.W.K.; Bressington, D. Experiences of Self-stigmatization and Parenting in Chinese Mothers with Severe Mental Illness. *Int. J. Ment. Health Nurs.* **2019**, *28*, 527–537. [CrossRef]
62. Lister, K.; McFarlane, R. Designing for Wellbeing: An Inclusive Learning Design Approach with Student Mental Health Vignettes. *Open Prax.* **2021**, *13*, 184–200. [CrossRef]
63. Törrönen, J. Using Vignettes in Qualitative Interviews as Clues, Microcosms or Provokers. *Qual. Res. J.* **2018**, *18*, 276–286. [CrossRef]
64. Braun, V.; Clarke, V. Reflecting on Reflexive Thematic Analysis. *Qual. Res. Sport. Exerc. Health* **2019**, *11*, 589–597. [CrossRef]
65. Braun, V.; Clarke, V. *Thematic Analysis: A Practical Guide*; SAGE Publishing: London, UK, 2022.
66. Braun, V.; Clarke, V. Using Thematic Analysis in Psychology. *Qual. Res. Psychol.* **2006**, *3*, 77–101. [CrossRef]
67. Daundasekara, S.S.; Beauchamp, J.E.; Hernandez, D.C. Parenting Stress Mediates the Longitudinal Effect of Maternal Depression on Child Anxiety/Depressive Symptoms. *J. Affect. Disord.* **2021**, *295*, 33–39. [CrossRef] [PubMed]
68. Bernard, K.; Nissim, G.; Vaccaro, S.; Harris, J.L.; Lindhiem, O. Association between Maternal Depression and Maternal Sensitivity from Birth to 12 Months: A Meta-Analysis. *Attach. Hum. Dev.* **2018**, *20*, 578–599. [CrossRef]
69. Grove, C.; Riebschleger, J.; Bosch, A.; Cavanaugh, D.; van der Ende, P.C. Expert Views of Children's Knowledge Needs Regarding Parental Mental Illness. *Child. Youth Serv. Rev.* **2017**, *79*, 249–255. [CrossRef]
70. In Focus: Talking with Children about Parental Mental Health Difficulties—Emerging Minds. Available online: https://emergingminds.com.au/resources/in-focus-talking-with-children-about-parental-mental-health-difficulties/ (accessed on 1 October 2025).
71. Talking to Your Primary School-Aged Child about Your Mental Health Difficulties—Emerging Minds. Available online: https://emergingminds.com.au/resources/talking-to-primary-school-aged-child-about-mh-difficulties/ (accessed on 1 October 2025).
72. Starting the Conversation About Your Mental Illness with Your Child—Emerging Minds. Available online: https://emergingminds.com.au/resources/starting-the-conversation-about-your-mental-illness-with-your-child/ (accessed on 1 October 2025).
73. Talking with Children About Their Parent's Mental Health—Satellite Foundation. Available online https://www.satellitefoundation.org.au/resources/talking-with-children-about-their-parents-mental-health/ (accessed on 1 October 2025).
74. Talking to Children of Primary School Age—COPMI. Available online: https://www.copmi.net.au/parents/helping-my-child-and-family/talking-about-mental-illness-with-your-child/talking-to-children-of-primary-school-age/ (accessed on 1 October 2025).
75. Riebschleger, J.; Grové, C.; Cavanaugh, D.; Costello, S. Mental Health Literacy Content for Children of Parents with a Mental Illness: Thematic Analysis of a Literature Review. *Brain Sci.* **2017**, *7*, 141. [CrossRef]
76. Cooklin, A. Promoting Children's Resilience to Parental Mental Illness: Engaging the Child's Thinking. *Adv. Psychiatr. Treat.* **2013**, *19*, 229–240. [CrossRef]

https://doi.org/10.3390/children13010129

77. Smout, A.; Melvin, G.; Cardamone-Breen, M.; Jorm, A.; Xie, J.; Bartindale, T.; Olivier, P.; Seguin, J.; Wu, L.; Yap, M.B.H. A Coach-Assisted, Online Parenting Programme to Support Parents of Adolescents Who Refuse School: Evidence of Acceptability and Feasibility. *BJPsych Open* **2025**, *11*, e115. [CrossRef]
78. Cao, A.; Melvin, G.; Breen, M.C.; Salvaris, C.; Olivier, P.; Wu, L.; Seguin, J.; Xie, J.; Basur, D.; Thompson, A.; et al. A Coach-Supported, Digital Parenting Program for Parents of Adolescents at Risk of Suicide: A Pilot Trial of Acceptability, Feasibility, Validity, and Short-Term Effects. *BJPsych Open* 2025, *submitted*.
79. Sekhon, M.; Cartwright, M.; Francis, J.J. Acceptability of Healthcare Interventions: An Overview of Reviews and Development of a Theoretical Framework. *BMC Health Serv. Res.* **2017**, *17*, 88. [CrossRef]
80. Sekhon, M.; Cartwright, M.; Francis, J.J. Development of a Theory-Informed Questionnaire to Assess the Acceptability of Healthcare Interventions. *BMC Health Serv. Res.* **2022**, *22*, 279. [CrossRef]
81. Motulsky, S. Is Member Checking the Gold Standard of Quality in Qualitative Research? *Qual. Psychol.* **2021**, *8*, 389–406. [CrossRef]
82. Cooper, C.; Tchernegovski, P.; Hine, R. "The Validation Is Not Enough": Australian Mothers' Views and Perceptions of Mental Health Support from Psychologists in Private Practice. *Clin. Psychol.* **2023**, *27*, 392–403. [CrossRef]
83. Maybery, D.; Goodyear, M.; Reupert, A.E.; Grant, A. Worker, Workplace or Families: What Influences Family Focused Practices in Adult Mental Health? *J. Psychiatr. Ment. Health Nurs.* **2016**, *23*, 163–171. [CrossRef] [PubMed]
84. Radley, J.; Sivarajah, N.; Moltrecht, B.; Klampe, M.-L.; Hudson, F.; Delahay, R.; Barlow, J.; Johns, L.C. A Scoping Review of Interventions Designed to Support Parents with Mental Illness That Would Be Appropriate for Parents with Psychosis. *Front. Psychiatry* **2022**, *12*, 787166. [CrossRef]
85. Overbeek, M.M.; Iozzia, G.; Maras, A.; Rijnberk, C. Interventions for Parents with Mental Illnesses: A Scoping Review. *Couple Fam. Psychol. Res. Pract.* **2022**, *12*, 233–264. [CrossRef]
86. van der Ende, P.C.; van Busschbach, J.T.; Nicholson, J.; Korevaar, E.L.; van Weeghel, J. Strategies for Parenting by Mothers and Fathers with a Mental Illness. *J. Psychiatr. Ment. Health Nurs.* **2016**, *23*, 86–97. [CrossRef]
87. Nicholson, J.; Albert, K.; Gershenson, B.; Williams, V.; Biebel, K. Family Options for Parents with Mental Illnesses: A Developmental, Mixed Methods Pilot Study. *Psychiatr. Rehabil. J.* **2009**, *33*, 106–114. [CrossRef]
88. Afzelius, M.; Plantin, L.; Östman, M. Families Living with Parental Mental Illness and Their Experiences of Family Interventions. *J. Psychiatr. Ment. Health Nurs.* **2018**, *25*, 69–77. [CrossRef]
89. Grove, C.; Reupert, A.; Maybery, D. Gaining Knowledge about Parental Mental Illness: How Does It Empower Children?: 'Family Focus': A DVD Intervention. *Child Fam. Soc. Work* **2015**, *20*, 377–386. [CrossRef]
90. Day, J.J.; Sanders, M.R. Do Parents Benefit from Help When Completing a Self-Guided Parenting Program Online? A Randomized Controlled Trial Comparing Triple P Online with and Without Telephone Support. *Behav. Ther.* **2018**, *49*, 1020–1038. [CrossRef]
91. Jones, M.; Pietilä, I.; Joronen, K.; Simpson, W.; Gray, S.; Kaunonen, M. Parents with Mental Illness—A Qualitative Study of Identities and Experiences with Support Services. *Psychiatr. Ment. Health Nurs.* **2016**, *23*, 471–478. [CrossRef]
92. Sanders, M.R.; Turner, K.M.T.; Metzler, C.W. Applying Self-Regulation Principles in the Delivery of Parenting Interventions. *Clin. Child. Fam. Psychol. Rev.* **2019**, *22*, 24–42. [CrossRef]
93. Dell, N.A.; Long, C.; Mancini, M.A. Models of Mental Health Recovery: An Overview of Systematic Reviews and Qualitative Meta-Syntheses. *Psychiatr. Rehabil. J.* **2021**, *44*, 238–253. [CrossRef] [PubMed]
94. Reupert, A.; Maybery, D. Programmes for Parents with a Mental Illness: Programmes for Parents with a Mental Illness. *J. Psychiatr. Ment. Health Nurs.* **2011**, *18*, 257–264. [CrossRef] [PubMed]
95. Al Sager, A.; Goodman, S.H.; Jeong, J.; Bain, P.A.; Ahun, M.N. Effects of Multi-Component Parenting and Parental Mental Health Interventions on Early Childhood Development and Parent Outcomes: A Systematic Review and Meta-Analysis. *Lancet Child Adolesc. Health* **2024**, *8*, 656–669. [CrossRef] [PubMed]
96. Oliver-Parra, A.; Dalmau-Bueno, A.; Ruiz-Muñoz, D.; García-Altés, A. Relationship between Parents' Mental Disorders and Socioeconomic Status and Offspring's Psychopathology: A Cross-Sectional Study. *PLoS ONE* **2020**, *15*, e0240681. [CrossRef]
97. Pierce, M.; Abel, K.M.; Muwonge, J.; Wicks, S.; Nevriana, A.; Hope, H.; Dalman, C.; Kosidou, K. Prevalence of Parental Mental Illness and Association with Socioeconomic Adversity among Children in Sweden between 2006 and 2016: A Population-Based Cohort Study. *Lancet Public Health* **2020**, *5*, e583–e591. [CrossRef]
98. Foster, K.; Maybery, D.; Reupert, A.; Gladstone, B.; Grant, A.; Ruud, T.; Falkov, A.; Kowalenko, N. Family-Focused Practice in Mental Health Care: An Integrative Review. *Child Youth Serv.* **2016**, *37*, 129–155. [CrossRef]

https://doi.org/10.3390/children13010129

children

MDPI

Article

COVID-19 Stress and Family Well-Being: The Role of Sleep in Mental Health Outcomes for Parents and Children

Alzena Ilie [1], Andy J. Kim [1], Danika DesRoches [1], Elizabeth Keys [2], Simon B. Sherry [1,3], Sherry H. Stewart [1,3], S. Hélène Deacon [1] and Penny V. Corkum [1,3,*]

[1] Department of Psychology and Neuroscience, Faculty of Science, Dalhousie University, Halifax, NS B3H 4R2, Canada; alzenailie@dal.ca (A.I.)
[2] School of Nursing, University of British Columbia Okanagan, Kelowna, BC V1V 1V7, Canada
[3] Department of Psychiatry, Faculty of Medicine, Dalhousie University, Halifax, NS B3K 6R8, Canada
* Correspondence: penny.corkum@dal.ca

Abstract

Background/Objectives: The COVID-19 pandemic introduced various stressors for families, including changes to daily routines, work, and schooling. Studies have linked these stressors to increased mental health challenges for parents and children. Sleep difficulties were also common during the pandemic, with some children and parents experiencing poorer sleep quality and shorter sleep duration. However, it remains unclear whether the effects of COVID-19 stress on mental health challenges are explained, at least in part, by effects of COVID-19 stress on child and/or parent sleep challenges. This study examined the impacts of COVID-19 stress on sleep and, in turn, mental health difficulties in school-aged children and their parents in Canada and the United States. Methods: Parents (N = 961) completed validated measures of COVID-19 stress, and of their own and their child's sleep and mental health. Path analyses tested direct and indirect effects of COVID-19 stress on mental health outcomes with sleep problems as the potential mediator. Results: Child sleep problems partially mediated COVID-19 stress effects on both parent (β = 0.33) and child (β = 0.20) mental health difficulties, while parent sleep problems contributed significantly but to a lesser degree (parent mental health: β = 0.07; child mental health: β = 0.03). There also remained significant direct effects of COVID-19 stress on both child and parent mental health difficulties that were not mediated through sleep difficulties. Conclusions: Our findings underscore the interconnected nature of sleep and mental health, demonstrating that stress-related disruptions in sleep (particularly children's sleep) can exacerbate mental health difficulties for both parents and children during crises like the COVID-19 pandemic.

Keywords: COVID-19 stress; mental health; sleep; well-being; family

1. Introduction

Throughout the world, public health recommendations related to the COVID-19 pandemic resulted in unprecedented changes to everyday life [1,2]. These changes aimed to urgently reduce the spread of the virus. Yet, they also led many families with school-aged children in Canada and the United States to experience significant disruptions to their routines [3]. For example, the closure of in-person schooling, the transition to remote learning, and closure of organized activities (e.g., sports, music lessons, organized social activities) significantly changed some children's routines, which impacted their learning, socialization, and extracurricular activities [3].

 https://doi.org/10.3390/children12080962

School-aged children are a population particularly vulnerable to the effects of disruptions in routine due to their developmental need for structure, consistency, and predictable daily schedules, which support both academic and social development [4]. Research underscores the importance of consistent daily routines, which are closely linked to positive child development and mental health outcomes [4]. Stability in routines provides a sense of predictability and security that supports emotional regulation and overall well-being in children. However, the pandemic disrupted this stability for many families, leading to varied outcomes. While some families found these disruptions to be positive, enabling more family time and a slower pace of life, others reported negative impacts such as heightened stress, problematic behaviours, and emotional challenges in both children and parents [5,6]. For instance, caregivers noted increases in children's anhedonia, anger, restlessness, sleep problems, appetite issues, and sadness after the COVID-19 pandemic started [3,7]. These behavioural and emotional challenges are critical indicators of broader mental health difficulties, as they may reflect disruptions in coping mechanisms, emotional dysregulation, and difficulties with overall psychological well-being. Observed behavioural changes, such as increased sedentary activities, later sleep timing, and heightened screen use, underscore the impact of the pandemic on daily routines [8]. During the COVID-19 pandemic, declines in physical activity, increases in screen time, later bedtimes, and unhealthy eating behaviours were reported in Canadian children [9]. These lifestyle disruptions may adversely interact with stress and sleep behaviours, compounding difficulties in maintaining healthy routines under pandemic conditions [10].

Insomnia and/or insomnia symptoms affect ~30% of typically developing children [11], and include difficulties with falling asleep, staying asleep, and/or having early morning awakenings [12]. Sleep has a reciprocal role in the mental well-being of children: after children have a good night's sleep, they tend to report higher positive affect and lower negative affect throughout the day [13]. In contrast, insufficient quantity and poor-quality sleep are associated with worse mood and emotion regulation in youth, as well as increased likelihood of developing a mood or anxiety disorder, and heightened risk of suicidal ideation [14]. Sleep duration and latency have been strongly correlated with internalizing (e.g., depression, anxiety) and externalizing (e.g., aggression, hyperactivity) behaviours in children [15].

The cyclical relationship between sleep and mental health is well established: poor sleep exacerbates mental health difficulties, while mental health challenges disrupt sleep [15]. The correlation between sleep and mental health difficulties becomes even more heightened under conditions of stress [16,17], such as COVID-19-specific stressors. For example, Mackenzie and colleagues found that disruptions to routines during the pandemic adversely affected the sleep and stress levels of parents and children with pre-existing insomnia [6]. Indeed, although some families reported improved sleep, many parents reported sleep disruptions for both themselves and their children: some 40% of parents indicated their child's sleep worsened, while 60% reported declines in their own sleep quality [6]. Similarly, Cellini and colleagues demonstrated that the majority of children experienced delayed sleep timing (e.g., later bedtime and wakeup times), worsened sleep quality, and increased psychological difficulties during the pandemic [18]. Cellini et al. found that these child sleep and mental health difficulties were associated with maternal psychological challenges, suggesting a reciprocal relationship between caregiver and child sleep and well-being [18]. COVID-19 stress has had significant impacts on parent and child mental health outside of North America, such as in Norway and Greece [19,20].

Poor mental health in children has been a persistent issue prior to the COVID-19 pandemic. In Canada, approximately one in five children and youth have a diagnosable mental health condition [21]. These challenges are associated with lower academic achievement, higher stress levels, increased risk of substance use, and diminished social support [22]. During the pandemic, mental health problems in children and youth worsened [23–25], likely exacerbated by heightened stressors and disrupted routines. Cost and colleagues surveyed school-aged children and their caregivers in Canada during the COVID-19 pandemic and found that over two-thirds of children experienced worsened mental health symptoms, which were linked to stress related to social isolation [23]. Similarly, parental mental health problems, which increased during the pandemic, were strongly associated with worse mental health outcomes in children [26]. For example, Canadian parents with children reported higher rates of stress, alcohol consumption, suicidal ideation, and negative parent–child interactions during the pandemic [5]. These findings underscore the cyclical nature of the stress–sleep–mental health relationship [27], wherein stress exacerbates sleep difficulties and mental health challenges, which in turn amplify stress.

Despite this knowledge, there are key remaining questions as to the specific relations between stress, sleep, and mental health in children in the context of COVID-19. Given the unprecedented and prolonged disruptions caused by the pandemic, including school closures, social isolation, and disruptions to daily routines, stress levels in children and parents were found to be amplified during the pandemic compared to typical stressors [3]. Evidence from pre-pandemic research suggests that sleep may mediate the relationship between stress and mental health, with sufficient sleep mitigating the adverse effects of stress, and poor sleep exacerbating these adverse effects [16,17]. For example, children with sufficient sleep report less negative affect and better emotion regulation following a stressful situation [28]. Conversely, insufficient sleep heightens the risk of emotional dysregulation and psychological disorders after experiencing a stressful event [28]. Since sleep is a more modifiable variable than broader pandemic-related stressors, identifying sleep as a key mechanism could inform targeted strategies to support child mental health through pandemics and other events that have broad societal impacts.

Understanding these relationships is particularly important, as sleep disruptions may contribute to reciprocal and cross-over effects within families [29], beyond their likely mediation in the link between COVID-19 stress and mental health difficulties. For instance, COVID-19 stress could worsen child sleep disruptions, and in turn worsen parental mental health, while parental sleep difficulties may contribute to dysregulation in children [5,6]. Previous research highlights associations between parent and child sleep and mental health, suggesting that disruptions in one family member's sleep can have cascading effects on the entire household [30]. Thus, studying both parent and child sleep within the context of pandemic-related stress is critical for capturing the full scope of its impact on family mental health. This is a novel contribution of our study design, as no studies to date have examined the relations of COVID-19-related stressors, sleep, and mental health in a sample of both parents and children.

The objectives of this study were to (a) describe sleep behaviours and mental health symptoms during the COVID-19 pandemic in school-aged children (aged 5 to 11 years) and their parents, (b) test sleep disruption as a mediator between COVID-19 stress and mental health outcomes, and (c) examine the relative mediating roles of parental and child sleep disruptions in predicting both parent and child mental health outcomes. By exploring these relationships, this study aimed to provide a deeper understanding of how stress, sleep, and mental health intersected during the COVID-19 pandemic.

This paper reports on secondary analysis of data from a larger study examining the effects of COVID-19 pandemic mandated homeschooling on families entitled *COVID-19 Pandemic: Factors that Support and Impede Family Well-Being During Mandatory Homeschooling* conducted by the Language and Literacy Lab and the Mood, Anxiety and Co-Morbidity Lab at

Dalhousie University [31–33]. This study included children engaging in one of three types of schooling (i.e., in-person learning, mandated homeschooling, and voluntary homeschooling).

2. Materials and Methods

2.1. Study Design and Sample

A total of 961 parents were recruited from March to May 2021 for this cross-sectional study. To be eligible for the larger study, participants were required to be (a) at least 19 years of age, (b) in a romantic relationship for 3 months or more, (c) with a partner who is at least 19 years of age, and (d) have a child at home in grades 1 to 5. These criteria ensured that only couples who were romantically involved for more than three months and who lived with a school-aged child participated in the larger study, as it looked at the effects of homeschooling on parental, child and couple-level variables. While couples were recruited for the larger study, only data from the first responding parent (who reported on themselves and their child) was utilized in the present study. When a parent had more than one child in grades 1 to 5 living at home, they reported on the youngest eligible child. No other inclusion or exclusion criteria were employed for our specific study.

2.2. Procedures

Participants completed a survey via Qualtrics Survey Panels (Qualtrics, Provo, UT, USA) between March and May 2021. Qualtrics Survey Panels is an online survey management service that recruits from a pool of potential participants based on eligibility criteria specified by the researcher. The participant was asked to think about the 30-day period between 15 January and 15 February 2021 as the reference for completing all measures except for demographics. Although the survey was open to all parents in the general population living in Canada and the United States, recruitment was targeted in specific geographical areas where in-person learning was occurring (i.e., Canada: Edmonton, Calgary, Vancouver, Halifax, Montreal; USA: Miami and Jacksonville) and where mandated homeschooling (i.e., children who learned at home due to reasons related to the COVID-19 pandemic) was in effect (i.e., Canada: Toronto; USA: Los Angeles, Philadelphia, San Diego, Boston) at the same time (from 15 January to 15 February 2021) [34].

About two-thirds of participants were recruited and compensated through Qualtrics Panels using their guidelines. Additional recruitment was needed, for reasons related to the parent study, of parents who schooled a child at home voluntarily irrespective of COVID-19 restrictive measures, due to low recruitment via Qualtrics Panels. For these additional participants, recruitment was performed via social media platforms and homeschooling groups, and these participants were compensated with CAD 10 Amazon e-gift cards. This study was approved by the Dalhousie University Social Sciences and Humanities Research Ethics Board (REB #2020-5336).

2.3. Measures

2.3.1. Demographics

The demographics questionnaire asked the respondent to self-report their age, gender, highest level of education completed, employment status, family income, and location (i.e., province or state). The parent also reported on their child's age, gender, ethnicity, and the number of children living in the home.

2.3.2. Pandemic-Related Stress

Parent COVID-19 stress. The presence of COVID-19 stressors was measured using an adapted version of the Coronavirus Stressor Survey [35]. The Coronavirus Stressor Survey [35] asks participants to rate their exposure to the following seven pandemic-related stressful experiences: "job requires possible exposure to coronavirus", "lost job, been laid off or furloughed, due to the coronavirus pandemic", "lost income due to the coronavirus pandemic", "difficulty getting food, medication, or other necessities due to the coronavirus pandemic", "had a loved one die due to confirmed or suspected coronavirus infection", "work has moved to work-from-home due to coronavirus pandemic", and "difficulty getting needed social support due to the coronavirus pandemic". The only adaptation to the list of COVID-19 stressors was that we also asked participants to indicate whether they have had/have COVID-19 [35].

Response options were adapted to allow participants to rate to what extent they have been affected by the seven pandemic-related stressful experiences on a scale of 0 ("it did not happen to me") to 6 ("affected me to a great extent") since the beginning of the pandemic. Consistent with past research [36,37], and because we were interested in exposure severity, we re-coded responses to indicate whether each stressful experience had or had not happened to them (0—no, it did not happen to the participant; 1—yes, it did happen to the participant). Anytime the participant rated an experience as anything other than 0, the response was recoded as a 1, regardless of severity. A total score ranging from 0 to 8 was computed by summing all eight items. The measure showed good internal consistency ($\alpha = 0.85$).

2.3.3. Child and Parent Mental Health

Child mental health. Child mental health was assessed using the internalizing and externalizing scales of the Strengths and Difficulties Questionnaire (SDQ) [38]. The parent indicated how true each item was of their child on a 3-point scale (0 = "Not true"; 1 = "Somewhat true"; 2 = "Certainly true"). Twenty items asked about internalizing problems, half of which assessed emotional problems (e.g., "Often unhappy, depressed or tearful"), and the other half of which assessed peer problems (e.g., "Has at least one good friend" [reverse scored]). Another twenty items asked about externalizing problems, half of which measured conduct problems (e.g., "Often fights with other children or bullies them") and the other half of which measured hyperactivity problems (e.g., "Restless, overactive, cannot stay still for long"). A total SDQ score, representing overall child mental health symptoms, was calculated by summing responses from both the internalizing and externalizing scales and could range from 0 to 40 following reverse scoring of any inversely keyed items. The SDQ has been standardized for 4- to 16-year-olds, and has shown both good convergent and discriminant validity with other child mental health scales [38] and internal consistency [39]. Similarly, the current sample demonstrated good internal consistency for the SDQ total ($\alpha = 0.83$).

Parent mental health. Participants self-reported on their own mental health by completing both the Patient Health Questionnaire-9 (PHQ-9) [40], a measure of depressive symptoms, and the Generalized Anxiety Disorder-7 (GAD-7) questionnaire [41], a measure of anxiety symptoms. Participants rated nine items on the PHQ-9 and seven items on the GAD-7. Both scales were on a 4-point Likert scale ranging from 0 (not at all) to 3 (nearly every day). Both the PHQ-9 ($\alpha = 0.89$) [40] and the GAD-7 ($\alpha = 0.92$) [41] have shown good internal consistency in past research.

A composite mental health score, known as the Anxiety–Depression Scale (ADS), was computed for the responding parent [42]. Previous research on the ADS has shown high internal reliability in three clinical trials (α ranging from 0.80 to 0.90) [42]. Two of the nine items of the PHQ-9 (i.e., Items 3 and 4) were dropped due to their redundancy with the parent sleep measure used in this study. As such, a modified ADS total score was computed by summing the remaining items of the PHQ-9 and the GAD-7, with higher scores indicating worse mental health through higher levels of depression and anxiety symptomology. The modified ADS demonstrated excellent internal reliability in this study ($\alpha = 0.95$).

2.3.4. Sleep

Child sleep. Child sleep problems were measured using the Patient-Reported Outcomes Measurement Information System (PROMIS) Parent Proxy Short Form v1.0—Sleep Disturbance—4a [43]. Participants rated four statements, such as "My child had difficulty falling asleep" on a scale from 1 (never) to 5 (always). The four items were then summed to compute a total score, ranging from 4 to 20, with a higher score indicating worse sleep. Research has indicated that this measure has excellent psychometric properties, including internal consistency ($\alpha > 0.90$) and content, structural and convergent validity with other child sleep and fatigue measures [44]. This measure had acceptable internal consistency within our own study ($\alpha = 0.75$).

Parent sleep. Parent sleep difficulties were assessed using the PROMIS Short Form v1.0—Sleep Disturbance—4a [43]. Participants self-reported on their own sleep by rating four statements on a 5-point Likert scale (e.g., "I had a problem with my sleep"), which were summed together to create a final score ranging from 4 to 20 (higher score indicating worse sleep). This scale has shown good convergent and discriminant validity with other adult sleep measures [45]. In our study, this measure showed acceptable internal consistency ($\alpha = 0.77$), falling in line with previous research ($\alpha = 0.88$) [45].

2.4. Data Analysis

Descriptive statistics, including means and standard deviations for continuous variables and percentages for categorical variables, were calculated for the demographic questionnaire. Bivariate correlations were conducted to examine the relationships among the predictor, mediator, and outcome variables. Correlation strength was interpreted using the following guidelines: a small correlation was defined as an r-value between 0.10 and 0.29, a moderate correlation was an r-value between 0.30 and 0.49, and a strong correlation was an r-value of 0.50 or higher [46]. A path model was fitted, with COVID-19 stress as the predictor, child and parent sleep problems as mediators, and child and parent mental health as outcomes, using R (version 4.2.1) with the *lavaan* package [47]. Given that parent and child scores were reported by the parent, we accounted for their interdependence by specifying correlations between the errors of child and parent sleep problems, as well as between child and parent mental health difficulties. To estimate the confidence intervals for all coefficients and the significance of indirect effects, bias-corrected standard errors were computed using bootstrapping with 5000 re-samples [48] The model was just identified, as all paths were required to estimate total effects and mediation effect sizes. Consequently, there are no fit indices to report.

3. Results

The parent and child demographic information is reported in Tables 1 and 2. Overall, parents' mean age was 38.21 years old, with an almost equal distribution of male and female participants. Most parents identified as White, were college/university graduates, were employed, had a family income of at least CAD 76,000 per year, and lived in Central Canada (i.e., Ontario and Quebec). The mean age of the child on whom participants were reporting was 8.64 years old. In terms of gender, the majority (57%) of children were male, with the majority reported to be White.

Table 1. Parental demographics (N = 961).

Variable	
Mean age (*SD*)	38.21 (6.61)
Gender	
Man	483 (50.26%)
Woman	475 (49.43%)
Non-Binary	2 (0.21%)
Prefer not to answer	1 (0.10%)
Parent ethnicity	
White	707 (73.60%)
Asian or Arab/West Asian (e.g., Armenian, Egyptian, Iranian, Lebanese, Moroccan) [a]	145 (15.09%)
Latin American or Black or Indigenous a	68 (7.07%)
Multiracial	32 (3.30%)
Other	4 (0.42%)
Prefer not to answer	5 (0.52%)
Highest level of education completed	
College or university graduate [b]	726 (75.55%)
Less than college or university completion [c]	235 (24.45%)
Employment status (15 January–15 February)	
Employed [d]	770 (80.13%)
Unemployed [e]	191 (19.87%)
Mean number of children living at-home (*SD*)	1.89 (0.89)
Family income	
CAD 25,000 or less per year	34 (3.54%)
Between CAD 26,000 and 50,000	113 (11.76%)
Between CAD 51,000 and 75,000	184 (19.15%)
Between CAD 76,000 and 100,000	203 (21.12%)
Between CAD 101,000 and 125,000	131 (13.63%)
Between CAD 126,000 and 150,000	127 (13.22%)
CAD 151,000 or more per year	138 (14.36%)
Prefer not to answer	31 (3.22%)
Location	
Canada	805 (83.77%)
Atlantic Provinces [f]	88 (10.93%)
Central Canada [g]	477 (59.26%)
Prairie Provinces [h]	169 (20.99%)
West Coast [i]	67 (8.32%)
Northern Territories	2 (0.25%)
Unspecified	2 (0.25%)
United States	156 (16.23%)
North-East [a]	24 (15.38%)
South [a]	41 (26.28%)
Mid-West [a]	8 (5.13%)
West [a]	83 (53.21%)

Notes. Canadian provinces and American states were separated into main regions [49,50]. [a] Combined to maintain confidentiality of respondents due to low numbers in one or more of these categories. [b] Includes participants who indicated being a college/university graduate, having completed some post-graduate education or having a post-graduate degree. [c] Includes participants who indicated that they completed elementary school, some high school, are a high school graduate or completed some college/university. [d] Includes participants who indicated being employed full or part-time. [e] Includes participants who indicated being unemployed, not in the labour force, or a full- or part-time student. [f] Includes Nova Scotia, New Brunswick, Prince Edward Island, and Newfoundland and Labrador. [g] Includes Ontario and Quebec. [h] Includes Manitoba and Saskatchewan. [i] Includes Alberta and British Columbia.

Table 2. Child demographics (*N* = 961).

Variable	
Mean child age in years (*SD*)	8.64 (2.63)
Child gender	
Boy	551 (57.3%)
Girl	408 (42.46%)
Non-binary	1 (0.10%)
Prefer not to answer	1 (0.10%)
Child ethnicity	
White	687 (71.49%)
Asian or Arab/West Asian (e.g., Armenian, Egyptian, Iranian, Lebanese, Moroccan) [a]	127 (13.21%)
Latin America or Black or Indigenous [a]	63 (6.55%)
Other	12 (1.25%)
Prefer not to answer	9 (0.94%)
Multiracial	63 (6.56%)

[a] Combined to maintain confidentiality of respondents due to low numbers in one or more of these categories.

Table 3 presents bivariate correlations and descriptive statistics. The bivariate correlations indicated moderate positive correlations between COVID-19 stress and child sleep problems, as well as between COVID-19 stress and parent mental health difficulties. There was a strong positive correlation between COVID-19 stress and child mental health difficulties, whereas a small correlation was found between COVID-19 stress and parent sleep problems. Child sleep problems showed strong positive correlations with both child and parent mental health difficulties, which were also strongly correlated with one another. Similarly, parent sleep problems were strongly and positively correlated with parent mental health difficulties and moderately correlated with child mental health difficulties and sleep problems.

Table 3. Bivariate correlations, means, standard deviations, and ranges.

Measure	1	2	3	4	5
1. COVID-19 stress	-				
2. Child sleep problems	0.45 ***	-			
3. Parent sleep problems	0.21 ***	0.38 ***	-		
4. Child mental health difficulties	0.51 ***	0.64 ***	0.39 ***	-	
5. Parent mental health difficulties	0.40 ***	0.52 ***	0.51 ***	0.58 ***	-
Mean	3.80	12.75	10.87	9.03	10.65
Standard deviation	2.55	7.34	9.34	3.36	3.63
Possible range	0–8	4–20	4–20	0–40	0–42
Observed range	0–7	0–31	0–42	4–19	4–20

Notes. *** $p < 0.001$.

The path model (Figure 1) tested the hypothesized relationships between COVID-19 stress (predictor) and both child mental health and parent mental health difficulties (outcomes)—both direct effects and indirect effects through child and parent sleep problems (mediators).

Significant indirect effects of COVID-19 stress on child mental health difficulties were observed through child sleep problems ($\beta = 0.20$, 95% CI [0.17; 0.24]) and, to a lesser extent, through parent sleep problems ($\beta = 0.03$, 95% CI [0.02; 0.05]). This suggests that for every 1 standard deviation increase in COVID-19 stress, child mental health difficulties increase by 0.20 and 0.03 standard deviations through child and parent sleep problems, respectively.

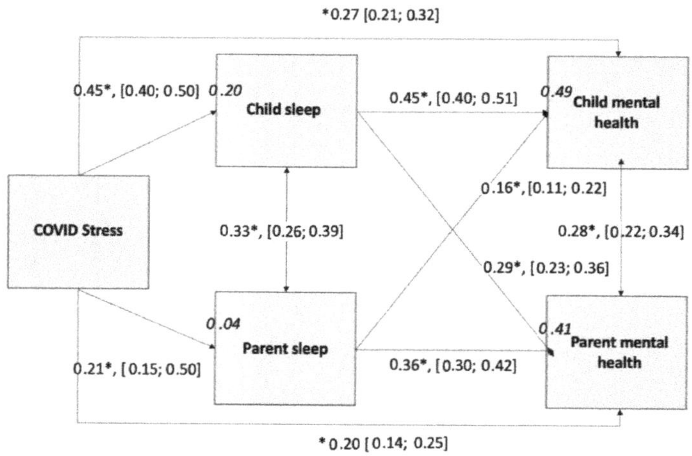

Figure 1. Path analysis of COVID-19 stress, sleep problems, and mental health. *Note.* $N = 961$. Double-headed arrows indicate correlations between error terms. Single-headed arrows indicate paths. All paths noted with asterisk are significant ($p < 0.001$). Path coefficients are standardized. Bracketed values indicate the lower and upper limits of confidence intervals. Italicized numbers appearing in the bubbles represent the R^2.

The mediation analysis also revealed significant indirect effects of COVID-19 stress on parent mental health difficulties through child sleep problems ($\beta = 0.13$, 95% CI [0.10; 0.16]) and through parent sleep problems ($\beta = 0.07$, 95% CI [0.05; 0.10]). Specifically, for every 1 standard deviation increase in COVID-19 stress, parent mental health difficulties increase by 0.13 and 0.07 standard deviations through child and parent sleep problems, respectively.

In terms of direct effects, the path coefficients indicated significant relationships between COVID-19 stress and both child and parent mental health difficulties. Additionally, the path coefficients indicated significant relationships between COVID-19 stress and both child and parent sleep problems. Significant relationships were also observed in the direct paths from child sleep problems to child mental health difficulties, from parent sleep problems to parent mental health difficulties, from child sleep problems to parent mental health difficulties, and from parent sleep problems to child mental health difficulties. The error variances for child and parent sleep problems were moderately correlated with one another, as were the error variances for child and parent mental health difficulties.

We examined the 95% CIs to determine which indirect effects were significantly stronger than other mediational pathways; a given set of mediational pathways was considered significantly different from one another if the 95% CIs were not overlapping. Child sleep problems was a stronger mediator than parent sleep problems in explaining the link between COVID-19 stress and child mental health difficulties; in contrast child and parent sleep problems were similar in magnitude as mediators in explaining the link between COVID-19 stress and parent mental health difficulties. Additionally, child sleep problems was a stronger mediator of the link between COVID-19 stress and mental health difficulties in the case of child mental health difficulties than in the case of parent mental health difficulties; in contrast, parent sleep problems showed a similar magnitude mediational effect in the link between COVID-19 stress and mental health difficulties for both child and parent.

The total effects of COVID-19 stress on parent mental health ($\beta = 0.40$, 95% CI [0.34; 0.46]) and child mental health ($\beta = 0.51$, 95% CI [0.46; 0.55]) were computed by summing their associated direct and indirect effects.

The percent mediation is the percentage of a total effect that is accounted for by indirect effect(s). We first calculated the percent mediation for parent mental health difficulties by dividing the sum of both its indirect effects by its total effect (51%). We did the same for child mental health difficulties (47%). This percentage was further broken down for parent mental health difficulties into the percent mediated by the individual indirect effects of parent sleep problems (18% of the 51%) and child sleep problems (33% of the 51%), as well as parent sleep problems (7% of the 47%) and child sleep problems (40% of the 47%) for child mental health difficulties.

4. Discussion

To our knowledge, this study is the first to examine the relationship between COVID-19 stress, parent and child mental health, and sleep behaviours in both children and parents, filling an important gap in the literature, and potentially providing intervention targets during times of high stress. In this large cohort of 961 parent and child dyads from Canada and the US who had experienced varying levels of COVID-19 related stress, we conducted a secondary analysis to determine the role of sleep in mediating the relationship between COVID-19 stress and mental health outcomes in parents and children. Overall, the path analysis found significant indirect effects between COVID-19 stress, sleep problems in children and parents, and their contributions to mental health difficulties. Additionally, there were significant direct effects of COVID-19 stress on parent and children mental health difficulties.

The path analysis revealed significant indirect effects: COVID-19 stress was linked to sleep problems in both children and parents, and these sleep problems, in turn, contributed to mental health difficulties. Specifically, both child and parent sleep were partial mediators of the effect of COVID-19 stress on mental health. For children, their own sleep was a stronger predictor of their mental health outcomes, while for parents, both their own sleep and their child's sleep were significant predictors. These findings suggest that sleep may serve as a key pathway through which external stressors impact psychological well-being across family members [51,52].

In the mediation analysis, COVID-19 stress indirectly affected parents' mental health through both their own sleep problems and their child's sleep problems. For children, COVID-19 stress indirectly impacted their mental health through their own sleep problems and their parent's sleep problems. While COVID-19 stress had direct effects on both parent and child mental health difficulties, a significant portion of these effects was mediated by sleep problems. Child sleep problems accounted for a larger portion of the mediation on parent mental health compared to parent sleep problems. Moreover, child sleep problems played a significantly stronger role in mediating the link between COVID-19 stress and parent mental health difficulties compared to parent sleep problems. Our findings are consistent with previous research that has shown when children have sleep difficulties, it can cause insomnia symptoms and higher pre-sleep arousal in parents [51], and that child sleep mediates the association between parent's sleep and mood. Additionally, another study found that children's sleep problems were significant predictors of sleep problems in parents, and subjective reports of children's sleep schedules impacted parents' mental health [52]. This demonstrates that disruption in children's sleep can increase both child behavioural difficulties and risk of parental burnout [53,54]. Therefore, the current study suggests that the association between COVID-19 stress and child mental health problems appear to be partially explained by the link between child sleep and mental health.

Interestingly, child sleep problems had a larger mediation effect on child mental health difficulties compared to parent sleep problems and their mediational effect on parent mental health. This may be because, according to Canadian and American sleep guidelines [55,56], children require more hours of sleep per night than adults do, and therefore, adults may be able to function better with less sleep. Furthermore, child sleep is directly linked to brain development across childhood and adolescence, mood, emotional regulation, and academic achievement, which further highlights the importance of children getting the recommended hours of sleep per night [57]. Aligning with our results, a meta-analysis by Bussières and colleagues found that the COVID-19 pandemic had a negative influence on children's mental health, with anxiety and depression symptoms being two times higher than pre-pandemic estimates [58]. In our results, parent sleep problems showed a small magnitude correlation with COVID-19 stress, though parent mental health difficulties were moderately correlated with child sleep problems, highlighting a broader interrelation between sleep and mental health outcomes. Previous research has demonstrated that child sleep problems impact parents' sleep by reducing their total sleep time [51], in turn, negatively impacting parents daytime functioning and mood [53,59]. This may explain why child sleep problems proved stronger mediators than parent sleep problems when examining the effect of COVID-19 stress on both child and parent mental health difficulties.

Consistent with the supporting literature [58,60,61], the path analysis found that COVID-19 stress directly impacted parent and child mental health, even after accounting for sleep problems. This suggests that COVID-19 stress may influence mental health through other factors, such as financial strain, increased caregiver burden, and disruption to routines. In addition, the presence of direct effects reinforces the robustness of the relationship between pandemic-related stressors and mental distress in children and parents, aligning with previous research on the impact of the COVID-19 pandemic on increased internalizing symptoms in both parents and children [5,23–27].

When examining the confidence intervals of the indirect effects, child sleep problems were a significantly stronger mediator of the relationship between COVID-19 stress and child mental health difficulties compared to parent sleep problems. This finding highlights the particularly important role of child sleep in shaping children's emotional and behavioural responses to stress. In contrast, child and parent sleep problems were comparable in their mediating roles when explaining the link between COVID-19 stress and parent mental health difficulties, suggesting that both self- and child-related sleep disruptions contribute meaningfully to parents' psychological well-being. Taken together, these results underscore the differential impact of sleep disruptions depending on whether the mental health outcomes pertain to the child or the parent. These findings also reinforce the need to consider both sleep and family dynamics when supporting mental health during periods of high stress.

When combining direct and indirect effects, COVID-19 stress had a large overall impact on both child and parent mental health difficulties. The strength of these associations suggests that COVID-19 stress functioned as a risk factor for family mental health difficulties, consistent with broader literature documenting heightened rates of depression, anxiety, and distress in both children and adults during the pandemic [58,62].

4.1. Strengths

The large sample size ($N = 961$) and relatively equal distribution between mothers ($n = 478$) and fathers ($n = 483$) in the sample is a strength, as it increased statistical power and enhanced the reliability of the findings. Path analysis was also used, which allowed for the examination of both direct effects of COVID-19 stress on child and parent mental health and indirect effects through sleep, providing a nuanced understanding of how COVID-19 stress impacts mental health in both children and parents. In addition, the current study sample was racially diverse, and was roughly representative of the Canadian and American population, with ~70% participants identifying as White, and ~30% of participants identifying as part of a non-majority racial/ethnic background [63,64]. The high R^2 values observed in the study indicate that a substantial portion of the variance in mental health outcomes was explained by the model regarding the impact of COVID-19 stress on both parent and child mental health. This suggests that the findings have a strong explanatory power in understanding how stressors during the pandemic affected child and parent well-being.

4.2. Limitations

The analyses included in this study were cross-sectional, so temporal precedence and causality cannot be determined between variables. A longitudinal analysis could have provided insight into the persistence of COVID-19 stress on sleep and mental health beyond the immediate pandemic context. While some researchers argue that mediation analyses should not be conducted on cross-sectional data since mediation is a process that unfolds over time [65], others suggest that such analyses can serve as a useful starting point for testing novel models, such as the path model examined in this study [66].

Due to the design of the larger study from which the data were drawn [31–33], all parents who participated in this study were in a romantic relationship and were co-parenting. This may have influenced the study's results and may limit our ability to generalize the findings to single-parent households. Given that single-parent households often have reduced social and parenting support [67], the effects of COVID-19 stress on parent and child sleep and mental health may be even more pronounced in this population. Additionally, this analysis could have been stronger if there were multiple indicators (i.e., three or more measures) that were being analyzed for each construct (i.e., child mental health, parent mental health, child sleep, parent sleep), which would have enhanced the reliability and robustness of these findings. Furthermore, the relationships between COVID-19 stress and child and parent mental health were not fully explained by child and parent sleep. Variables such as hopelessness, lack of social support, and family conflict may have played a role in the results.

While the large R^2 values suggest that the model explains a significant portion of variance in mental health outcomes, it is possible that other unmeasured factors, such as socio-economic status, other (non-COVID-19-related) environmental stressors, or pre-existing health conditions may have contributed to these outcomes. Lastly, all measures were reported by parents (i.e., COVID-19 stress, child sleep, child mental health), which may have introduced bias or limitations in capturing the full scope of stress experienced within the household [68].

4.3. Implications

Clinicians should be aware of the adverse effects of heightened stress on both child and parent sleep and mental health. The findings of this study underscore the interrelated nature of these issues, highlighting that child and parent sleep problems can significantly exacerbate family mental health difficulties. Therefore, it is essential for health care providers to assess sleep quality and duration alongside mental health, especially in families experiencing heightened stress, as the treatment of sleep problems may reduce the impact of stress on mental health.

Though emergency measures from the COVID-19 pandemic have ended, wait times to see physicians and other clinicians remain high. The average wait time to see a physician in Canada is at an average of 27.7 weeks; wait times in the province of Ontario are ~22 weeks, and waitlists in Nova Scotia are up to 57 weeks [69]. Given the observed effects of parent and child sleep on stress and mental health during the COVID-19 pandemic, online intervention programs targeting both child sleep and mental health could be beneficial. Online programs are cost-effective, easily accessible, and scalable, especially during pandemics when in-person contact is diminished.

4.4. Future Directions

As the COVID-19 pandemic has ended, future research should focus on assessing the long-term effects of pandemic-related stress on both parent and child sleep and mental health. While the current study provides valuable insights into immediate impacts, a longitudinal approach could offer a deeper understanding of these effects over time. Though the current study sample had to be living in an area where COVID-19 emergency measures (e.g., lockdowns) were or were not occurring in the period of interest, no comparison was performed in the present study between children who were being home-schooled/going through virtual learning and children who were still attending in-person learning. COVID-19 stress, child and parent sleep, and child and parent mental health may differ between these two groups, as children attending in-person learning may have had increased stress during this time and lower sleep duration. Furthermore, having children self-report on their mental health symptoms, sleep, and stress regarding the COVID-19 pandemic in addition to parent report would help researchers understand children's perspectives and allow for the assessment of the convergence or divergence of the results across reporting sources. Moreover, intervention studies focusing on mitigating the effects of pandemic-related stress are also needed. For instance, Better Nights, Better Days for COVID-19 has been developed to help parents/caregivers improve sleep in school-aged children [6]. Given the strong relationship between sleep and mental health found in this study, developing and testing sleep-focused interventions that target both parents and children could help alleviate ongoing stress and potentially prevent or reduce mental health difficulties.

Finally, it may be valuable to explore broader societal and environmental impacts on sleep and mental health during the COVID-19 pandemic. For example, future research could investigate how factors such as work-from-home policies, changes in social interaction, and public health messaging may have influenced family dynamics, stress, sleep, and mental health in children and parents. Understanding these broader contexts can help policymakers design better support systems for families in the event of future global crises.

5. Conclusions

In summary, the current study found that COVID-19 stress significantly impacted both parent and child mental health, with these effects partially mediated by child and parent sleep problems. For children, their own sleep was a better predictor of their own mental health outcomes, while for parents, both their own sleep and their child's sleep equally predicted their mental health outcomes. This was observed in a sample of parents from Canada and the US who experienced various levels of emergency measures and restrictions during the COVID-19 pandemic. These findings underscore the need for targeted interventions that address sleep disturbances within families as part of a broader approach to mitigating the mental health impacts of the pandemic. Clinicians and policymakers must prioritize sleep as a key component of mental health care, particularly in the context of long-term COVID-19 pandemic recovery and similar future crises.

Author Contributions: Conceptualization, A.I., A.J.K., D.D., E.K., S.H.S., S.B.S., S.H.D. and P.V.C.; methodology, A.I., A.J.K., D.D., E.K., S.H.S., S.B.S., S.H.D. and P.V.C.; validation, S.H.S., S.H.D., S.B.S. and P.V.C.; formal analysis, A.I., D.D. and A.J.K.; investigation, S.H.D. and S.H.S.; resources, S.H.S., S.H.D., S.B.S. and P.V.C.; writing—original draft preparation, A.I., A.J.K. and D.D.; writing—review and editing, E.K., S.H.S., S.B.S., S.H.D. and P.V.C.; visualization, A.I. and P.V.C.; supervision, P.V.C., S.H.S., S.B.S. and S.H.D.; funding acquisition, S.H.S. and S.H.D. All authors have read and agreed to the published version of the manuscript.

Funding: This research was funded by the Social Science and Humanities Research Council of Canada (SSHRC) Partnership Engagement Grant (#1008-2020-0220).

Institutional Review Board Statement: This study was approved by the Dalhousie University Social Sciences and Humanities Research Ethics Board (REB #2020-5336, 5 May 2021).

Informed Consent Statement: Informed consent was obtained from all participants involved in the study.

Data Availability Statement: The datasets generated and analyzed during the current study are not publicly available due to keeping participant's identity and information confidential. The researchers do not have ethical approval to share the data.

Acknowledgments: The authors would like to thank the Language and Literacy Lab and the Mood, Anxiety, and Addiction Co-Morbidity Lab at Dalhousie University for making available the dataset used in this secondary analysis. We also thank the participants for their time and contributions to the original study.

Conflicts of Interest: The authors declare no conflicts of interest. The funders had no role in the design of the study; in the collection, analyses, or interpretation of data; in the writing of the manuscript; or in the decision to publish the results.

Abbreviations

The following abbreviations are used in this manuscript:

COVID-19	Coronavirus Disease of 2019

References

1. Filip, R.; Gheorghita Puscaselu, R.; Anchidin-Norocel, L.; Dimian, M.; Savage, W.K. Global Challenges to Public Health Care Systems during the COVID-19 Pandemic: A Review of Pandemic Measures and Problems. *J. Pers. Med.* **2022**, *12*, 1295. [CrossRef] [PubMed]
2. Miyah, Y.; Benjelloun, M.; Lairini, S.; Lahrichi, A. COVID-19 Impact on Public Health, Environment, Human Psychology, Global Socioeconomy, and Education. *Sci. World J.* **2022**, *2022*, 5578284. [CrossRef] [PubMed]
3. Gassman-Pines, A.; Ananat, E.O.; Fitz-Henley, J.; Leer, J. Effect of Daily School and Care Disruptions during the COVID-19 Pandemic on Child Behavior Problems. *Dev. Psychol.* **2022**, *58*, 1512–1527. [CrossRef] [PubMed]
4. Selman, S.B.; Dilworth-Bart, J.E. Routines and Child Development: A Systematic Review. *J. Fam. Theory Rev.* **2024**, *16*, 272–328. [CrossRef]
5. Gadermann, A.C.; Thomson, K.C.; Richardson, C.G.; Gagné, M.; McAuliffe, C.; Hirani, S.; Jenkins, E. Examining the Impacts of the COVID-19 Pandemic on Family Mental Health in Canada: Findings from a National Cross-Sectional Study. *BMJ Open* **2021**, *11*, e042871. [CrossRef] [PubMed]
6. MacKenzie, N.E.; Keys, E.; Hall, W.A.; Gruber, R.; Smith, I.M.; Constantin, E.; Godbout, R.; Stremler, R.; Reid, G.J.; Hanlon-Dearman, A.; et al. Children's Sleep During COVID-19: How Sleep Influences Surviving and Thriving in Families. *J. Pediatr. Psychol.* **2021**, *46*, 1051–1062. [CrossRef] [PubMed]
7. Büber, A.; Aktaş Terzioğlu, M. Caregiver's Reports of Their Children's Psychological Symptoms after the Start of the COVID-19 Pandemic and Caregiver's Perceived Stress in Turkey. *Nord. J. Psychiatry* **2022**, *76*, 215–224. [CrossRef] [PubMed]
8. Burkart, K.G.; Brauer, M.; Aravkin, A.Y.; Godwin, W.W.; Hay, S.I.; He, J.; Iannucci, V.C.; Larson, S.L.; Lim, S.S.; Liu, J.; et al. Estimating the Cause-Specific Relative Risks of Non-Optimal Temperature on Daily Mortality: A Two-Part Modelling Approach Applied to the Global Burden of Disease Study. *Lancet* **2021**, *398*, 685–697. [CrossRef] [PubMed]
9. Maximova, K.; Khan, M.K.A.; Dabravolskaj, J.; Maunula, L.; Ohinmaa, A.; Veugelers, P.J. Perceived Changes in Lifestyle Behaviours and in Mental Health and Wellbeing of Elementary School Children during the First COVID-19 Lockdown in Canada. *Public Health* **2022**, *202*, 35–42. [CrossRef] [PubMed]
10. Olive, L.S.; Sciberras, E.; Berkowitz, T.S.; Hoare, E.; Telford, R.M.; O'Neil, A.; Mikocka-Walus, A.; Evans, S.; Hutchinson, D.; McGillivray, J.A.; et al. Child and Parent Physical Activity, Sleep, and Screen Time During COVID-19 and Associations With Mental Health: Implications for Future Psycho-Cardiological Disease? *Front. Psychiatry* **2022**, *12*, 774858. [CrossRef] [PubMed]
11. Lunsford-Avery, J.R.; Bidopia, T.; Jackson, L.; Sloan, J.S. Behavioral Treatment of Insomnia and Sleep Disturbances in School-Aged Children and Adolescents. *Child Adolesc. Psychiatr. Clin. N. Am.* **2021**, *30*, 101–116. [CrossRef] [PubMed]

12. American Psychiatric Association. *Diagnostic and Statistical Manual of Mental Disorders*; DSM-5-TR; American Psychiatric Association Publishing: Washington, DC, USA, 2022; ISBN 978-0-89042-575-6.
13. Könen, T.; Dirk, J.; Leonhardt, A.; Schmiedek, F. The Interplay between Sleep Behavior and Affect in Elementary School Children's Daily Life. *J. Exp. Child Psychol.* **2016**, *150*, 1–15. [CrossRef] [PubMed]
14. Uccella, S.; Cordani, R.; Salfi, F.; Gorgoni, M.; Scarpelli, S.; Gemignani, A.; Geoffroy, P.A.; De Gennaro, L.; Palagini, L.; Ferrara, M.; et al. Sleep Deprivation and Insomnia in Adolescence: Implications for Mental Health. *Brain Sci.* **2023**, *13*, 569. [CrossRef] [PubMed]
15. Blok, E.; Koopman-Verhoeff, M.E.; Dickstein, D.P.; Saletin, J.; Luik, A.I.; Rijlaarsdam, J.; Hillegers, M.; Kocevska, D.; White, T.; Tiemeier, H. Sleep and Mental Health in Childhood: A Multi-Method Study in the General Pediatric Population. *Child Adolesc. Psychiatry Ment. Health* **2022**, *16*, 11. [CrossRef] [PubMed]
16. Meng, R.; Xu, J.; Luo, Y.; Mastrotheodoros, S.; Jiang, C.; Garofalo, C.; Mazzeschi, C.; Nielsen, T.; Fong, D.Y.T.; Dzierzewski, J.M.; et al. Perceived Stress Mediates the Longitudinal Effect of Sleep Quality on Internalizing Symptoms. *J. Affect. Disord.* **2025**, *373*, 51–59. [CrossRef] [PubMed]
17. Zhang, L.; Cui, Z.; Huffman, L.G.; Oshri, A. Sleep Mediates the Effect of Stressful Environments on Youth Development of Impulsivity: The Moderating Role of within Default Mode Network Resting-State Functional Connectivity. *Sleep Health* **2023**, *9*, 503–511. [CrossRef] [PubMed]
18. Cellini, N.; Di Giorgio, E.; Mioni, G.; Di Riso, D. Sleep and Psychological Difficulties in Italian School-Age Children During COVID-19 Lockdown. *J. Pediatr. Psychol.* **2021**, *46*, 153–167. [CrossRef] [PubMed]
19. Myhr, A.; Naper, L.R.; Samarawickrema, I.; Vesterbekkmo, R.K. Impact of COVID-19 Pandemic Lockdown on Mental Well-Being of Norwegian Adolescents During the First Wave—Socioeconomic Position and Gender Differences. *Front. Public Health* **2021**, *9*, 717747. [CrossRef] [PubMed]
20. Papadopoulos, D. Impact of Child and Family Factors on Caregivers' Mental Health and Psychological Distress during the COVID-19 Pandemic in Greece. *Children* **2023**, *11*, 7. [CrossRef] [PubMed]
21. Mental Health Commission of Canada. Mental Health Commission of Canada: Ottawa, ON, Canada, 2025. Available online: https://mentalhealthcommission.ca/ (accessed on 15 March 2025).
22. Bond, L.; Butler, H.; Thomas, L.; Carlin, J.; Glover, S.; Bowes, G.; Patton, G. Social and School Connectedness in Early Secondary School as Predictors of Late Teenage Substance Use, Mental Health, and Academic Outcomes. *J. Adolesc. Health* **2007**, *40*, 357.E9–357.E18. [CrossRef] [PubMed]
23. Cost, K.T.; Crosbie, J.; Anagnostou, E.; Birken, C.S.; Charach, A.; Monga, S.; Kelley, E.; Nicolson, R.; Maguire, J.L.; Burton, C.L.; et al. Mostly Worse, Occasionally Better: Impact of COVID-19 Pandemic on the Mental Health of Canadian Children and Adolescents. *Eur. Child Adolesc. Psychiatry* **2022**, *31*, 671–684. [CrossRef] [PubMed]
24. Lee, C.M.; Cadigan, J.M.; Rhew, I.C. Increases in Loneliness Among Young Adults During the COVID-19 Pandemic and Association With Increases in Mental Health Problems. *J. Adolesc. Health* **2020**, *67*, 714–717. [CrossRef] [PubMed]
25. Wu, T.; Jia, X.; Shi, H.; Niu, J.; Yin, X.; Xie, J.; Wang, X. Prevalence of Mental Health Problems during the COVID-19 Pandemic: A Systematic Review and Meta-Analysis. *J. Affect. Disord.* **2021**, *281*, 91–98. [CrossRef] [PubMed]
26. Pierce, M.; Hope, H.F.; Kolade, A.; Gellatly, J.; Osam, C.S.; Perchard, R.; Kosidou, K.; Dalman, C.; Morgan, V.; Di Prinzio, P.; et al. Effects of Parental Mental Illness on Children's Physical Health: Systematic Review and Meta-Analysis. *Br. J. Psychiatry* **2020**, *217*, 354–363. [CrossRef] [PubMed]
27. Kalmbach, D.A.; Anderson, J.R.; Drake, C.L. The Impact of Stress on Sleep: Pathogenic Sleep Reactivity as a Vulnerability to Insomnia and Circadian Disorders. *J. Sleep Res.* **2018**, *27*, e12710. [CrossRef] [PubMed]
28. Lollies, F.; Schnatschmidt, M.; Bihlmeier, I.; Genuneit, J.; In-Albnon, T.; Holtmann, M.; Legenbauer, T.; Schlarb, A.A. Associations of Sleep and Emotion Regulation Processes in Childhood and Adolescence—A Systematic Review, Report of Methodological Challenges and Future Directions. *Sleep Sci.* **2022**, *15*, 490–514. [CrossRef] [PubMed]
29. Ng, C.S.M.; Ng, S.S.L. Impact of the COVID-19 Pandemic on Children's Mental Health: A Systematic Review. *Front. Psychiatry* **2022**, *13*, 975936. [CrossRef] [PubMed]
30. Peltz, J.S.; Rogge, R.D. The Moderating Role of Parents' Dysfunctional Sleep-Related Beliefs Among Associations Between Adolescents' Pre-Bedtime Conflict, Sleep Quality, and Their Mental Health. *J. Clin. Sleep Med.* **2019**, *15*, 265–274. [CrossRef] [PubMed]
31. Deacon, S.H.; Rodriguez, L.M.; Elgendi, M.; King, F.E.; Nogueira-Arjona, R.; Sherry, S.B.; Stewart, S.H. Parenting through a Pandemic: Mental Health and Substance Use Consequences of Mandated Homeschooling. *Couple Fam. Psychol. Res. Pract.* **2021**, *10*, 281–293. [CrossRef]
32. Elgendi, M.M.; Stewart, S.H.; DesRoches, D.I.; Corkum, P.; Nogueira-Arjona, R.; Deacon, S.H. Division of Labour and Parental Mental Health and Relationship Well-Being during COVID-19 Pandemic-Mandated Homeschooling. *Int. J. Environ. Res. Public Health* **2022**, *19*, 17021. [CrossRef] [PubMed]

33. Groff, L.V.M.; Elgendi, M.M.; Stewart, S.H.; Deacon, S.H. Long-Term Mandatory Homeschooling during COVID-19 Had Compounding Mental Health Effects on Parents and Children. *Children* **2024**, *11*, 1072. [CrossRef] [PubMed]
34. Statistics Canada. 2022. Available online: https://www.statcan.gc.ca/o1/en/plus/2210-homeschool-enrollment-doubled-canada-during-covid-19-lockdowns (accessed on 15 March 2025).
35. McLean, C.P.; Wachsman, T.; Morland, L.; Norman, S.B.; Hooper, V.; Cloitre, M. The Mental Health Impact of COVID-19–Related Stressors among Treatment-seeking Trauma-exposed Veterans. *J. Trauma. Stress* **2022**, *35*, 1792–1800. [CrossRef] [PubMed]
36. Kaniuka, A.R.; Kelliher Rabon, J.; Brooks, B.D.; Sirois, F.; Kleiman, E.; Hirsch, J.K. Gratitude and Suicide Risk among College Students: Substantiating the Protective Benefits of Being Thankful. *J. Am. Coll. Health* **2021**, *69*, 660–667. [CrossRef] [PubMed]
37. Langhinrichsen-Rohling, J.; Montanaro, E.; Mennicke, A.; Ybarra, M.L. Cybervictimization in Relation to Self and Other Protection and Response Behaviors: A Cross-Sectional Look at an Age-Diverse National Sample. *J. Interpers. Violence* **2024**, *39*, 3062–3087. [CrossRef] [PubMed]
38. Goodman, A.; Lamping, D.L.; Ploubidis, G.B. When to Use Broader Internalising and Externalising Subscales Instead of the Hypothesised Five Subscales on the Strengths and Difficulties Questionnaire (SDQ): Data from British Parents, Teachers and Children. *J. Abnorm. Child Psychol.* **2010**, *38*, 1179–1191. [CrossRef] [PubMed]
39. Borg, A.-M.; Kaukonen, P.; Salmelin, R.; Joukamaa, M.; Tamminen, T. Reliability of the Strengths and Difficulties Questionnaire among Finnish 4–9-Year-Old Children. *Nord. J. Psychiatry* **2012**, *66*, 403–413. [CrossRef] [PubMed]
40. Kroenke, K.; Spitzer, R.L.; Williams, J.B.W. The PHQ-9: Validity of a Brief Depression Severity Measure. *J. Gen. Intern. Med.* **2001**, *16*, 606–613. [CrossRef] [PubMed]
41. Spitzer, R.L.; Kroenke, K.; Williams, J.B.W.; Löwe, B. A Brief Measure for Assessing Generalized Anxiety Disorder: The GAD-7. *Arch. Intern. Med.* **2006**, *166*, 1092. [CrossRef] [PubMed]
42. Kroenke, K.; Wu, J.; Yu, Z.; Bair, M.J.; Kean, J.; Stump, T.; Monahan, P.O. Patient Health Questionnaire Anxiety and Depression Scale: Initial Validation in Three Clinical Trials. *Psychosom. Med.* **2016**, *78*, 716–727. [CrossRef] [PubMed]
43. Stallwood, E.; Elsman, E.B.M.; Monsour, A.; Baba, A.; Butcher, N.J.; Offringa, M. Measurement Properties of Patient Reported Outcome Scales: A Systematic Review. *Pediatrics* **2023**, *152*, e2023061489. [CrossRef] [PubMed]
44. Forrest, C.B.; Meltzer, L.J.; Marcus, C.L.; De La Motte, A.; Kratchman, A.; Buysse, D.J.; Pilkonis, P.A.; Becker, B.D.; Bevans, K.B. Development and Validation of the PROMIS Pediatric Sleep Disturbance and Sleep-Related Impairment Item Banks. *Sleep* **2018**, *41*, zsy054. [CrossRef] [PubMed]
45. Buysse, D.J.; Yu, L.; Moul, D.E.; Germain, A.; Stover, A.; Dodds, N.E.; Johnston, K.L.; Shablesky-Cade, M.A.; Pilkonis, P.A. Development and Validation of Patient-Reported Outcome Measures for Sleep Disturbance and Sleep-Related Impairments. *Sleep* **2010**, *33*, 781–792. [CrossRef] [PubMed]
46. Schober, P.; Boer, C.; Schwarte, L.A. Correlation Coefficients: Appropriate Use and Interpretation. *Anesth. Analg.* **2018**, *126*, 1763–1768. [CrossRef] [PubMed]
47. Ivanenko, Y.P.; Poppele, R.E.; Lacquaniti, F. Motor Control Programs and Walking. *Neuroscientist* **2006**, *12*, 339–348. [CrossRef] [PubMed]
48. Shrout, P.E.; Bolger, N. Mediation in Experimental and Nonexperimental Studies: New Procedures and Recommendations. *Psychol. Methods* **2002**, *7*, 422–445. [CrossRef] [PubMed]
49. World Atlas. 2025. Available online: https://www.worldatlas.com/ (accessed on 15 March 2025).
50. Government of Canada. World Atlas. 2025. Available online: https://natural-resources.canada.ca/maps-tools-publications/maps/atlas-canada (accessed on 15 March 2025).
51. Varma, P.; Conduit, R.; Junge, M.; Jackson, M.L. Examining Sleep and Mood in Parents of Children with Sleep Disturbances. *Nat. Sci. Sleep* **2020**, *12*, 865–874. [CrossRef] [PubMed]
52. Wearick-Silva, L.E.; Richter, S.A.; Viola, T.W.; Nunes, M.L. Sleep Quality among Parents and Their Children during COVID-19 Pandemic. *J. De Pediatr.* **2022**, *98*, 248–255. [CrossRef] [PubMed]
53. Kerr, M.L.; Fanning, K.A.; Huynh, T.; Botto, I.; Kim, C.N. Parents' Self-Reported Psychological Impacts of COVID-19: Associations With Parental Burnout, Child Behavior, and Income. *J. Pediatr. Psychol.* **2021**, *46*, 1162–1171. [CrossRef] [PubMed]
54. Wauters, A.; Vervoort, T.; Dhondt, K.; Soenens, B.; Vansteenkiste, M.; Morbée, S.; Waterschoot, J.; Haerynck, F.; Vandekerckhove, K.; Verhelst, H.; et al. Mental Health Outcomes Among Parents of Children With a Chronic Disease During the COVID-19 Pandemic: The Role of Parental Burn-Out. *J. Pediatr. Psychol.* **2022**, *47*, 420–431. [CrossRef] [PubMed]
55. Canadian Society for Exercise Physiology. *24-Hour Movement Guidelines*; Canadian Society for Exercise Physiology: Ottawa, ON, Canada, 2025; Available online: https://csepguidelines.ca (accessed on 15 March 2025).
56. Paruthi, S.; Brooks, L.J.; D'Ambrosio, C.; Hall, W.A.; Kotagal, S.; Lloyd, R.M.; Malow, B.A.; Maski, K.; Nichols, C.; Quan, S.F.; et al. Recommended Amount of Sleep for Pediatric Populations: A Consensus Statement of the American Academy of Sleep Medicine. *J. Clin. Sleep Med.* **2016**, *12*, 785–786. [CrossRef] [PubMed]

57. Dutil, C.; Walsh, J.J.; Featherstone, R.B.; Gunnell, K.E.; Tremblay, M.S.; Gruber, R.; Weiss, S.K.; Cote, K.A.; Sampson, M.; Chaput, J.-P. Influence of Sleep on Developing Brain Functions and Structures in Children and Adolescents: A Systematic Review. *Sleep Med. Rev.* **2018**, *42*, 184–201. [CrossRef] [PubMed]
58. Bussières, E.-L.; Malboeuf-Hurtubise, C.; Meilleur, A.; Mastine, T.; Hérault, E.; Chadi, N.; Montreuil, M.; Généreux, M.; Camden, C.; PRISME-COVID Team. Consequences of the COVID-19 Pandemic on Children's Mental Health: A Meta-Analysis. *Front. Psychiatry* **2021**, *12*, 691659. [CrossRef] [PubMed]
59. McArthur, B.A.; Racine, N.; McDonald, S.; Tough, S.; Madigan, S. Child and Family Factors Associated with Child Mental Health and Well-Being during COVID-19. *Eur. Child Adolesc. Psychiatry* **2021**, *32*, 223–233. [CrossRef] [PubMed]
60. Neculicioiu, V.S.; Colosi, I.A.; Costache, C.; Sevastre-Berghian, A.; Clichici, S. Time to Sleep?—A Review of the Impact of the COVID-19 Pandemic on Sleep and Mental Health. *Int. J. Environ. Res. Public Health* **2022**, *19*, 3497. [CrossRef] [PubMed]
61. Sharma, M.; Aggarwal, S.; Madaan, P.; Saini, L.; Bhutani, M. Impact of COVID-19 Pandemic on Sleep in Children and Adolescents: A Systematic Review and Meta-Analysis. *Sleep Med.* **2021**, *84*, 259–267. [CrossRef] [PubMed]
62. Racine, N.; McArthur, B.A.; Cooke, J.E.; Eirich, R.; Zhu, J.; Madigan, S. Global Prevalence of Depressive and Anxiety Symptoms in Children and Adolescents During COVID-19: A Meta-Analysis. *JAMA Pediatr.* **2021**, *175*, 1142. [CrossRef] [PubMed]
63. Statistics Canada Population and Demography Statistics. 2025. Available online: https://www.statcan.gc.ca/en/subjects-start/population_and_demography (accessed on 15 March 2025).
64. United States Census Bureau Race. 2025. Available online: https://www.census.gov/topics/population/race.html (accessed on 15 March 2025).
65. O'Laughlin, K.D.; Martin, M.J.; Ferrer, E. Cross-Sectional Analysis of Longitudinal Mediation Processes. *Multivar. Behav. Res.* **2018**, *53*, 375–402. [CrossRef] [PubMed]
66. Hayes, A.F. Beyond Baron and Kenny: Statistical Mediation Analysis in the New Millennium. *Commun. Monogr.* **2009**, *76*, 408–420. [CrossRef]
67. Martin-West, S. The Role of Social Support as a Moderator of Housing Instability in Single Mother and Two-Parent Households. *Soc. Work Res.* **2019**, *43*, 31–42. [CrossRef]
68. Freisthler, B.; Gruenewald, P.J.; Tebben, E.; Shockley McCarthy, K.; Price Wolf, J. Understanding At-the-Moment Stress for Parents during COVID-19 Stay-at-Home Restrictions. *Soc. Sci. Med.* **2021**, *279*, 114025. [CrossRef] [PubMed]
69. OurCare Primary Care Needs. 2025. Available online: https://www.ourcare.ca/ (accessed on 15 March 2025).

children

MDPI

Article

Parenting Under Pressure: The Transformative Impact of PCIT on Caregiver Depression and Anxiety and Child Outcomes

Abigail Peskin *, Alexis Landa, Juliana Acosta, William Andrew Rothenberg, Rachel Levi, Eileen Davis, Dainelys Garcia, Jason F. Jent and Elana Mansoor

Miller School of Medicine, University of Miami, Miami, FL 33136, USA; all162@med.miami.edu (A.L.); jxa840@med.miami.edu (J.A.); war37@miami.edu (W.A.R.); rachlevi24@gmail.com (R.L.); exm305@miami.edu (E.D.); ngarcia09@med.miami.edu (D.G.); jjent@med.miami.edu (J.F.J.); emansoor@med.miami.edu (E.M.)

* Correspondence: a.pooch@umiami.edu

Abstract

Background Objectives: Parental anxiety and depression demonstrate bidirectional connections with child developmental outcomes (e.g., disruptive behavior). Directly targeting child development through behavioral parent training (BPT) has potential for reversing this cycle. Parent–Child Interaction Therapy (PCIT), a BPT with robust research evidence for decreasing child disruptive behaviors, has demonstrated promise in also decreasing caregiver anxiety and depression. However, the mechanisms that explain this relationship are less understood. **Methods:** The current study examined whether caregivers (N = 840) completing time-limited PCIT experienced significant reductions in depression and anxiety symptoms and improvements in child disruptive behaviors at each time point. Generalized estimate equation analyses assessed whether caregiver anxiety and depression moderated changes in child disruptive behavior. Mediation analyses explored the extent that changes in caregiver–child interactions over time explained changes in family outcomes. **Results:** Child disruptive behavior and caregiver depression and anxiety symptoms improved significantly at each time point of PCIT. Change in child behavioral outcomes was significantly moderated by caregiver race. Caregivers with higher anxiety reported fewer improvements in child disruptive behavior compared to other caregivers. Changes in caregiver anxiety and depression over the course of treatment were partially mediated by improvement in caregiver–child interaction skills. Changes in child disruptive behavior were not mediated by improvement in caregiver–child interaction skills. **Conclusions:** Results demonstrate that time-limited PCIT could significantly improve caregiver anxiety and depression, and some PCIT-taught parenting skills are direct drivers of this process. Further research is needed to understand other mechanisms underlying the relationship between PCIT and improved family outcomes.

Keywords: Parent–Child Interaction Therapy; caregiver mental health; child disruptive behaviors; caregiver–child interactions

1. Introduction

Caregiver distress is a common experience, as caregivers must continually adapt to the changes in their child's development, manage competing demands, and navigate emotional, financial, and social challenges [1]. When caregivers lack the resources to cope with these challenges, caregiver distress can negatively impact both their well-being and their child's behavior and development. High and persistent caregiving distress has been linked to an increased risk of caregiver depression, marital conflict, maladaptive parenting strategies, strained caregiver–child relationships, and a higher likelihood of child behavior problems [1].

Caregiver distress, which can be heightened by a child's mental health needs [2], increases the likelihood of disengagement, criticism, and inconsistent parenting strategies [3]. Caregivers who report greater anxiety and depression often have fewer positive interactions with their children, use ineffective parenting strategies, fail to model healthy emotional regulation, and, consequently, may develop strained relationships with their children [4]. Indeed, caregivers' depression and distress not only transmit genetic vulnerabilities but also create an environmental context more prone to coercive interactions [4]. Mothers with higher levels of life satisfaction and well-being may have children with better developmental outcomes, prosocial behavior, and emotional regulation [4].

This relationship between child and caregiver mental health is reciprocal. Child mental health concerns can significantly increase caregiver emotional burden and risk for psychological distress [2]. Given these transactional dynamics between caregiver and child mental health, active caregiver participation in child mental health prevention programs has been linked to improved child and caregiver outcomes, such as reductions in stress and improved caregiver–child relationship quality [5]. However, caregiver mental health challenges, particularly anxiety and depression, can negatively impact engagement in treatment (e.g., treatment attendance, retention) [6]. Caregivers experiencing psychological distress may face difficulties attending treatment sessions and completing home assignments, which are critical components of an effective intervention. This, in turn, can hinder treatment progress and outcomes for the child [5,6].

The well-established Patterson's Coercive Family Process Model [7,8] explains how child mental health difficulties often emerge and are maintained through escalating cycles of negative caregiver–child interactions. In these coercive cycles, caregivers and children unintentionally reinforce each other's aversive behaviors through negative reinforcement. For example, a child escalates problem behavior to escape demands, and a caregiver withdraws the demand to avoid conflict, strengthening the problematic cycle [7]. Over time, this bidirectional dynamic contributes to worsening mental health in both the caregiver and child as distress in one often intensifies problems in the other [2,9]. These compounding interactions create a harmful feedback loop that exemplifies the core mechanisms described in Patterson's model (see Figure 1).

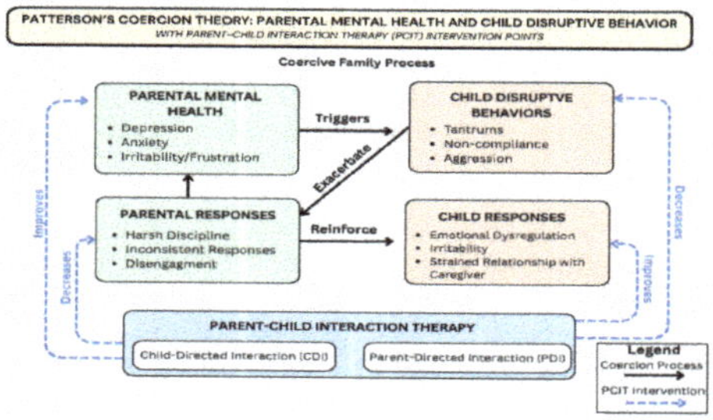

Figure 1. The role of PCIT in addressing coercive caregiver–child interactions and parental mental health

Behavioral parent training (BPT) programs such as Parent–Child Interaction Therapy (PCIT) are designed to interrupt this cycle by teaching caregivers more effective ways to interact with their children (see Figure 1). That is, it is believed that as caregivers adopt more positive relational practices and more consistent effective discipline practices, children's disruptive behavior will improve. As a result, caregivers' own anxiety and depression symptoms may decrease, which research suggests may be due to changes in how caregivers interpret their child's behavior [10]. For example, caregivers participating in BPT often gain deeper insights into the environmental, emotional, and developmental factors influencing their child's behavior. By fostering this nuanced understanding, caregivers may respond more effectively with tailored support.

Importantly, these changes create a positive feedback loop within the parent–child relationship. As caregivers respond more effectively, children may exhibit improved behavior. In turn, witnessing these positive changes in their children reinforces caregivers' use of positive practices and enhances their confidence in managing behavioral challenges. This mutual reinforcement strengthens the parent–child bond and supports ongoing improvements in both child behavior and caregiver mental health.

1.1. Behavioral Parent Training

PCIT is a form of BPT that uses live coaching to teach caregivers effective parenting techniques, discipline strategies, and methods for reducing parenting distress [11,12]. PCIT consists of two treatment phases. The first phase, Child-Directed Interaction (CDI), teaches caregivers to use their attention to reinforce positive behaviors while decreasing negative behaviors (see Figure 1). It also aims to enhance the caregiver–child relationship through child-led play. The second phase, Parent-Directed Interaction (PDI), teaches caregivers how to give effective commands and set limits through the consistent use of time-out. Through live coaching of their caregiver–child interactions, therapists teach caregivers to be predictable, consistent, and proactive in their responses to child behavior, which can help reduce caregiver distress by instilling a greater sense of control and simultaneously improving child emotion regulation [12,13]. Although PCIT was originally developed to conclude when specific criteria for caregiver observable skills and child behavior had been met [14], this sometimes means that PCIT can last longer than 7 months, which often makes it difficult for families to officially "graduate" from treatment because they need to terminate earlier. However, time-limited PCIT that ends after a specific number of weeks or sessions has shown promise in accomplishing similar behavioral improvements to traditional competency-based PCIT [15,16].

PCIT was designed to target child disruptive behaviors. Due to the reciprocal effects between child behavior and caregiver mental health, prior research has explored whether traditional (i.e., not time-limited) PCIT could improve caregiver anxiety and depression [11]. Results showed that despite the intervention focusing solely on child behavior, both caregiver anxiety and depression reduced significantly [11]. In addition to addressing caregiver–child interactions, PCIT may also target negative caregiver cognitions regarding their children's behavior. Research indicates that negative caregiver attributions often contribute to problematic behaviors in children, particularly when paired with ineffective parenting strategies [17]. PCIT's in vivo coaching of the caregiver–child dyad creates added benefits in targeting negative parental cognitions by reframing negative or unhelpful attributions, encouraging mindful attention to positive child behaviors, and ultimately enhancing the caregiver–child relationship. In addition, consideration of cultural values of minoritized caregivers is essential in BPT for effectively reducing parenting distress and improving child outcomes [18]. Parenting distress can be influenced by socioeconomic status as well, with economic challenges linked to increased risk for maladaptive parenting and child maltreatment [19].

1.2. Current Study

Building on these findings, the present study examined whether time-limited PCIT can produce similar improvements in caregiver anxiety and depression and child disruptive behavior. We first sought to examine how caregiver anxiety and depression were associated with treatment processes.

Hypothesis 1: *Specifically, we hypothesized that higher levels of caregiver pre-treatment anxiety and depression would be associated with reduced treatment engagement, as evidenced by attending fewer PCIT sessions and a lower likelihood of treatment completion. We sought to replicate prior PCIT research by examining the effects of PCIT on caregiver mental health, parenting skills, and child disruptive behaviors.*

Hypothesis 2: *Second, we sought to examine the extent that families demonstrated clinically significant levels of caregiver depression and anxiety and child disruptive behavior at each time point in PCIT (pre-, mid-, and post-treatment).*

Hypothesis 3: *Specifically, we assessed whether participation in PCIT was associated with reductions in caregiver anxiety and depression, reductions in child disruptive behaviors, and improvement in parenting skills at each time point in PCIT (i.e., pre- to mid-treatment, mid- to post-treatment, and pre- to post-treatment).*

Time-limited PCIT has demonstrated clinically and statistically significant decreases in caregivers' total stress levels [12], indicating that it may have potential to affect caregiver mental health as well. Prior researchers have suggested that the effectiveness of PCIT in alleviating caregiver distress and improving mental health may be enhanced by providing caregivers with psychoeducation on emotions, offering strategies for coping skills, encouraging modeling of effective emotion regulation, and discussing the advantages of using selective attention for minor disruptive behaviors [12]. However, most PCIT research to date [20] has only examined the direct effects of PCIT on caregiver and child outcomes and very little attention has been provided to exploring the mechanisms that are proposed to promote these changes in family outcomes [13,21]. Therefore, further exploration of potential mediating and moderating mechanisms involving caregiver functioning and parenting skills in relation to key treatment outcomes, including child disruptive behavior and caregiver mental health, is warranted.

Hypothesis 4: *Specifically, we explored potential moderators of treatment effects, including pre-treatment caregiver mental health (i.e., parental anxiety and depression) and/or sociodemographic characteristics (i.e., caregiver race, ethnicity, household income, education), to identify for whom PCIT may be most effective.*

Hypothesis 5: *Finally, we explored mechanisms of change by examining whether changes in parenting skills (i.e., observed Do/Avoid skills) mediated the relationship between PCIT participation and both child behavioral (i.e., disruptive behaviors) and caregiver mental health outcomes (i.e., anxiety, depression). Through these objectives, we aimed to provide a comprehensive evaluation of the direct effects of time-limited PCIT, clarify contextual factors that may influence treatment response, and identify mechanisms through which PCIT promotes positive family outcomes.*

2. Materials and Methods

2.1. Participants

Participants consisted of children (N = 840) aged 2–8 years (M = 4.77, SD = 1.50, 68.2% male) and their primary caregivers (88.2% female) who received in-person PCIT services at six university-affiliated clinics or via telehealth. Telehealth PCIT (i.e., I-PCIT) involved meeting via HIPAA-compliant teleconferencing software and a therapist coaching the caregiver in their home instead of the clinic via Bluetooth or wired headset. Session fidelity to the PCIT model was retained, but instead of being behind a one-way mirror (i.e., clinic coaching), the therapist coached through the videoconferencing platform. IPCIT has been studied extensively in randomized and open trials and has demonstrated robust evidence as being equally efficacious to in-person PCIT for improving child behavior outcomes [22,23]. Two clinic locations were in academic centers, and the remaining four clinics were within a large metropolitan community in the Southeast United States. Services were grant-funded and therefore free to families. Demographic information was collected through the online Research Electronic Data Capture (REDCap) [24] database management system. For additional demographic characteristics, see Table 1.

Table 1. PCIT participant demographics.

Characteristic (N = 840)	*n*	%	*n*	%
Child Gender (*n* = 808)				
Male			573	70.9
Female			235	29.1
Language PCIT was Delivered in (*n* = 775)				
English			545	70.3
Spanish			159	20.5
English and Spanish			70	9.0
Portuguese			1	0.1
Caregiver Education Level (*n* = 804)				
Some grade school			11	1.4
High school diploma/GED			61	7.6
Some college			86	10.7
Associate degree			58	7.2
Bachelor's degree			282	35.1
Graduate degree			306	38.1
Household Income (*n* = 762)				
Less than USD 20,000			62	8.1
USD 20,000 to USD 34,999			76	10.0
USD 35,000 to USD 49,999			74	9.7
USD 50,000 to USD 74,999			92	12.1
USD 75,000 to USD 99,999			106	13.9
$\geq$ USD 100,000			352	46.2
Child Race by Ethnicity (*n* = 807)	**Hispanic (*n* = 567)**		**Non-Hispanic (*n* = 240)**	
White	494	87.1	147	61.3
Biracial or Multiracial	47	8.3	36	15.0
Prefer to Self-Describe	18	3.2	6	2.5
Black or African American	6	1.1	42	17.5
American Indian or Alaskan Native	2	0.4	2	1.0
Asian	0	0.0	6	2.5
Pacific Islander	0	0.0	1	0.04

Note: Total sample N = 840. Sample sizes vary due to missing data.

Study inclusion criteria consisted of child age between 2 and 8 years; primary caregiver being fluent in English, Spanish, or Portuguese; and elevated child disruptive behavior scores on the Eyberg Child Behavior Inventory Intensity Scale (ECBI; Intensity Raw Score $\geq$ 131) [25] or on the Externalizing Problems subscales or composite of the Behavior Assessment System for Children, Third Edition (BASC-3; T-Score $\geq$ 60) [26]. Children were also eligible if they had a history of involvement with child protective services. Children were excluded from this sample if they had received a diagnosis of autism spectrum disorder (ASD), as children with this diagnosis received a longer course of time-limited PCIT. Institutional Review Board (IRB) approval was obtained from the university on 24 January 2021. All study procedures were conducted in accordance with the ethical standards of the IRB.

2.2. Procedure

Following screening, families meeting inclusion criteria were contacted by a PCIT therapist to schedule an intake session (i.e., pre-treatment assessment), during which written consent was obtained (and child assent, for children ages 7 years or older) and an adapted Cultural Formulation Interview (CFI) was administered [27]. Additionally, a 20 min behavioral observation was conducted. Caregiver-report questionnaires about child and family functioning were sent electronically following this session.

Of the 840 families who completed the pre-treatment assessment, 632 completed the mid-treatment assessment (75.24% of families who started treatment), and 567 completed the post-treatment assessment (67.50% of families who started treatment). At post-treatment, families completed treatment outcome and satisfaction questionnaires and another 10 min behavioral observation.

Parent–Child Interaction Therapy

Families received 18 weeks of weekly, one-hour individual PCIT sessions. While the caregiver–child dyad played together, therapists provided live coaching to caregivers on parenting skills via headset, either from behind a one-way mirror or via telehealth. PCIT was delivered by master's and doctoral-level therapists with training in clinical psychology and mental health. While some PCIT clinics may video record sessions for fidelity, this clinic utilizes a training co-therapy model so that trainers can rate therapist competence live to ensure treatment fidelity. Caregivers completed assessments (e.g., caregiver report measures and behavioral observation) at each time point (i.e., pre-, mid-, and post-treatment). Employing a family-centered approach, assessment procedures integrated a brief cultural assessment (adapted from the CFI) [27] to better meet individual needs and foster more culturally responsive services [28]. Further, caregivers participated in didactic sessions for both CDI and PDI, and up to five CDI coaching sessions. The remaining sessions focused on PDI coaching. Families could progress through CDI in fewer sessions upon demonstrating skill proficiency (i.e., 10 labeled praises, 10 reflections, 10 descriptions, and 3 or fewer questions, commands, and criticisms). Families were eligible to graduate in fewer than 18 weeks if they met graduation criteria (i.e., CDI [see above] and PDI skill proficiency [75% effective command rate and 75% correct follow-through], ECBI Intensity Raw Score $\leq$ 114, and caregiver-reported confidence in their ability to manage their child's behaviors) [14]. Therapists received PCIT training and weekly supervision from a Certified PCIT International Within-Agency or Regional Trainer and licensed therapist.

2.3. Measures

2.3.1. Family and Treatment Characteristics

Caregivers completed an online survey to provide demographic information, including child gender (male, female, non-binary, transgender), child age, caregiver education level (less than bachelor's degree, bachelor's degree or higher), caregiver race (American Indian or Alaskan, Asian, Black or African American, Pacific Islander, Prefer to Self-Describe. Other, Biracial or Multiracial) and ethnicity (Hispanic, Haitian, Non-Hispanic). In addition, therapists recorded the primary language(s) in which services were delivered (English, Spanish, Portuguese, or multiple languages).

2.3.2. Treatment Variables

A few treatment process variables were included in these analyses to ensure that any detected caregiver improvement over the course of treatment was not due to attrition of more severe cases. The variable "Treatment Completion" indicated whether a family completed 18 weeks of PCIT or prematurely terminated treatment. The other treatment variable was the number of sessions the family attended, meant to indicate the family's engagement in treatment above and beyond whether they completed the 18 weeks of treatment or not.

2.3.3. Child Behavior Measure

The Eyberg Child Behavior Inventory (ECBI) is a 36-item caregiver-report measure designed to assess disruptive behaviors in children ages 2–16 years [25]. The Intensity Scale evaluates the frequency of behavior problems, with a raw score of 131 or higher (T-score > 60) indicating clinically significant levels of disruptive behavior (1 = clinically elevated, 0 = within normal limits). Caregivers rate items such as "has temper tantrums," "argues with parents about rules," "hits parents," and "fails to finish tasks or chores," reflecting a range of externalizing behaviors. The ECBI has demonstrated reliability ($\alpha = 0.94$, test–retest = 0.75) [29] and validity (e.g., positive associations with other measures of disruptive behavior and emotion dysregulation) [13,30,31]. It has been validated across racially and ethnically diverse populations, demonstrated stability over time, and proven sensitive to treatment effects. In the current study, the ECBI Intensity Scale raw score was used for both eligibility screening and as an outcome measure of child disruptive behavior problems. The ECBI was administered to caregivers at pre-treatment, mid-treatment, and post-treatment.

2.3.4. Caregiver Skills

The Dyadic Parent–Child Interaction Coding System, Fourth Edition (DPICS-IV) [32] is a behavioral coding system used to assess caregiver verbalizations, behaviors, and overall quality of caregiver and child interactions. PCIT therapists, trained to an interrater agreement of at least 80% on the DPICS-IV, coded three five-minute caregiver–child interaction tasks which consisted of (1) child-led play (CLP) during which the caregiver follows the child's lead, (2) caregiver/parent-led play (PLP), in which the caregiver leads the play, and (3) clean-up (CU), in which the child is instructed to clean up the activity independently. The DPICS-IV has demonstrated acceptable reliability and validity for its coding categories in English-speaking populations [33]. In this study, the DPICS-IV served as an outcome measure of caregiver skill acquisition. Specifically, composite ratio scores were created for "Do" skills defined as the sum of labeled praises (e.g., "Nice job stacking those blocks"), reflections (e.g., child says "I made a tower," and caregiver repeats, "You made a tower"), and descriptions (e.g., "You're coloring the flower") divided by total frequency of all verbalizations. "Avoid" skills included the sum of questions (e.g., "What are you building?"), commands (e.g., "Put that piece there"), and negative talk (e.g., "You're doing it wrong"). This ratio has been established by previous studies as a more concise strategy of examining both the "Do" and "Avoid" skills from the DPICS-IV [34]. Correct follow-through percentages were calculated by the total number of times that caregivers followed through an effective command with a labeled praise for child compliance or a discipline sequence for noncompliance divided by their total direct commands that have an opportunity for child compliance. The frequency of "Do" skills and "Avoid" skills was coded during CLP observations at pre-treatment, mid-treatment and post-treatment. Child compliance was assessed during the five-minute PLP and CU tasks at pre- and post-treatment. Both caregiver skill variables are continuous variables.

2.3.5. Caregiver Anxiety Symptoms

The Generalized Anxiety Disorder 7-item scale (GAD-7) [35] is a brief, self-report screening tool designed to assess the severity of generalized anxiety symptoms over the past two weeks. Respondents rate how often they have been bothered by symptoms such as "feeling nervous, anxious, or on edge," "not being able to stop or control worrying," and "trouble relaxing," using a 4-point Likert scale ranging from 0 ("not at all") to 3 ("nearly every day"). Total raw scores range from 0 to 21, with clinical cutoffs commonly interpreted as follows: 5 (mild anxiety), 10 (moderate anxiety), and 15 (severe anxiety) [35]. Scores of $\geq$10 were coded as 1 (clinically elevated) and scores < 10 were coded as 0 (within normal limits). The GAD-7 was administered at pre-, mid-, and post-treatment to track caregiver anxiety over the course of PCIT. Total raw scores were used for analyses. Internal consistency for the GAD-7 was good in this sample (α = 0.892).

2.3.6. Caregiver Depressive Symptoms

The Patient Health Questionnaire-8 (PHQ-8) [36] is an eight-item self-report measure designed to assess depressive symptoms over the past two weeks. Caregivers rate how often they have experienced symptoms such as "little interest or pleasure in doing things," "feeling down, depressed, or hopeless," and "trouble concentrating on things, such as reading the newspaper or watching television". Each item is rated on a four-point scale (0 = not at all to 3 = nearly every day), with a total score ranging from 0 to 24. A score of 10 or higher indicates clinically significant depression (1 = clinically elevated, 0 = within normal limits). The scale was administered at pre-, mid-, and post-treatment to track changes in caregiver depression throughout the intervention. It has been validated across diverse populations and is widely used in research and public health settings, particularly in large-scale epidemiological studies. Internal consistency for the PHQ-8 was good in this sample (α = 0.849).

2.4. Data Analytic Plan

All analyses were conducted using IBM SPSS Statistics (Version 29). Missing data were analyzed in more detail. Chi square and independent *t* test analyses were completed to determine whether caregivers with complete data (i.e., no missing pre- or post-assessments for ECBI, PHQ, or GAD) differed from those with incomplete data on sociodemographic variables or levels of any of the pre-treatment assessments of interest in the current study (i.e., pre-treatment ECBI intensity, GAD-7 total score, PHQ-8 total score, Do/Avoid skill ratio, or correct follow-through).

2.4.1. Research Hypothesis 1 Analytic Plan

Correlation analyses were completed for treatment engagement variables (i.e., number of sessions in treatment and whether the family completed treatment or not) comparing them to caregiver pre-treatment anxiety and depression to determine whether caregiver mental health impacted the family's ability to attend treatment (i.e., number of sessions) as well as their ability to complete PCIT (i.e., treatment completion).

2.4.2. Research Hypothesis 2 Analytic Plan

Descriptive statistics were calculated for sample demographic characteristics, clinically elevated caregiver depression and anxiety, and child disruptive behavior levels (1 = clinically elevated, 0 = mild or within normal limits) at pre-, mid-, and post-treatment.

2.4.3. Research Hypothesis 3 Analytic Plan

A series of generalized estimating equation (GEE) models were conducted to examine the direct effects of PCIT participation on the following dependent (i.e., outcome) variables:

caregiver anxiety (GAD-7) and depression (PHQ-8), positive parenting skills (DPICS-IV Do/Avoid skill ratio and correct follow-through), and child disruptive behaviors (ECBI). Time (pre-, mid-, post-treatment) was entered as a within-subject factor predicting each outcome variable separately. We used GEE to account for repeated measurements within participants over time. An exchangeable correlation structure was specified, which assumes that all time points are equally correlated. An identity link function was used so that the estimated effects could be interpreted directly in the original units of each outcome (e.g., raw scores on behavior measures).

2.4.4. Research Hypothesis 4 Analytic Plan

To evaluate whether caregiver sociodemographic characteristics (race, ethnicity, education, and income), anxiety, and/or depression moderated changes in child disruptive behavior over the course of PCIT, we also used GEE with repeated measures across three time points (pre-, mid-, and post-treatment). These GEE models started with the aforementioned measure of time in PCIT (1 = pre-treatment, 2 = mid-treatment, 3 = post-treatment) as the main independent variable predicting the main dependent variable, changes in child disruptive behavior over the course of PCIT. Additionally, the main effects of each potential moderator, including caregiver depression (PHQ-8), anxiety (GAD-7), race, ethnicity, education [dichotomized as less than a bachelor's degree vs. bachelor's or higher (coded as 0 and 1, respectively)], and income [dichotomized as below vs. above the 100K household income threshold (coded as 0 and 1, respectively)], were included in the model to ensure that interaction terms could be calculated appropriately. Finally, interaction terms between time in PCIT (the main IV) and each moderator were calculated. These interaction terms captured the moderating effect of each potential moderator on the association between time in PCIT and child disruptive behavior. Given that caregiver depression and anxiety were both measured at multiple time points over the course of treatment, GEE interaction terms were also able to capture whether caregiver depression and anxiety at pre-treatment, mid-treatment, and post-treatment each moderated associations between time in PCIT and child disruptive behavior. Household income was dichotomized as below or $\geq$100K, as a recent 2023 report indicated that a minimum household income of 100K or higher was needed to not be rent-burdened in Miami [37]. Significant time in PCIT $\times$ moderator interactions were followed by pairwise comparisons to interpret differences in outcome trajectories based on moderator levels. These analyses allowed us to assess whether changes in child behavior varied based on caregiver mental health or sociodemographic characteristics.

2.4.5. Research Hypothesis 5 Analytic Plan

To examine whether changes in Do/Avoid skill ratio and correct follow-through (both continuous variables) mediated the effects of PCIT on caregiver mental health, within-subject mediation analyses were conducted using the MEMORE macro (Version 2.1) in SPSS 29.0 [38] (see Figure 2). Similarly, we examined whether changes in Do/Avoid skill ratio mediated the effects of PCIT on child disruptive behavior. In these within-subject mediation models, PCIT is operationalized as the change over time from pre-treatment to mid-treatment to post-treatment. Because all participants received the intervention, the model does not include a between-subject contrast (e.g., treatment vs. control). Instead, the analysis examines whether within-person changes in parenting skills from pre- to mid- to post-treatment mediate within-person changes in caregiver mental health outcomes (i.e., anxiety, depression) and child disruptive behavior over the same period. Thus, the path representing the effect of "PCIT" reflects the temporal change associated with participation in the intervention, rather than a comparison between exposed and unexposed groups. Put another way, the independent variable in these mediation analyses was time in PCIT

(1 = pre-treatment, 2 = mid-treatment, 3 = post-treatment), the mediators were changes in Do/Avoid skill ratio and correct follow-through over the course of PCIT, and the dependent variable in these mediation analyses was changes in GAD-7, PHQ-8, and ECBI scores. Pre- to mid- or post-treatment change time points in parenting skills (i.e., Do/Avoid skill ratio, correct follow-through) were entered as the mediator within each analysis, and pre- to mid- or post-treatment time points in GAD-7, PHQ-8, or ECBI scores were entered as outcome variables. Bootstrapping with 5000 resamples was used to estimate the confidence intervals for indirect effects. Step 1 estimated the total effect (Path C) of time in PCIT on caregiver or child mental health (see Figure 2). Step 2 estimated the effect of time in PCIT on parenting skills (Path A). Step 3 included both time in PCIT and the mediator to estimate the direct effect of treatment (Path C) and the mediator's effect on the outcome (Path B). Mediation was classified as full, partial, or none based on the significance of the indirect effect and comparison between total and direct effects. Full mediation was defined as a statistically significant indirect effect accompanied by a nonsignificant direct effect, indicating that the mediator fully explains the treatment–outcome relationship. Partial mediation was defined as both the indirect and direct effects being significant, suggesting that the mediator accounts for part, but not all, of the intervention's effect.

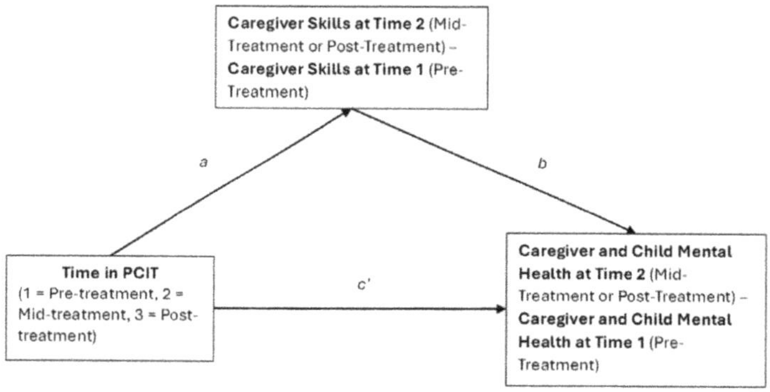

Figure 2. Mediation model illustrating the proposed mediating effect of PCIT on changes in caregiver and child mental health over the course of PCIT treatment through changes in parenting skills. Each of the mediational models described in the results examined these mediational analyses over the course of two time points for caregiver skills (e.g., Do skill/Avoid skill ratio and correct follow-through) and caregiver (depressive symptoms on PHQ-9, anxiety symptoms on GAD-7) and child (disruptive behavior based on ECBI intensity scores) mental health (from pre-treatment to either mid-treatment or post-treatment, depending on the model). This conceptual model is adapted from Montoya, 2024 [39].

3. Results

3.1. Missing Data

Measure completers and non-completers differed significantly in the language of their treatment. Specifically, Spanish-speaking and bilingual families were more likely to complete their paperwork ($\chi^2(4) = 9.752$, $p = 0.045$). Measure completers also differed significantly from non-completers in caregiver race ($\chi^2(5) = 11.526$, $p = 0.042$). Specifically, Black caregivers were significantly less likely to have completed pre- and post-assessments compared to other caregivers ($\chi^2(1) = 4.941$, $p = 0.026$). Completer caregivers also differed significantly from non-completers in their educational attainment ($\chi^2(5) = 17.851$, $p = 0.003$). Caregivers with a bachelor's degree or higher were more likely to have completed their pre- and post-assessments than those with lower levels of educational attainment. Completers and non-completers also demonstrated significant differences in correct follow-through, with non-completers reporting higher pre-treatment rates of correct follow-through ($M = 3.217$, $SD = 15.226$) than completers ($M = 1.841$, 9.407) ($t(1012) = 12.181$, $p < 0.001$, $d = 0.107$). Completers and non-completers also differed significantly in the age of the child enrolled in PCIT, with younger ages for completers ($M = 4.604$, $SD = 1.42$) than non-completers ($M = 4.845$, $SD = 1.548$) ($t(1053) = 5.008$, $p = 0.025$, $d = 0.162$). Completion of pre- and post-assessments did not significantly differ by caregiver ethnicity, child sex, intake Do/Avoid skill ratio, ECBI raw intensity score, or caregiver depression or anxiety symptoms. Findings related to differences between completers and non-completers should be interpreted with caution due to the potential for bias introduced by non-random patterns of missingness.

3.2. *Hypothesis 1: Attendance/Attrition*

Caregiver pre-treatment depression was not correlated with any of the markers of engagement in treatment, including treatment completion ($r[650] = -0.020$, $p = 0.610$) and total PCIT sessions completed ($r[712] = 0.041$, $p = 0.278$; see Table 2). Additionally, caregiver pre-treatment anxiety was not correlated with any of the markers of treatment engagement, including treatment completion ($r[651] = -0.001$, $p = 0.984$) and total PCIT sessions attended ($r[712] = 0.047$, $p = 0.209$; see Table 2).

3.3. *Hypothesis 2: Clinically Significant Changes in Family Outcomes over Time*

Child disruptive behavior, caregiver anxiety, and caregiver depression scores at all three time points (pre-, mid-, post-treatment) were transformed into binary variables indicating whether caregiver-reported levels of anxiety or depression symptoms and child disruptive behaviors were above or below the clinical cutoff.

3.3.1. Clinically Significant Caregiver Depression Changes

At pre-treatment, 8.2% ($n = 69$) of caregivers reported scores at or above 10, the clinical cutoff for the PHQ-8. At mid-treatment, 5.0% ($n = 42$) of caregivers reported clinically elevated scores for depression. At post-treatment, 2.9% ($n = 24$) of caregivers reported clinically elevated scores.

3.3.2. Clinically Significant Caregiver Anxiety Changes

With regard to clinical significance, at pre-treatment 14.3% ($n = 120$) of caregivers reported clinically elevated scores (i.e., at or above 10) on the GAD-7. At mid-treatment, 8.6% ($n = 72$) of caregivers reported clinically elevated anxiety scores. At post-treatment, 4.8% ($n = 40$) of caregivers reported clinically elevated anxiety.

3.3.3. Clinically Significant Child Behavior Changes

At pre-treatment, 72.87% ($n = 752$) of children had caregiver-reported clinically elevated disruptive behavior as measured by the clinical cutoff of a raw intensity score of 131 on the ECBI. At mid-treatment, 36.0% ($n = 295$) of children demonstrated clinical elevations in disruptive behavior. At post-treatment, this decreased to 11.8% ($n = 86$).

Next, using the total scores, GEE models were utilized to examine changes in child outcomes, as measured by the ECBI Intensity Scale, caregiver depression, as measured by the PHQ-8, caregiver anxiety, as measured by the GAD-7, caregiver Do/Avoid skill ratio as measured by the DPICS-IV, and caregiver correct follow-through rate as measured by the DPICS-IV across three time points: pre-, mid-, and post-treatment.

Table 2. Correlation table.

	1	2	3	4	5	6	7	8	9	10	11	12	13	14
1. PCIT Language	1													
2. Drop Status	0.007	1												
3. PCIT Completion	0.043	–	1											
4. # of PCIT Sessions	0.025	0.728 **	0.752 **	1										
5. Do Skills	0.100 **	0.040	0.045	0.056	1									
6. Avoid Skills	0.019	−0.026	−0.011	0.051	0.149 **	1								
7. ECBI Intensity Score	−0.034	0.086	−0.034	−0.007	−0.026	−0.036	1							
8. ECBI Problem Score	−0.057	0.111	−0.024	0.024	−0.050	−0.059	0.754 **	1						
9. Intake PHQ-8 Total Score	0.000	−0.028	−0.020	0.041	−0.018	−0.042	0.290 **	0.244 **	1					
10. Intake GAD-7 Total Score	−0.019	−0.007	−0.001	0.047	0.031	−0.033	0.255 **	0.211 **	0.715 **	1				
11. Caregiver Ethnicity	−0.355 **	0.027	0.033	0.092 **	−0.064	−0.006	−0.036	−0.087 *	−0.056	−0.061	1			
12. Caregiver Race	0.138 **	−0.053	−0.016	−0.003	0.076 *	−0.021	0.027	0.011	0.055	0.068	−0.288 **	1		
13. Child Sex	−0.003	−0.001	0.029	0.028	−0.017	−0.057	−0.057	−0.055	0.006	−0.015	−0.032	0.039	1	
14. Child Age	−0.122 **	−0.014	−0.085 *	−0.112 **	−0.290 **	0.300 **	0.048	0.121 **	0.059	0.022	0.019	−0.026	−0.060	1

Note: * $p < 0.05$, ** $p < 0.01$.

3.4. Hypothesis 3: Family Outcome Main Effects

3.4.1. Child Behavior

The overall effect of time was significant, indicating that ECBI scores changed across the intervention period (Wald $\chi^2(2) = 1446.92$, $p < 0.001$). Estimated marginal means showed that average ECBI scores decreased from $M = 148.70$ ($SE = 1.05$) at pre-treatment to M = 121.97 ($SE = 1.29$) at mid-treatment, and further to $M = 97.92$ ($SE = 1.22$) at post-treatment. Pairwise comparisons revealed that all time-point contrasts were statistically significant after Bonferroni correction. Specifically, ECBI scores decreased significantly from pre- to mid-treatment ($B = -26.73$, $SE = 1.21$, $p < 0.001$), from mid- to post-treatment ($B = -24.05$, $SE = 1.14$, $p < 0.001$), and from pre- to post-treatment ($B = -50.78$, $SE = 1.34$, $p < 0.001$; see Table 3). These findings suggest substantial and consistent caregiver-reported reductions in child disruptive behavior over the course of PCIT.

Table 3. Pairwise comparisons of parent and child outcome measures across time points.

Outcome	Time Comparison	Mean Difference (B)	*SE*	95% CI	*p*-Value (Bonferroni)
ECBI (Child Behavior)	Pre vs. Mid	−26.73	1.21	[−29.62, −23.84]	<0.001
	Mid vs. Post	−24.05	1.14	[−26.77, −21.33]	<0.001
	Pre vs. Post	−50.78	1.34	[−53.98, −47.59]	<0.001
GAD-7 (Caregiver Anxiety)	Pre vs. Mid	−0.77	0.18	[−1.20, −0.34]	<0.001
	Mid vs. Post	−1.31	0.18	[−1.73, −0.89]	<0.001
	Pre vs. Post	−2.08	0.19	[−2.54, −1.62]	<0.001
PHQ-8 (Caregiver Depression)	Pre vs. Mid	−0.42	0.16	[−0.81, −0.04]	0.027
	Mid vs. Post	−0.75	0.15	[−1.11, −0.40]	<0.001
	Pre vs. Post	−1.17	0.16	[−1.57, −0.78]	<0.001
Do/Avoid Skill Ratio	Pre vs. Mid	4.08	0.26	[3.45, 4.70]	<0.001
	Mid vs. Post	1.00	0.34	[0.19, 1.80]	0.009
	Pre vs. Post	5.07	0.33	[4.27, 5.87]	<0.001
Correct Follow-Through Rate	Pre vs. Post	35.37	1.45	[32.53, 38.21]	<0.001

3.4.2. Caregiver Depression

Using the GEE model, the overall effect of time was statistically significant (Wald $\chi^2(2) = 54.91$, $p < 0.001$), indicating that PHQ-8 scores changed significantly over the course of treatment. Estimated marginal means revealed that PHQ-8 scores decreased from M = 3.75 (SE = 0.16) at pre-treatment to $M = 3.33$ ($SE = 0.16$) at mid-treatment and to $M = 2.57$ ($SE = 0.15$) at post-treatment. Pairwise comparisons with Bonferroni correction showed statistically significant reductions from pre- to mid-treatment ($B = -0.42$, $SE = 0.16$, $p = 0.027$), mid- to post-treatment ($B = -0.75$, $SE = 0.15$, $p < 0.001$), and pre- to post-treatment ($B = -1.17$, $SE = 0.16$, $p < 0.001$; see Table 3).

3.4.3. Caregiver Anxiety

The overall time effect was statistically significant (Wald $\chi^2(2) = 123.01$, $p < 0.001$), indicating a reduction in anxiety symptoms across the course of PCIT. Estimated marginal means showed that GAD-7 scores decreased from $M = 5.36$ ($SE = 0.18$) at pre-treatment to $M = 4.59$ ($SE = 0.18$) at mid-treatment, and further to $M = 3.28$ ($SE = 0.17$) at post-treatment. Pairwise comparisons using Bonferroni correction revealed significant reductions between all time points: pre- to mid-treatment ($B = -0.77$, $SE = 0.18$, $p < 0.001$), mid- to post-treatment ($B = -1.31$, $SE = 0.18$, $p < 0.001$), and pre- to post-treatment ($B = -2.08$, $SE = 0.19$, $p < 0.001$; see Table 3).

3.4.4. Caregiver Do/Avoid Parenting Skill Ratio

The overall effect of time was statistically significant (Wald $\chi^2(2) = 343.67$, $p < 0.001$), indicating a significant increase in the ratio of positive parenting verbalization skills to Avoid skills over the course of PCIT. Estimated marginal means showed that the total Do/Avoid skill ratio increased from $M = 0.27$ (SE = 0.01) at pre-treatment to $M = 4.35$ (SE = 0.26) at mid-treatment, and to $M = 5.34$ ($SE = 0.33$) at post-treatment. Pairwise comparisons revealed significant improvements at each time point. Specifically, there was a significant increase from pre- to mid-treatment ($B = 4.08$, $SE = 0.26$, $p < 0.001$), from mid- to post-treatment ($B = 1.00$, $SE = 0.34$, $p = 0.009$), and from pre- to post-treatment ($B = 5.07$, $SE = 0.33$, $p < 0.001$; see Table 3).

3.4.5. Caregiver Correct Follow-Through

An additional GEE model examined changes in caregiver correct follow-through rates from pre- to post-treatment. Results showed a statistically significant increase in rates from pre- to post-treatment (Wald $\chi^2(1) = 595.34$, $p < 0.001$). Estimated marginal means showed that correct follow-through rates increased from M = 2.60% ($SE = 0.39$) at pre-treatment to $M = 37.97\%$ ($SE = 1.43$) at post-treatment. Pairwise comparisons revealed significant improvements from pre- to post-treatment in observed caregiver correct follow-through rates ($B = 35.37$, $SE = 1.45$, $p < 0.001$; see Table 3)

3.5. Hypothesis 4 Moderator Analysis

A GEE model was used to examine whether child disruptive behavior outcomes (ECBI scores) varied by caregiver characteristics and their interactions with time (see Table 4). Significant main effects were found for time, indicating reductions in ECBI scores from pre-treatment ($B = 53.26$, $p < 0.001$) and mid-treatment ($B = 31.28$, $p < 0.001$), relative to post-treatment.

Table 4. Moderators of child disruptive behavior change on the ECBI over time.

Independent Variable	*B*	*SE*	95% CI	Wald χ^2	*p*-Value
Intercept	95.24	6.63	[82.23, 108.24]	206.17	<0.001
Time: Pre-treatment	53.26	8.06	[37.46, 69.05]	43.67	<0.001
Time: Mid-treatment	31.28	7.41	[16.75, 45.81]	17.80	<0.001
Parental Depression (PHQ-8)	0.17	0.63	[−1.05, 1.40]	0.08	0.78
Parental Anxiety (GAD-7)	1.30	0.51	[0.30, 2.30]	6.47	0.01
Household Income (<100K)	−2.07	2.81	[−7.57, 3.44]	0.54	0.46
Education (Less than Bachelor's degree)	−4.90	3.41	[−11.58, 1.77]	2.07	0.15
Race: Asian	−5.30	9.53	[−23.99, 13.38]	0.31	0.58
Race: Black/African American	13.75	9.28	[−4.43, 31.93]	2.20	0.14
Race: White	−0.47	6.08	[−12.39, 11.44]	0.01	0.94
Race: Other	3.11	10.01	[−16.51, 22.73]	0.31	0.76
Ethnicity: Hispanic	0.00	2.85	[−5.58, 5.59]	0.00	0.99
Ethnicity: Haitian	−16.19	12.52	[−40.73, 8.36	1.67	0.20
Pre-treatment X PHQ-8	1.28	0.71	[−0.12, 2.68]	3.23	0.07
Mid-treatment X PHQ-8	0.56	0.82	[−1.05, 2.17]	0.47	0.49
Pre-treatment X GAD-7	−0.73	0.61	[−1.93, 0.47]	1.43	0.23
Mid-treatment X GAD-7	−0.31	0.68	[−1.64, 1.02]	0.21	0.65
Household Income (<100K) X Pre-treatment	2.60	3.20	[−3.67, 8.87]	0.66	0.42
Household Income (<100K) X Mid-treatment	2.92	2.74	[−2.46, 8.30]	1.13	0.29

Table 4. Cont.

Independent Variable	B	SE	95% CI	Wald χ^2	p-Value
Education (Less than Bachelor's degree) X Pre-treatment	4.18	3.71	[−3.09, 11.44]	1.27	0.26
Education (Less than Bachelor's degree) X Mid-treatment	−0.05	3.28	[−6.49, 6.39]	0.00	0.99
Race: Asian X Pre-treatment	−5.31	10.73	[−26.34, 15.71]	0.25	0.62
Race: Asian X Mid-treatment	−6.76	10.32	[−26.99, 13.48]	0.43	0.51
Race: Black/African American X Pre-treatment	−13.43	−13.43	[−34.35, 7.50]	1.582	0.21
Race: Black/African American X Mid-treatment	−17.51	8.41	[−33.99, −1.03]	4.337	0.04
Race: White X Pre-treatment	−11.31	7.41	[−25.84, 3.22]	2.33	0.13
Race: White X Mid-treatment	−12.14	6.91	[−25.69, 1.41]	3.08	0.08
Race: Other X Pre-treatment	−3.72	9.63	[−22.60, 15.16]	0.15	0.70
Race: Other X Mid-treatment	4.90	9.18	[−13.01, 22.90]	0.28	0.59
Ethnicity: Hispanic X Pre-treatment	2.04	3.18	[−4.20, 8.27]	0.41	0.52
Ethnicity: Hispanic X Mid-treatment	0.33	2.59	[−4.75, 5.41]	0.02	0.90
Ethnicity: Haitian X Pre-treatment	−0.84	15.10	[−30.45, 28.67]	0.00	0.96
Ethnicity: Haitian X Mid-treatment	7.96	19.72	[−30.69, 46.61]	0.16	0.69

Note. Sample cell sizes were too small for some caregiver races to be included in moderator analyses. Reference categories for predictor variables include time (post-treatment), household income (≥100K), education (bachelor's degree or higher), race (Biracial/Multiracial), ethnicity (Non-Hispanic).

Among caregiver characteristics, parental anxiety (GAD-7) emerged as a significant main effect predictor of child disruptive behavior (B = 1.30, p = 0.01), suggesting that children of more anxious caregivers rated their children as displaying more frequent child disruptive behaviors across time points. No significant main effects were found for parental depression (PHQ-8), caregiver income, education, race, or ethnicity.

A significant time × moderator interaction emerged for caregiver race: Black/African American. Specifically, caregivers who identified as Black/African American reported significantly lower child disruptive behavior scores relative to Biracial caregivers at mid-treatment (B = –17.51, SE = 8.41, 95% CI [–33.99, –1.03], Wald $\chi^2(1)$ = 4.34, p = 0.037). This suggests that child behavior trajectories differed modestly by caregiver race, with Black/African American caregivers reporting greater decreases in child disruptive behaviors relative to Biracial caregivers.

No significant moderation effects were found for caregiver depression, anxiety, household income, education, or ethnicity, suggesting that PCIT may be equally effective across these caregiver subgroups in this sample.

3.6. Hypothesis 5 Mediation Analyses

3.6.1. Mediation Analyses for Caregiver Anxiety and Depression

A series of within-subject mediation models using MEMORE were conducted to evaluate whether improvements in parenting skills, as measured by the Do/Avoid skill ratio, mediated reductions in caregiver anxiety (GAD-7) across different phases of PCIT. Results consistently supported partial mediation at each interval (see Table 5). For the pre-to-mid model, the indirect effect of PCIT on anxiety through parenting skill change was significant (B = –0.58, 95% CI [–1.16, –0.15]), with a remaining direct effect (B = –0.91, 95% CI [–1.59, –0.22]). Similarly, the pre-to-post model revealed a significant indirect effect (B = –0.77, 95% CI [–1.39, –0.23]) and a significant direct effect (B = –1.29, 95% CI [–2.10, –0.48]). Finally, the mid-to-post model yielded a significant indirect effect (B = –0.45, 95% CI [–0.94, –0.06]) with a continued direct effect (B = –0.78, 95% CI [–1.46, –0.12]).

Table 5. Mediators of caregiver mental health outcomes.

Caregiver Mental Health	Effect	Pre to Mid (B)	95% CI Pre to Mid	Mid to Post (B)	95% CI Mid to Post	Pre to Post (B)	95% CI Pre to Post
Caregiver Anxiety (GAD-7)	a (Change in Caregiver Do/Avoid Ratio Skills)	0.72	[0.35, 1.09]	0.65	[0.22, 1.09]	0.82	[0.42, 1.23]
	b (Change in Caregiver Do/Avoid Ratio Skills x Anxiety)	−0.81	[−1.35, −0.27]	−0.69	[−1.26, −0.11]	−0.94	[−1.50, −0.34]
	Indirect Effect (a × b)	−0.58	[−1.16, −0.15]	−0.45	[−0.94, −0.06]	−0.77	[−1.39, −0.23]
	Direct Effect (c′)	−0.91	[−1.59, −0.22]	−0.78	[−1.46, −0.12]	−1.29	[−2.10, −0.48]
Caregiver Anxiety (GAD-7)	a (Change in Caregiver Correct Follow-Through Rate)					0.68	[0.32, 1.03]
	b (Caregiver Correct Follow-Through Rate × Anxiety)					−0.69	[−1.25, −0.11]
	Indirect Effect (a × b)					−0.47	[−0.90, −0.12]
	Direct Effect (c′)					−0.92	[−1.57, −0.28]
Caregiver Depression (PHQ-8)	a (Change in Caregiver Do/Avoid Ratio Skills	0.64	[0.29, 1.01]	0.6	[0.20, 1.01]	0.74	[0.37, 1.12]
	b (Change in Caregiver Do/Avoid Ratio Skills × Depression)	−0.81	[−1.38, −0.27]	−0.68	[−1.26, −0.11]	−0.91	[−1.50, −0.34]
	Indirect Effect (a × b)	−0.52	[−1.08, −0.13]	−0.41	[−0.91, −0.04]	−0.68	[−1.28, −0.21]
	Direct Effect (c′)	−1.05	[−1.79, −0.30]	−0.89	[−1.58, −0.18]	−1.24	[−2.02, −0.45]
Caregiver Depression (PHQ-8)	a (Change in Caregiver Correct Follow-Through Rate)					0.69	[0.31, 1.07]
	b (Caregiver Correct Follow-Through Rate × Anxiety)					−0.72	[−1.31, −0.12]
	Indirect Effect (a × b)					−0.5	[−1.09, −0.10]
	Direct Effect (c′)					−1.22	[−2.02, −0.44]

Similarly, a within-subject mediation model using MEMORE was conducted to evaluate whether improvements in caregiver behavior management (i.e., correct follow-through after effective commands) mediated reductions in caregiver anxiety from pre- to post-treatment. Results of this pre-to-post model supported partial mediation (see Table 5). The indirect effect of PCIT on anxiety through changes in correct follow-through was significant ($B = -0.47$, 95% *CI* [−0.90, −0.12]), and the direct effect remained significant ($B = -0.92$, 95% *CI* [−1.57, −0.28]). These findings suggest that greater discipline consistency in caregiver responses to child behavior partially explains reductions in caregiver anxiety observed over the course of PCIT. Together, these findings suggest that improvements in positive and discipline-focused parenting skills partially explain reductions in caregiver anxiety across the full course of PCIT.

To examine whether improvements in parenting skills mediated reductions in caregiver depression, three within-subject mediation analyses were conducted using MEMORE, with pre-to-mid, pre-to-post, and mid-to-post change intervals modeled separately (see Table 5). Parenting skills were assessed using the Do-to-Avoid skill ratio, and caregiver depression was measured using the PHQ-8. For the pre-to-mid model, the indirect effect of PCIT on PHQ-8 scores through changes in parenting skills was statistically significant ($B = -0.52$, 95% *CI* [−1.08, −0.13]). The direct effect remained significant ($B = -1.05$, 95% *CI* [−1.79, −0.30]), indicating partial mediation. Similarly, in the pre-to-post model, the indirect effect was also significant ($B = -0.68$, 95% *CI* [−1.28, −0.21]), with a retained direct effect ($B = -1.24$, 95% *CI* [−2.02, −0.45]), again supporting partial mediation. Finally, for the mid-to post model, the mediation pathway remained significant ($B = -0.41$, 95% *CI* [−0.91, −0.04]), with a direct effect of $B = -0.89$, 95% *CI* [−1.58, −0.18].

Similarly, a within-subject mediation model was conducted to test whether improvements in caregiver correct follow-through skills mediated reductions in caregiver depressive symptoms from pre- to post-treatment (see Table 5). The pre-to-post analysis revealed a significant indirect effect of PCIT on depression through improved correct follow-through ($B = -0.50$, 95% *CI* [−1.09, −0.10]), indicating that increases in follow-through behaviors were associated with decreased caregiver depressive symptoms. The direct effect of PCIT on depression remained significant after accounting for the mediator ($B = -1.22$, 95% *CI* [−2.02, −0.44]), suggesting partial mediation. Together, these findings indicate that improvements in parenting skills contribute meaningfully to reductions in caregiver depression across all stages of the intervention, supporting the role of positive parenting behaviors and consistent responding as a mechanism of change in PCIT. Mediation was observed at each stage of PCIT, suggesting that improvements in use of effective parenting skills are potentially a consistent mechanism for reducing caregiver depressive symptoms over the course of PCIT.

3.6.2. Mediation Analysis for Child Disruptive Behavior

A within-subject mediation model using MEMORE was conducted to examine whether improvements in caregiver Do/Avoid skill ratio mediated reductions in parent reported child disruptive behavior, from pre- to post-treatment. Results showed a significant total effect of PCIT on ECBI improvement ($B = -48.96$, $SE = 1.42$, 95% *CI* [−51.75, −46.17], $p < 0.001$), indicating a large reduction in child behavior problems over the course of treatment (see Table 6). Caregivers demonstrated a significant increase in Do/Avoid skill ratio from pre- to post-treatment ($B = 5.02$, $SE = 0.34$, 95% *CI* [4.36, 5.68], $p < 0.001$). However, the path from changes in Do/Avoid skill ratio to ECBI improvement was not statistically significant ($B = -0.74$, $SE = 3.12$, $p = 0.813$, 95% *CI* [−6.86, 5.38]). The indirect effect of PCIT on ECBI through Do/Avoid skill ratio was also nonsignificant ($B = -1.35$, $SE = 8.08$, 95% *CI* [−15.38, 19.63]). These results indicate that although caregivers significantly improved in their relative use of positive parenting behaviors and child disruptive behaviors decreased, changes in the total ratio of positive parenting skills did not significantly mediate the relationship.

Table 6. Mediators of child disruptive behavior.

Child Disruptive Behavior	Effect	Pre to Mid (B)	95% CI Pre to Mid	Mid to Post (B)	95% CI Mid to Post	Pre to Post (B)	95% CI Pre to Post
Child Disruptive Behavior (ECBI)	a (Change in Caregiver Do/Avoid Skill Ratio)	4.15	[3.61, 4.69]	0.87	[0.14, 1.60]	5.02	[4.36, 5.68]
	b (Change in Caregiver Do/Avoid Skill Ratio × Child Disruptive Behavior)	−3.69	[−9.10, 1.72]	−0.05	[−0.39, 0.28]	−0.74	[−6.86, 5.38]
	Indirect Effect (a × b)	−15.32	[−39.97, 8.38]	−0.05	[−0.38, 0.22]	−1.35	[−15.38, 19.63]
	Direct Effect (c′)	−12.98	[−35.57, 9.61]	−22.46	[−24.91, −20.00]	−47.61	[−63.29, −31.94]

Similarly, a within-subject mediation model was conducted to examine whether changes in the CDI phase of caregiver Do/Avoid skill ratio mediated improvements in child disruptive behavior from pre- to mid-treatment. Caregivers showed a significant reduction in child behavior problems during this period, with ECBI scores decreasing by an average of 28 points ($B = -28.30$, $SE = 1.32$, 95% CI [−30.90, −25.70], $p < 0.001$). Caregivers also significantly increased the ratio of their use of Do/Avoid skills ($B = 4.15$, $SE = 0.28$, 95% CI [3.61, 4.69], $p < 0.001$). However, the indirect effect of treatment on ECBI improvement through Do/Avoid skill ratio was not statistically significant ($B = -15.32$, SE = 12.45, 95% CI [−39.97, 8.38]). The direct effect of PCIT on child disruptive behavior remained nonsignificant after controlling for Do/Avoid skill ratio changes ($B = -12.98$, $SE = 11.50$, $p = 0.259$). These findings suggest that while child behavior and parenting skills improved early in treatment, changes in Do/Avoid skill ratio did not significantly mediate child behavior improvement during this early phase.

Finally, a within-subject mediation model was conducted to examine whether changes in caregiver Do/Avoid skill ratio from mid- to post-treatment mediated improvements in child disruptive behavior during PDI. Results indicated continued reductions in ECBI scores during the second half of PCIT ($B = -22.50$, $SE = 1.24$, 95% CI [−24.94, −20.07], $p < 0.001$; see Table 6). Caregivers also demonstrated a significant increase in Do/Avoid skill ratio over this period ($B = 0.87$, $SE = 0.37$, 95% CI [0.14, 1.60], $p = 0.020$). However, the indirect effect of PCIT on ECBI improvement through Do/Avoid skill ratio was not statistically significant ($B = -0.05$, SE = 0.15, 95% CI [−0.38, 0.22]), indicating that changes in positive parenting behavior ratios did not mediate changes in child behavior during the PDI. The direct effect of PCIT on ECBI remained significant even after accounting for the mediator ($B = -22.46$, $SE = 1.25$, $p < 0.001$).

4. Discussion

This study evaluated the impact of time-limited PCIT on caregiver mental health, parenting practices, and child behavior. Consistent with expectations, caregiver anxiety and depression and child disruptive behavior demonstrated significant improvement over the course of PCIT. Importantly, caregiver anxiety and depression reduced significantly at each time point (mid- and post-), indicating that caregivers who stay in PCIT exhibit mental health improvements consistently over both phases of treatment. These findings reflect those of Agazzi and colleagues [11] and reiterate the positive impact of PCIT without adaptations on caregiver mental health [40], as well as the promise of time-limited PCIT [16] in improving caregiver-specific wellness. Similar to existing PCIT research [20], caregivers rated their children's disruptive behaviors as showing significant improvement over the course of treatment, and caregivers also demonstrated observed positive changes in effective parenting skills.

The findings highlight the role of caregiver anxiety in shaping child behavior trajectories during PCIT. Higher caregiver anxiety was associated with greater reports of child disruptive behavior across time points. It may be that anxious caregivers inadvertently escalate coercive interactions (e.g., through heightened reactivity or inconsistent discipline), thereby reinforcing child disruptive behaviors. It is also possible that caregivers who begin treatment with higher anxiety are more likely to demonstrate a negative attributional style (e.g., a tendency to attribute the negative to internal factors and positive to external factors outside their control) about their child's behavioral difficulties [41]. Therefore, they may have difficulty seeing child behavior improvement as caused by their actions instead of caused by factors outside their control.

These findings underscore the importance of considering caregiver mental health not only as an outcome within PCIT, but also as an important contextual factor that can shape the effectiveness of parenting interventions. Clinically, this suggests the importance of screening parental mental health as a standard part of PCIT. In addition, caregivers with elevated anxiety may benefit from additional support early in treatment to maximize the benefits of PCIT for child outcomes (e.g., discussions of caregiver cognitions and attributions). By identifying caregiver mental health as an important influence on child outcomes in PCIT, this study highlights the importance of tailoring interventions to meet the emotional and behavioral needs of both caregivers and their children.

Interestingly, caregiver race emerged as a significant moderator, with Black/African American caregivers reporting significantly greater reductions in child disruptive behavior by mid-treatment relative to Biracial/Multiracial caregivers. One possible interpretation is that cultural differences in parenting expectations or interpretations of child behavior may influence perceived improvements in child disruptive behavior. However, parenting cultural expectations were not systematically assessed beyond the used of the Cultural Formulation Interview. Importantly, no moderation effects were found for caregiver ethnicity, income, or education, indicating that PCIT yielded similar benefits across sociodemographic groups, reinforcing the generalizability of PCIT for those who complete treatment and its applicability across diverse family contexts [16].

The skills caregivers learned over the course of PCIT played a significant role in the improvement of their self-reported anxiety and depression symptoms. Specifically, caregivers learning to attend more verbally to their child's positive, prosocial behaviors and attend less to behaviors that needed to be changed or directed partially explained caregivers reporting fewer of their own symptoms of anxiety and depression over the course of treatment. These results bolster Patterson's coercion theoretical model proposing that parenting behavior is a key leverage point not only for child behavior change but also for improving caregiver functioning. Attentional bias (e.g., focus on the negative or threatening) is often the focus of intervention for anxiety and depression and implicated in the cause of long-term depressive symptoms [42]. Parenting interventions like PCIT that teach caregivers to shift their attention from the "problem" or behavior that needs to be addressed to the positive behavior that can be reinforced and increased may serve the same function as cognitive therapies that teach a shift in this negative attentional bias. Similarly, caregivers who demonstrate less skill growth may have more difficulty shifting their negative attentional bias more generally, which in this case impacts both their skill learning and their anxiety and depression symptoms.

Mindfulness-based interventions are also often profoundly impactful in decreasing symptoms of adult anxiety and depression [43]. The unique delivery of PCIT prescribes that caregivers are intentionally present with their children for at least five minutes per day and paying deliberate attention to their child's appropriate behaviors. Through this close attention for five minutes, caregivers comment on these child prosocial behaviors frequently. This present-moment awareness mirrors many practices recommended in mindfulness-based interventions, so it is possible that similar mechanisms may underlie the caregiver anxiety and depression improvements in PCIT as those mechanisms that underlie improvements in mindfulness-based treatments [44]. Furthermore, incorporating caregiver-only sessions (i.e., the CDI and PDI Teach sessions) within PCIT creates an opportunity to explore cognitive barriers that may hinder progress by promoting cognitive restructuring, providing opportunities for practice of mindfulness techniques, and allowing parents to process new learning [17].

Similarly, caregivers increasing their consistent responses after giving their child effective commands partially explained caregivers reporting fewer anxiety and depression symptoms over the course of PCIT. Self-efficacy, or the ability to feel like you are in control of valued outcomes, also plays an impactful role in decreasing symptoms of depression [45]. In PCIT, caregivers are taught to be the vehicle for child behavior change via the skills learned in the intervention. It may be that improved caregiver skills increase caregiver ownership of their child's improvements in PCIT, and this self-efficacy further impacted caregiver improvements in anxiety and depression symptoms.

In the mediation models examined, Do/Avoid skill ratio and caregiver correct follow-through only partially mediated the change in caregiver anxiety and depression over PCIT. Therefore, other factors remain to further explicate the decreased symptoms of caregiver anxiety and depression. Given the theory of change proposed for PCIT combined with Patterson's coercive cycle, several possible explanations exist. Increased warmth in the caregiver–child relationship has the potential to improve caregiver mental health and decrease child combativeness. Selective attention, a skill taught in PCIT but non-specifically measured (i.e., not captured in the Do/Avoid skill ratio or correct follow-through), also has the potential to reverse Patterson's coercive cycle as the caregiver chooses to ignore child arguing/escalating rather than engage. Caregivers ignoring or focusing attention away from the child's disruptive behavior also possibly could shift caregiver mental health by focusing their attention away more regularly from the negative.

Overall, both caregiver anxiety and depression were associated with greater child behavioral difficulties at specific time points. Then improvements in caregiver mental health outcomes were partially explained by the improvements in their parenting skills—skills that are known to decrease the escalating conflict between caregiver and child [2,46].

Surprisingly, improvements in caregivers' Do/Avoid skill ratio did not mediate the relationship between participation in PCIT and reductions in child disruptive behaviors. These findings do not support the mechanisms of action proposed within Patterson's coercive cycle model. While increased use of positive parenting strategies (e.g., labeled praise, behavior descriptions, reflections) and decreased use of negative or directive statements are widely recognized as core mechanisms of change in PCIT [14], this anticipated mediation pathway was not supported in the current study. One possible explanation is that other unmeasured dimensions of the parent–child relationship, such as emotional attunement, warmth, or the reduction in coercive cycles, may better account for child behavior improvements. Further, children may have responded to broader structural changes in the home, such as increased predictability, routines, and/or reduced family conflict, that were not measured in the current study. These findings highlight the importance of examining multiple and potentially interacting mechanisms of change within evidence-based parenting interventions.

Importantly, child and caregiver outcomes did not differ significantly across family sociodemographic characteristics. This could indicate that across race, ethnicity, and income, families benefit similarly from the therapeutic impact of PCIT. Should these results continue to be replicated, they provide further support for PCIT as an efficacious treatment for reducing negative family interaction patterns for families with diverse lived experiences.

Limitations

Several limitations deserve mention for consideration of the conclusions that can be drawn from these findings. First, caregiver reports of child disruptive behavior as well as caregiver mental health can lead to reporter bias. Caregivers who experience depression and anxiety can sometimes report higher levels of behavioral challenges for their children, implying that if their symptoms of depression and anxiety reduced, perhaps they would report fewer child behavioral concerns due to their own mental health improvements and not necessarily due solely to an improvement in their child [47,48].

Another limitation regarding caregiver reports of mental health is that the GAD-7 and PHQ-8 are meant to serve clinically as screeners for symptoms of anxiety and depression relatively, and not comprehensive diagnostic assessments. A screener is simply meant to be a way to indicate if further assessment is needed, and not a definitive diagnostic tool [49].

The study did not include a control or comparison group, which limits our ability to conclude definitively that PCIT caused the observed improvements. For example, primary caregivers who self-enrolled in PCIT for this study were disproportionately female, which means that male caregivers were not as evenly represented, and generalization of findings is most clear for female rather than male caregivers given this imbalance. It is possible that some reduction in caregiver distress or child problems could occur over time with maturation or other outside influences. However, the magnitude of improvements and the established efficacy of PCIT for child behavior make it likely that the intervention played a key role in the changes.

A notable limitation of this study is the presence of systematic differences between participants who completed both pre- and post-treatment assessments and those who did not. Specifically, assessment non-completers were more likely to be Black/African American, have lower educational attainment, and report higher pre-treatment correct follow-through rates. These patterns suggest that missingness may not be completely random and could introduce bias into the interpretation of findings. The potential for non-random attrition to influence effect estimates should be considered when interpreting the findings.

In interpreting the findings of this study, we demonstrated a temporal relationship between improvements in caregiver symptoms, reductions in child disruptive behaviors, and growth in caregiver behavioral skills. However, these conclusions are contingent on the validity of our measurement tools, including observational assessments of parenting behavior and caregiver self-reports of symptoms and child behaviors. While prior literature supports the connection between observable parenting behaviors and internal processes such as caregiver cognitions, we did not directly assess cognitive or affective mechanisms in this study. As such, we cannot draw definitive conclusions about the extent to which changes in caregiver beliefs, attributions, or emotion regulation contributed to treatment outcomes.

Further, a relatively small portion of the sample of caregivers reported elevated depression (8%) and anxiety (14%) at the beginning of treatment. Caregivers with more significant symptoms may have more difficulty seeing improvements with only behavioral parent training and no additional component directly specifically targeting their own mental health concerns, which likely extend beyond the caregiver–child relationship. Additionally, caregiver anxiety and/or depression is often comorbid with a number of other concerns (e.g., trauma, substance use, ADHD, autism, chronic health conditions) that were not systematically screened within this study, and caregivers with more complex psychiatric and/or medical concerns may experience even more difficulty benefiting from BPT alone [50]. It is also likely that alternate, unmeasured caregiver–child factors played a role in the changes witnessed in this study in caregiver mental health and child disruptive behavior over the course of PCIT. Indeed, several known factors could have been at play in decreasing child disruptive behavior as well as improving caregiver mental health, including differences in child temperament, and caregiver sensory processing sensitivity, which can affect caregiver response to child behavior [51,52].

5. Conclusions

Overall, this study supports PCIT as a valuable two-generation therapy approach, yielding benefits for the caregiver–child dyad. PCIT, although primarily designed to treat child disruptive behavior, proved beneficial for caregivers' mental health as well. By coaching caregivers in positive interaction and effective discipline techniques to reduce child disruptive behavior, therapists may simultaneously alleviate some caregiver anxiety and depressive symptoms. From a service delivery perspective, these findings encourage practitioners to routinely monitor caregiver mental health during caregiver-training programs. The empirical evidence that caregiver mental health may partially improve because of PCIT may increase caregiver buy-in and motivation for PCIT. Caregivers may feel more hopeful and engaged knowing that PCIT stands to help not only their child but also themselves. Future research should examine whether the reductions in caregiver anxiety and depression over the course of PCIT are maintained over time. Sustained improvements would strengthen the conclusion that caregiver training promotes lasting caregiver mental health benefits. Alternately, reductions in improvement over time would indicate the possible need for additional supports (e.g., caregiver individual therapy or further follow-up sessions following graduation from PCIT). Future research should also examine additional mechanisms of change (e.g., parenting self-efficacy, parental attributions/cognitions, parenting-related stress, other parental mental and physical health concerns) in caregiver and child mental health outcomes. Finally, the current study did not examine potential moderators that might alter the strength of mediational processes. For instance, it may be that progression through PCIT treatment improves Do/Avoid skill ratio, which subsequently improves parent anxiety symptoms, but that the strength of this mediational process depends upon whether caregivers experience high or low levels of anxiety (i.e., a moderator). Future studies could combine the moderation and mediational findings here to examine these moderated mediational processes [39].

Author Contributions: Conceptualization, A.P., A.L., J.A., J.F.J. and E.M.; data curation, A.P.; formal analysis, A.P. and J.F.J.; funding acquisition, E.D., D.G. and J.F.J.; investigation, A.P.; methodology, W.A.R., J.F.J. and E.M.; project administration, E.D. and D.G.; resources, R.L. and E.M.; software, A.P.; supervision, J.F.J. and E.M.; validation, A.P.; visualization, E.M.; writing—original draft, A.P., A.L., J.A., W.A.R., R.L., J.F.J. and E.M.; writing—review and editing, A.P., A.L., J.A., W.A.R., R.L., E.D., D.G., J.F.J. and E.M. All authors have read and agreed to the published version of the manuscript.

Funding: This research was funded by The Children's Trust (Grant Number: 2410-7572).

Institutional Review Board Statement: The study was conducted in accordance with the Declaration of Helsinki and approved by the Institutional Review Board (or Ethics Committee) of The University of Miami Miller School of Medicine (protocol code: 20161163; date of approval for this study: 21 July 2022) for studies involving humans.

Informed Consent Statement: Informed consent was obtained from all subjects involved in the study.

Data Availability Statement: The original contributions presented in this study are included in the article. Further inquiries can be directed to the corresponding author.

Acknowledgments: We extend our deepest appreciation to the participating families whose invaluable contributions made this study possible. We also thank the dedicated therapists who provided expert services and support throughout this project.

Conflicts of Interest: The authors declare no conflicts of interest. The funders had no role in the design of the study; in the collection, analyses, or interpretation of data; in the writing of the manuscript; or in the decision to publish the results.

Abbreviations

The following abbreviations are used in this manuscript:

BPT	Behavioral Parent Training
PCIT	Parent–Child Interaction Therapy
CDI	Child-Directed Interaction
PDI	Parent-Directed Interaction
I-PCIT	Telehealth Parent–Child Interaction Therapy
REDCap	Research Electronic Data Capture
ECBI	Eyberg Child Behavior Inventory
BASC-3	Behavior Assessment System for Children, Third Edition
IRB	Institutional Review Board
CFI	Culture Formulation Interview
DPICS-IV	Dyadic Parent–Child Interaction Coding System, Fourth Version
CLP	Child-Led Play
PLP	Caregiver/Parent-Led Play
CU	Clean-Up
GAD-7	Generalized Anxiety Disorder 7-item scale
PHQ-8	Patient Health Questionnaire-8
GEE	Generalized Estimating Equations
CI	Confidence Interval

References

1. Hosokawa, R.; Katura, T. Association among parents' stress recovery experiences, parenting practices, and children's behavioral problems: A cross-sectional study. *BMC Psychol.* **2025**, *13*, 124. [CrossRef] [PubMed]
2. Wirehag Nordh, E.-L.; Grip, K.; Axberg, U. The patient and the family: Investigating parental mental health problems, family functioning, and parent involvement in child and adolescent mental health services (CAMHS). *Eur. Child Adolesc. Psychiatry* **2024**. *online ahead of print*. [CrossRef]
3. Piro-Gambetti, B.; Greenlee, J.; Hickey, E.J.; Putney, J.M.; Lorang, E.; Hartley, S.L. Parental Depression Symptoms and Internalizing Mental Health Problems in Autistic Children. *J. Autism. Dev. Disord.* **2023**, *53*, 2373–2383. [CrossRef]
4. Quigley, A.N.; Lickenbrock, D.M.; Bailes, L.G. Infant Affect Regulation with Mothers and Fathers: The Roles of Parent Mental Health and Marital Satisfaction. *J. Child Fam. Stud.* **2025**, *34*, 502–517. [CrossRef]
5. Haine-Schlagel, R.; Dickson, K.S.; Lind, T.; Kim, J.J.; May, G.C.; Walsh, N.E.; Lazarevic, V.; Crandal, B.R.; Yeh, M. Caregiver Participation Engagement in Child Mental Health Prevention Programs: A Systematic Review. *Prev. Sci.* **2022**, *23*, 321–339. [CrossRef] [PubMed]
6. Haine-Schlagel, R.; Dickson, K.S.; Shapiro, A.F.; May, G.C.; Cheng, P. Parent Mental Health Problems and Motivation as Predictors of Their Engagement in Community-Based Child Mental Health Services. *Child. Youth Serv. Rev.* **2019**, *104*, 104370. [CrossRef]
7. Patterson, G.R. *Coercive Family Process*; Castalia Publishing Company: Detroit, MI, USA, 1982.
8. Patterson, G.R. Dishion, T.J., Snyder, J.J., Eds.; *Coercion Theory: The Oxford Handbook of Coercive Relationship Dynamics The Study of Change*; Oxford University Press: Oxford, UK, 2016; pp. 7–22.
9. Yan, N.; Ansari, A.; Peng, P. Reconsidering the relation between parental functioning and child externalizing behaviors: A meta-analysis on child-driven effects. *J. Fam. Psychol.* **2021**, *35*, 225–235. [CrossRef]
10. Snarr, J.; Slep, A.; Grande, V. Validation of a New Self-Report Measure of Parental Attributions. *Psychol. Assess.* **2009**, *21*, 390–401. [CrossRef]

11. Agazzi, H.; Yin, T.S.; Julia, O.; Kathleen, A.; Kirby, R.S. Does Parent-Child Interaction Therapy Reduce Maternal Stress, Anxiety, and Depression Among Mothers of Children with Autism Spectrum Disorder? *Child Fam. Behav. Ther.* **2017**, *39*, 283–303. [CrossRef]
12. Patel, Z.; Maylott, S.; Rothenberg, W.; Jent, J.; Garcia, D. Parenting Stress across Time-Limited Parent-Child Interaction Therapy. *J. Child Fam. Stud.* **2022**, *31*, 3069–3084. [CrossRef]
13. Rothenberg, W.; Weinstein, A.; Dandes, E.; Jent, J. Improving Child Emotion Regulation: Effects of Parent–Child Interaction-therapy and Emotion Socialization Strategies. *J. Child Fam. Stud.* **2019**, *28*, 720–731. [CrossRef]
14. Eyberg, S.M.; Funderburk, B.W. *Parent-Child Interaction Therapy Protocol*; PCIT International: Kalispell, MT, USA, 2011.
15. Jent, J.; Funderburk, B.; N'zi, A.; Best, K.; Garcia, D.; Rothenberg, W.; Peskin, A.; Parlade, M.; Abner, J.P. Is perfect fidelity the enemy of good treatment? In Proceedings of the 2024 Parent Child Interaction Therapy Conference, Knoxville, TN, USA, 4–6 September 2024.
16. Jent, J.F.; Rothenberg, W.A.; Peskin, A.; Acosta, J.; Weinstein, A.; Concepcion, R.; Dale, C.; Bonatakis, J.; Sobalvarro, C.; Chavez, F.; et al. An 18-week model of Parent-Child Interaction Therapy: Clinical approaches, treatment formats, and predictors of success for predominantly minoritized families. *Front. Psychol.* **2023**, *14*, 1233683. [CrossRef]
17. Fleming, G.E.; Sawrikar, V.; Kaouar, S.; Neo, B.; McDonogh, C.; Kimonis, E.R. The Impact of Parental Cognitions on Outcomes of Behavioral Parent Training for Children With Conduct Problems. *Behav. Ther.* 2025, *in press*. [CrossRef]
18. Blanchet, B.H.; Hayes, T.; Gillenson, C.; Neuman, K.; Heymann, P.; Comer, J.S.; Bagner, D.M. Caregiver Distress and Child Behavior Problems in Children with Developmental Delay from Predominantly Minoritized Backgrounds. *J. Clin. Child. Adolesc. Psychol.* 2024, *online ahead of print*. [CrossRef]
19. Parkes, A.; Sweeting, H.; Wight, D. Parenting stress and parent support among mothers with high and low education. *J. Fam. Psychol.* **2015**, *29*, 907–918. [CrossRef]
20. Thomas, R.; Abell, B.; Webb, H.J.; Avdagic, E.; Zimmer-Gembeck, M.J. Parent-Child Interaction Therapy: A Meta-analysis. *Pediatrics* **2017**, *140*, e20170352. [CrossRef] [PubMed]
21. Campbell, S.M.; Hawes, T.; Swan, K.; Thomas, R.; Zimmer-Gembeck, M.J. Evidence-Based Treatment in Practice: PCIT Research on Addressing Individual Differences and Diversity Through the Lens of 20 Years of Service. *Psychol. Res. Behav. Manag.* **2023**, *16*, 2599–2617. [CrossRef] [PubMed]
22. Comer, J.S.; Furr, J.M.; Miguel, E.M.; Cooper-Vince, C.E.; Carpenter, A.L.; Elkins, R.M.; Kerns, C.E.; Cornacchio, D.; Chou, T.; Coxe, S.; et al. Remotely delivering real-time parent training to the home: An initial randomized trial of internet-delivered parent-child interaction therapy (I-PCIT). *J. Consult. Clin. Psychol.* **2017**, *85*, 909–917. [CrossRef]
23. Peskin, A.; Barth, A.; Andrew Rothenberg, W.; Turzi, A.; Formoso, D.; Garcia, D.; Jent, J. New Therapy for a New Normal: Comparing Telehealth and in-Person Time-Limited Parent-Child Interaction Therapy. *Behav. Ther.* **2024**, *55*, 106–121. [CrossRef]
24. Harris, P.A.; Taylor, R.; Thielke, R.; Payne, J.; Gonzalez, N.; Conde, J.G. Research electronic data capture (REDCap)—A metadata-driven methodology and workflow process for providing translational research informatics support. *J. Biomed. Inform.* **2009**, *42*, 377–381. [CrossRef]
25. Eyberg, S.M.; Pincus, D. *Eyberg Child Behavior Inventory and Sutter-Eyberg Student Behavior Inventory: Professional Manual*; Psychological Assessment Resources: Lutz, FL, USA, 1999.
26. Reynolds, C.R.; Kamphaus, R.W. *Behavior Assessment System for Children*, 3rd ed.; Pearson: London, UK, 2015.
27. American Psychiatric Association. *Diagnostic and Statistical Manual of Mental Disorders (DSM-5)*, 5th ed.; American Psychiatric Association Publishing: Washington, DC, USA, 2013.
28. Sanchez, A.L.; Jent, J.; Aggarwal, N.K.; Chavira, D.; Coxe, S.; Garcia, D.; La Roche, M.; Comer, J.S. Person-Centered Cultural Assessment Can Improve Child Mental Health Service Engagement and Outcomes. *J. Clin. Child. Adolesc. Psychol.* **2022**, *51*, 1–22. [CrossRef]
29. Gross, D.; Fogg, L.; Young, M.; Ridge, A.; Cowell, J.; Sivan, A.; Richardson, R. Reliability and validity of the Eyberg Child Behavior Inventory with African-American and Latino parents of young children. *Res. Nurs. Health* **2007**, *30*, 213–223. [CrossRef]
30. Garcia, D.; Barnett, M.L.; Rothenberg, W.A.; Tonarely, N.A.; Perez, C.; Espinosa, N.; Salem, H.; Alonso, B.; San Juan, J.; Peskin, A.; et al. A Natural Helper Intervention to Address Disparities in Parent Child-Interaction Therapy: A Randomized Pilot Study. *J. Clin. Child. Adolesc. Psychol.* **2023**, *52*, 343–359. [CrossRef] [PubMed]
31. Davis, E.M.; Schmidt, E.; Rothenberg, W.A.; Davidson, B.; Garcia, D.; Barnett, M.L.; Fernandez, C.; Jent, J.F. Universal Teacher-Child Interaction Training in early childhood special education: A cluster randomized control trial. *J. Sch. Psychol.* **2023**, *97*, 171–191. [CrossRef] [PubMed]
32. Eyberg, S.M.; Nelson, M.M.; Ginn, N.C.; Bhuiyan, N.; Boggs, S.R. *Dyadic Parent-Child Interaction Coding System (DPICS): Comprehensive Manual for Research and Training*, 4th ed.; PCIT International: Kalispell, MT, USA, 2013.
33. Eyberg, S.M.; Nelson, M.M.; Ginn, N.C.; Bhuiyan, N.; Boggs, S.R. *Dyadic Parent-Child Interaction Coding System (DPICS): Clinical Manual*, 4th ed.; PCIT International: Kalispell, MT, USA, 2014.

34. Graziano, P.A.; Ros-Demarize, R.; Hare, M.M. Condensing parent training: A randomized trial comparing the efficacy of a briefer, more intensive version of Parent-Child Interaction Therapy (I-PCIT). *J. Consult. Clin. Psychol.* **2020**, *88*, 669–679. [CrossRef]
35. Spitzer, R.L.; Kroenke, K.; Williams, J.B.W.; Löwe, B. A Brief Measure for Assessing Generalized Anxiety Disorder: The GAD-7. *Arch. Intern. Med.* **2006**, *166*, 1092–1097. [CrossRef]
36. Kroenke, K.; Strine, T.W.; Spitzer, R.L.; Williams, J.B.W.; Berry, J.T.; Mokdad, A.H. The PHQ-8 as a measure of current depression in the general population. *J. Affect. Disord.* **2009**, *114*, 163–173. [CrossRef]
37. Glanzer, J. Report: Average Renter in Much of U.S. Needs $100,000 Salary. 2023. Available online: https://www.fau.edu/newsdesk/articles/april2023-rental-numbers (accessed on 1 May 2025).
38. Montoya, A.K.; Hayes, A.F. Two-condition within-participant statistical mediation analysis: A path-analytic framework. *Psychol. Methods* **2017**, *22*, 6–27. [CrossRef]
39. Montoya, A.K. Conditional Process Analysis for Two-Instance Repeated-Measures Designs. *Psychol. Methods* **2024**, preprint. [CrossRef]
40. Timmer, S.G.; Ho, L.K.; Urquiza, A.J.; Zebell, N.M.; Fernandez, Y.G.E.; Boys, D. The effectiveness of parent-child interaction therapy with depressive mothers: The changing relationship as the agent of individual change. *Child. Psychiatry Hum. Dev.* **2011**, *42*, 406–423. [CrossRef]
41. Skowron, E.A.; Nekkanti, A.K.; Skoranski, A.M.; Scholtes, C.M.; Lyons, E.R.; Mills, K.L.; Bard, D.; Rock, A.; Berkman, E.; Bard, E.; et al. Randomized trial of parent-child interaction therapy improves child-welfare parents' behavior, self-regulation, and self-perceptions. *J. Consult. Clin. Psychol.* **2024**, *92*, 75–92. [CrossRef]
42. Bar-Haim, Y.; Lamy, D.; Pergamin, L.; Bakermans-Kranenburg, M.J.; van IJzendoorn, M.H. Threat-related attentional bias in anxious and nonanxious individuals: A meta-analytic study. *Psychol. Bull.* **2007**, *133*, 1–24. [CrossRef] [PubMed]
43. Khoury, B.; Sharma, M.; Rush, S.E.; Fournier, C. Mindfulness-based stress reduction for healthy individuals: A meta-analysis. *J. Psychosom. Res.* **2015**, *78*, 519–528. [CrossRef]
44. Rothenberg, W.A.; Anton, M.T.; Gonzalez, M.; Lafko Breslend, N.; Forehand, R.; Khavjou, O.; Jones, D.J. BPT for Early-Onset Behavior Disorders: Examining the Link Between Treatment Components and Trajectories of Child Internalizing Symptoms. *Behav. Modif.* **2020**, *44*, 159–185. [CrossRef]
45. Goodman, S.H.; Simon, H.; McCarthy, L.; Ziegler, J.; Ceballos, A. Testing Models of Associations Between Depression and Parenting Self-efficacy in Mothers: A Meta-analytic Review. *Clin. Child. Fam. Psychol. Rev.* **2022**, *25*, 471–499. [CrossRef]
46. Patterson, G.R.; Dishion, T.J.; Bank, L. Family interaction: A process model of deviancy training. *Aggress. Behav.* **1984**, *10*, 253–267. [CrossRef]
47. Najman, J.M.; Williams, G.M.; Nikles, J.; Spence, S.; Bor, W.; O'Callaghan, M.; Le Brocque, R.; Andersen, M.J. Mothers' mental illness and child behavior problems: Cause-effect association or observation bias? *J. Am. Acad. Child. Adolesc. Psychiatry* **2000**, *39*, 592–602. [CrossRef]
48. Ringoot, A.P.; Tiemeier, H.; Jaddoe, V.W.; So, P.; Hofman, A.; Verhulst, F.C.; Jansen, P.W. Parental depression and child well-being: Young children's self-reports helped addressing biases in parent reports. *J. Clin. Epidemiol.* **2015**, *68*, 928–938. [CrossRef]
49. Zimmerman, M. The value and limitations of self-administered questionnaires in clinical practice and epidemiological studies. *World Psychiatry* **2024**, *23*, 210–212. [CrossRef]
50. Cuijpers, P.; Miguel, C.; Ciharova, M.; Quero, S.; Plessen, C.Y.; Ebert, D.; Harrer, M.; van Straten, A.; Karyotaki, E. Psychological treatment of depression with other comorbid mental disorders: Systematic review and meta-analysis. *Cogn. Behav. Ther.* **2023**, *52*, 246–268. [CrossRef]
51. Hartman, C.A.; Larsson, H.; Vos, M.; Bellato, A.; Libutzki, B.; Solberg, B.S.; Chen, Q.; Du Rietz, E.; Mostert, J.C.; Kittel-Schneider, S.; et al. Anxiety, mood, and substance use disorders in adult men and women with and without attention-deficit/hyperactivity disorder: A substantive and methodological overview. *Neurosci. Biobehav. Rev.* **2023**, *151*, 105209. [CrossRef] [PubMed]
52. Christou, A.I.; Fanti, K.; Mavrommatis, I.; Soursou, G.; Pergantis, P.; Drigas, A. Social affiliation and attention to angry faces in children: Evidence for the contributing role of parental sensory processing sensitivity. *Children* **2025**, *12*, 524. [CrossRef] [PubMed]

children

MDPI

Article

Mediating Role of Parental Support in the Relationship Between Immigrant Mothers' Mental Health and Adolescents' Self-Esteem

Yeseul Jeong [1,2] and Sangyoun Jang [3,*]

[1] College of Nursing, Keimyung University, Daegu 42601, Republic of Korea; yeseuljeong@kmu.ac.kr
[2] Research Institute of Nursing Science, Keimyung University, Daegu 42601, Republic of Korea
[3] Department of Nursing, Catholic Kwandong University, Gangneung 25601, Republic of Korea
* Correspondence: syjang@cku.ac.kr; Tel.: +82-33-649-7490

Abstract: Background/Objectives: This study aimed to identify the mediating effect of parental support on the relationship between immigrant mothers' mental health and adolescents' self-esteem. Methods: This study utilized data from 1077 Korean multicultural adolescents and their immigrant mothers from the 9th Multicultural Adolescents Panel data obtained in 2019. The data were analyzed using descriptive statistics, Pearson's correlation, Baron and Kenny's regression analysis, and bootstrapping using the process macro. Results: Immigrant mothers' mental health was significantly and positively associated with their adolescents' self-esteem (r = 0.14, $p < 0.001$), and parental support was also significantly and positively associated with adolescents' self-esteem (r = 0.50, $p < 0.001$). Parental support had a mediating effect on immigrant mothers' mental health and adolescents' self-esteem. Conclusions: The self-esteem of adolescents from multicultural families was found to be influenced by the mental health and support of their immigrant mothers. These findings highlight the mediating role of parental support in the relationship between immigrant mothers' mental health and adolescents' self-esteem, contributing to a deeper theoretical understanding of family dynamics in multicultural contexts. Therefore, these factors should be considered when developing parent education programs for immigrant mothers.

Keywords: immigrant; parental mental health; parental support; adolescent; self-esteem

1. Introduction

The transition from adolescence to adulthood is an important developmental period that requires the achievement of developmental tasks in various areas, such as career planning, forming social relationships, and establishing personal beliefs [1]. In particular, this stage offers freedom and hope to explore various possibilities, leading to a rapid increase in self-esteem. However, it is also marked by heightened anxiety due to uncertainty about the future, which can threaten the formation of a stable self-identity [1,2].

For adolescents approaching the transition to adulthood, self-esteem serves as an internal factor that protects against the psychological stress experienced during this transition process. Major life changes, such as changes in status to adulthood, progression to higher education, entry into the workforce, and expansion of social relationships, demand new roles and responsibilities from adolescents. The pressure caused by these life events can lead to maladaptive outcomes such as anxiety and depression, but self-esteem can act as an important protective factor that prevents these negative effects [3,4]. Since high

https://doi.org/10.3390/children12060677

self-esteem is closely related to an individual's overall quality of life and long-term psychological health [3,5], it is necessary to identify the factors and pathways that support or hinder its development during this sensitive period as adolescents approach the transition to adulthood.

1.1. Challenges to Self-Esteem Development in Immigrant Adolescents: The Korean Context

In immigrant families in Korean society, adolescents face not only significant transitional events in the development of their self-esteem but also additional challenges. Korea has long maintained a homogeneous society, but since the mid-1990s, the sharp increase in international marriages has diversified Korean society ethnically, presenting new challenges for social integration [6–8]. In 1990, the proportion of international marriages among all marriages was just 1.2%, but by 2005, it had surged to 13.5% and has remained at 10.1% up to the present [9]. Notably, 80.3% of international marriages involve Korean men and immigrant women [10], a trend driven by women's educational advancement, expanded social participation, and the resulting marriage difficulties for low-income men. As women's education levels and social participation have increased, low-income men in rural areas who emphasize traditional values and gender roles have found it more difficult to find spouses domestically, leading to a sharp increase in international marriages facilitated by commercial marriage brokers [6,7]. Amid this increase in international marriages and immigrant populations, immigrant families and their members in Korea have been exposed to social discrimination and prejudice [8,11], which negatively impacts the development of self-esteem in adolescents from immigrant backgrounds [12,13].

In cultures where the mother's role is crucial in child-rearing, the development of self-esteem in immigrant adolescents is significantly influenced by immigrant mothers. Parental support is essential for the development of children's self-esteem, but immigrant mothers often face difficulties in providing sufficient support due to cultural differences, language barriers, and social discrimination. For instance, in East Asian cultures influenced by Confucianism, parental, especially maternal, involvement in education is highly valued [14,15]. However, immigrant mothers often face challenges due to differences in values between their home and host countries, language barriers, discrimination, and difficulties in accessing informal information channels such as parent–teacher meetings [16–18]. Competence and recognition in areas that adolescents prioritize play a key role in the formation of self-esteem [19]. Therefore, at a time when adolescents are facing important transitions, such as entering higher education and planning their career paths, limited support due to their mothers' immigration background can lower the self-esteem of teenage children, which can threaten a smooth and healthy transition into adulthood.

1.2. Immigrant Mothers' Mental Health and Adolescents' Self-Esteem

The psychological difficulties faced by immigrant mothers pose an additional threat to the development of their children's self-esteem. A previous systematic review [20] has shown that marriage immigrant women in South Korea experience higher rates of overall mental health problems compared to native Korean women and are particularly vulnerable to specific conditions such as depression, postpartum depression, and anxiety. These mental health issues are understood to result from the combined effects of various factors, including socioeconomic conditions (e.g., income and education level), social factors (e.g., marital satisfaction, family relationships, and social support), and cultural factors related to immigration, such as acculturative stress and limited Korean language proficiency [20].

Mental health problems in immigrant parents are not confined to the parents themselves, but are also associated with lower self-esteem in their children [21,22]. The self-esteem, behavioral problems, and depression of youths with immigrant mothers were predicted by the mothers' sociocultural adaptation, acculturative stress, and perceived discrimination [21]. However, empirical research on the specific pathways linking these issues remains limited.

1.3. Potential Mediation by Parental Support

Some studies suggest that the lack of parental support, as perceived by children, may play a crucial mediating role in the relationship between parental mental health problems and the development of children's self-esteem. Parents with mental health issues tend to have a diminished capacity to provide appropriate support to their children [23], a finding consistently observed in qualitative studies exploring both parent and child experiences. Parents with serious mental health problems often become dependent on their children to meet their needs, failing to respond adequately when their children require support [24]. Additionally, adult children of parents with mental health issues tend to prioritize their parents' needs over their own, which can lower their self-esteem [25–27]. A study by No [28] suggested that the cultural adaptation stress experienced by immigrant mothers reduces parental support and consequently lowers their children's self-concept. Although this research focused on elementary school children, it suggested that immigrant mothers' mental health could also impact the self-esteem development of adolescents approaching the transition to adulthood.

1.4. In This Study

Previous research has provided fragmented knowledge on the effects of immigrant mothers' mental health and parental support on the self-esteem development of immigrant adolescents in Korea. Furthermore, empirical studies specifically investigating the pathways through which self-esteem develops in adolescents facing the transition to adulthood, and the protective effects of healthy self-esteem are scarce.

Therefore, this study aims to analyze in detail the impact of immigrant mothers' mental health, mediated by parental support, on the self-esteem development of adolescents approaching the transition to adulthood. The results of this study could serve as important foundational data for developing policies and interventions aimed at improving the self-esteem of adolescents from immigrant families and supporting their successful transition into adulthood.

2. Materials and Methods

2.1. Research Design

This study aimed to identify the mediating effect of parental support on the association between immigrant mothers' mental health and self-esteem among multicultural adolescents and their mothers, using raw data from the 9th year of the Multicultural Adolescent Panel Study in Korea.

2.2. Data Source and Study Population

The National Youth Policy Institute collects data from multicultural youths and their parents to improve their school life, social adaptation, physical and psychological health, and parent–child relationships. The Multicultural Adolescents Panel Study, conducted by the National Youth Policy Institute, targets multicultural 4th-grade elementary school students and their mothers in Korea as of 2011. Using stratified random sampling and probability proportional sampling across 16 cities/provinces, the first panel was established in 2011, with data collected annually through the 12th wave in 2023. In this study, the 9th wave of the 1st panel survey of the Multicultural Adolescents Panel Study was used

The 9th wave of the survey was conducted on 1146 multicultural adolescents and 1114 mothers (1105 foreign mothers). This study included data from immigrant mothers, excluding responses from Korean mothers and cases with missing data. The final sample consisted of 1077 third-year high school students and their immigrant mothers who completed questionnaires regarding key variables: maternal mental health, parental support, and adolescents' self-esteem.

The process for recruiting panel participants and collecting data was as follows. The National Youth Policy Institute sent an official document to schools with multicultural adolescents requesting their cooperation in recruiting households to participate in the panel survey. The school sent each household a multicultural panel survey-related household newsletter and consent form. Afterwards, the survey was conducted after obtaining voluntary consent from households that wished to participate in the panel survey. This survey was conducted with the approval of the Research Ethics Committee of the National Youth Policy Institute (IRB No. 201904-HR-Goyu-002-01), and this study was approved by the Institutional Review Board of Keimyung University, to which the researcher is affiliated (IRB No. 40525-202502-HR-105-01 and 14 March 2025, of approval). It was conducted by downloading raw data from the National Youth Policy Institute's data archive after agreeing to the "Data Request Agreement" and "Data Use and Analysis Compliance Guidelines". The raw data were guaranteed anonymity.

2.3. *Study Variables*

2.3.1. Immigrant Mothers' Mental Health

The mental health of immigrant mothers was assessed with a modified instrument that Hwang [29] reorganized into 12 items—covering physical and psychological health—from 20 items that Cawte [30] had selected from the Cornell Medical Index Test. A factor analysis conducted on 12 items revealed two factors, 'physical health' and 'mental health'. Most items demonstrated factor loadings of 0.50 or higher, indicating acceptable construct validity. Therefore, all 12 items were retained in the instrument [31]. Six psychological health items were used to assess mental health. The tool uses a 5-point Likert scale. Cronbach's alpha coefficient was 0.85 in Hwang [29] and 0.88 in our study. In a previous study that used the same instrument with identical participants [32], Cronbach's alpha was 0.88, the same as in this study.

2.3.2. Parental Support

Parental support was measured using nine items from the Parental Support Tool developed by Kim and Park [33] and extracted from the Multicultural Adolescent Panel Study. The tool consists of emotional, informational, and economic support. Emotional support items include statements such as 'My parents comfort me when I am having a hard time', informational support items include 'My parents give me advice on my future studies', and financial support items include 'My parents buy me things I need to study'. The tool was evaluated using a 5-point Likert scale. The scores ranged from 9 to 45, with higher scores indicating higher parental support. Cronbach's alpha coefficients for each subscale were 0.92 for emotional support, 0.87 for informational support, and 0.82 for economic support. The internal consistency of the overall parental support was 0.93 in Kim and Park [33] and 0.92 in our study. Similarly, a previous study [34], which examined parental support for multicultural adolescents, reported that Cronbach's alpha was 0.93.

2.3.3. Adolescents' Self-Esteem

Self-esteem was measured using nine items (five positive and four negative) from the Self-Esteem Scale developed by Rosenberg [35] and extracted from the Multicultural Adolescents Panel Study. It consists of items such as 'On the whole, I am satisfied with myself' and 'I feel that I have a number of good qualities', 'I feel that I'm a person of worth', and 'I take a positive attitude toward myself'. This tool is measured using a 5-point Likert scale, and negative items are reverse-coded and analyzed. The scores ranged from 9 to 45, with a higher score indicating higher self-esteem. In Rosenberg [35], Cronbach's alpha ranged from 0.85 to 0.88, whereas it was 0.88 in our study. In a study conducted by Lee and Yoo [36] examining the self-esteem of multicultural adolescents, Cronbach's alpha coefficient was reported to be 0.88.

2.4. Data Analysis

Statistical analyses were performed using SPSS Statistics for Windows, version 29 0 (IBM Corp., New York, NY, USA). The participants' general characteristics were analyzed by frequency and percentile. Differences in parental support and adolescents' self-esteem according to general characteristics were analyzed using a *t*-test and analysis of variance. Correlations between immigrant mothers' mental health, parental support, and adolescents' self-esteem were analyzed using Pearson's correlation coefficients.

To assess the mediating effect of parental support on the relationship between immigrant mothers' mental health and adolescents' self-esteem, Baron and Kenny's [37] three-step mediation analysis procedure was employed. The steps were as follows: (1) regression analysis of the mediator on the independent variables, (2) regression analysis of the dependent variable on the independent variables, and (3) regression analysis of the dependent variable on both the independent variables and the mediator. To confirm the statistical significance of the mediating effect, a bootstrapping test was performed using the SPSS Process macro (model 4) with a bootstrap sample size of 1000 and a 95% confidence interval.

3. Results

3.1. Differences in Parental Support and Adolescents' Self-Esteem by General Characteristics

The study included 1077 adolescents and their parents. The sex distribution of the adolescents was 49.6% male and 50.4% female. The education levels of mothers and fathers were mostly high school graduates (47.4% and 52.2%, respectively), and 66.7% of the mothers were employed. A significant difference in parental support was observed based on the mother's education level ($p = 0.021$) and monthly average income ($p < 0.001$). Additionally, adolescents' self-esteem showed a significant difference based on monthly average income ($p = 0.036$) (Table 1).

Table 1. General characteristics of the participants ($N = 1077$).

Variable	Category	n (%)	Parental Support ($n = 1077$)			Adolescents' Self-Esteem ($n = 1077$)		
			Mean ± SD	t/F	*p*	Mean ± SD	t/F	*p*
Sex	Male adolescent	534 (49.6)	35.56 ± 6.56	0.98	0.326	34.62 ± 5.89	1.75	0.080
	Female adolescent	543 (50.4)	35.18 ± 6.18			33.98 ± 6.13		
Mother's education	Middle school or below [a]	114 (10.6)	34.04 ± 6.77	2.90	0.021 a < e [†]	33.26 ± 6.62	2.32	0.055
	High school [b]	510 (47.4)	35.65 ± 6.17			34.19 ± 6.04		
	College [c]	284 (26.4)	35.13 ± 6.64			34.51 ± 5.87		
	University [d]	164 (15.2)	35.65 ± 6.10			34.80 ± 5.63		
	Graduate school [e]	5 (0.5)	41.60 ± 4.51			39.80 ± 6.72		
Father's education *	Middle school or below	335 (32.4)	35.05 ± 6.55	0.74	0.563	34.43 ± 6.07	0.39	0.819
	High school	540 (52.2)	35.50 ± 6.15			34.29 ± 6.03		
	College	59 (5.7)	35.92 ± 6.91			34.64 ± 5.37		
	University	91 (8.8)	36.22 ± 6.54			34.81 ± 6.21		
	Graduate school	9 (0.9)	35.44 ± 6.75			36.22 ± 5.09		
Mother's occupation	Yes	718 (66.7)	35.46 ± 6.26	−0.68	0.499	34.46 ± 5.92	−1.23	0.219
	No	359 (33.3)	35.18 ± 6.59			33.98 ± 6.21		
Father's occupation *	Yes	888 (86.0)	35.50 ± 6.44	−0.73	0.469	34.50 ± 6.02	−1.25	0.211
	No	145 (14.0)	35.08 ± 6.09			33.83 ± 5.89		

Table 1. *Cont.*

Variable	Category	n (%)	Parental Support (n = 1077)			Adolescents' Self-Esteem (n = 1077)		
			Mean ± SD	t/F	p	Mean ± SD	t/F	p
Monthly household income (KRW 10,000) *	<100 [a]	16 (1.5)	35.38 ± 6.52	4.71	<0.001 a < f [‡]	34.94 ± 5.11	2.40	0.036 b < f [‡]
	100~< 200 [b]	198 (18.4)	33.82 ± 6.99			33.49 ± 6.63		
	200~<300 [c]	308 (28.6)	35.18 ± 6.26			34.06 ± 5.73		
	300~<400 [d]	310 (28.8)	35.55 ± 6.28			34.20 ± 5.90		
	400~<500 [e]	152 (14.1)	36.22 ± 6.02			35.02 ± 6.08		
	≥500 [f]	92 (8.6)	37.27 ± 5.42			35.75 ± 5.70		

* Excludes non-responses. [†] Tukey HSD post hoc test; the mean difference is significant at the 0.10 level. [‡] Tukey HSD post hoc test; the mean difference is significant at the 0.05 level. The footnotes in a–f were used to indicate the results of the post-analysis.

3.2. The Degree of Immigrant Mothers' Mental Health, Parental Support, and Adolescents' Self-Esteem

The mean score for immigrant mothers' mental health was 4.23 ± 0.73 out of 5 points; the mean score for parental support was 3.93 ± 0.71 out of 5 points, and the mean score for adolescents' self-esteem was 3.81 ± 0.67 out of 5 points. The normality of the data was assessed using skewness and kurtosis, and all variables were found to follow a normal distribution.

3.3. Correlations Among Immigrant Mothers' Mental Health, Parental Support, and Adolescents' Self-Esteem

The mental health of immigrant mothers showed a significant positive correlation with parental support (r = 0.11, p < 0.001) and adolescents' self-esteem (r = 0.14, p < 0.001). Parental support had a significant positive correlation with adolescents' self-esteem (r = 0.50, p < 0.001) (Table 2).

Table 2. Correlations among the variables (N = 1077).

Variable	Immigrant Mothers' Mental Health	Parental Support
Parental support	0.11 (<0.001)	
Adolescent self-esteem	0.14 (<0.001)	0.50 (<0.001)

3.4. Mediating Effect of Parental Support in the Relationships Between Immigrant Mothers' Mental Health and Adolescents' Self-Esteem

To verify the mediating effect of parental support on the relationship between immigrant mothers' mental health and adolescents' self-esteem, we performed the three-step mediation effect verification procedure outlined by Baron and Kenny [37] and conducted the Process macro to assess the statistical significance of the mediation effect.

During the regression analysis, we checked for multicollinearity. The tolerance limit was 0.95 to 0.96, which was above the threshold of 0.1, and the variance inflation factor (VIF) was 1.014, well below the cutoff of 10, indicating that multicollinearity was not a concern. In the test for the autocorrelation of errors, the Durbin–Watson index was 1.952, which is close to 2, indicating that there was no autocorrelation. After verifying the assumptions of normality and homoscedasticity of the residuals, the normal P-P plot of the standardized residuals satisfied normality. The residuals were evenly distributed above and below zero in the scatter plot, satisfying the equal variance of the residuals. Therefore, all the basic assumptions of the regression analysis were satisfied.

In the mediation effect analysis, to more clearly confirm the mediating effect of parental support on the immigrant mothers' mental health and the adolescents' self-esteem, the mothers' education level and monthly household income—identified as statistically significant variables in the univariate analyses—were included as control variables in the mediation model.

Table 3 presents the results of the three-step mediation effect verification procedure based on Baron and Kenny's [37] model. In the first step, the effect of the independent variable, immigrant mothers' mental health, on the mediator, parental support, was statistically significant (β = 0.09, p = 0.003). In the second step, the independent variable, immigrant mothers' mental health, on the dependent variable, adolescents' self-esteem, was also statistically significant (β = 0.15. p < 0.001). In the third step, parental support significantly affected the adolescents' self-esteem (β = 0.48, p < 0.001). Notably, the β value for the effect of immigrant mothers' mental health on adolescents' self-esteem in the third step was 0.11 (p < 0.001), which was lower than the β value in the second step (β = 0.15, p < 0.001), indicating that parental support partially mediated the relationship between immigrant mothers' mental health and adolescents' self-esteem (Figure 1).

Table 3. Mediating effect of parental support on the relationship between immigrant mothers' mental health and adolescents' self-esteem (N = 1077).

Variable	B	SE	β	t	p	95% CI	R^2	Adj.R^2	F	p
Step 1. Immigrant mother's mental health → parental support	0.13	0.04	0.09	3.02	0.003	[0.05, 0.22]	0.040	0.032	4.64	<0.001
Step 2. Immigrant mother's mental health → adolescent self-esteem	0.21	0.04	0.15	5.02	<0.001	[0.13, 0.29]	0.041	0.032	4.65	<0.001
Step 3. Immigrant mother's mental health, parental support → adolescent self-esteem							0.260	0.253	35.16	<0.001
Immigrant mother' mental health → adolescent self-esteem	0.15	0.04	0.11	4.06	<0.001	[0.08, 0.22]				
Parental support → adolescent self-esteem	0.45	0.03	0.48	18.07	<0.001	[0.40, 0.50]				

Note. CI = confidence interval.

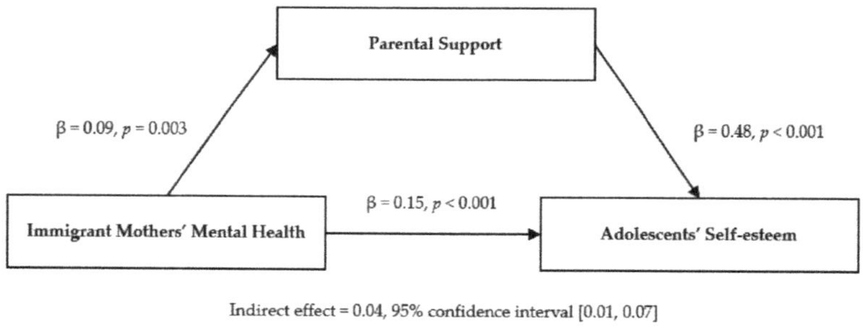

Figure 1. Mediating effect of parental support in the association between immigrant mothers' mental health and adolescents' self-esteem.

The significance of the indirect mediation effect was tested using bootstrapping analysis. The effect size was 0.04, which was found to be statistically significant because zero was not included between the 95% lower limit confidence interval (BootLLCI = 0.01) and the upper limit confidence interval (BootULCI = 0.07).

4. Discussion

This study examined the level of immigrant mothers' mental health, parental support, and adolescents' self-esteem and investigated whether parental support mediates the relationship between immigrant mothers' mental health and adolescents' self-esteem.

4.1. Influrence of Socioeconomic Factors on Parental Support and Adolescents' Self-Esteem

Significant differences in parental support and adolescents' self-esteem were observed based on their general characteristics. Parental support differed significantly depending on the mother's education level and the household's average monthly income. This study found that parental support was higher among mothers who had completed a four-year college degree or had higher income levels. This finding aligns with previous studies indicating that parents with higher educational attainment tend to provide better emotional support than those with lower education levels [38].

Also, adolescents' self-esteem showed significant differences by average monthly household income. In this study, higher income levels were associated with higher self-esteem among adolescents. These results are consistent with meta-analysis studies showing that parents with higher household income have more positive parenting behaviors [39], as well as prior research showing that children from families with higher socioeconomic status tend to exhibit greater self-esteem [40]. These results suggest that adolescents from higher-income families may benefit from greater financial stability and access to resources, which in turn contribute to enhanced self-esteem.

In contrast, parents with lower educational and socioeconomic status often face constraints due to long working hours, limited time for family interaction, and challenges in fulfilling supportive roles for their children [38]. In light of these results, immigrant mothers should be offered regular educational programs and counseling to improve their communication skills and ability to provide positive support for their children. Furthermore, it is essential to prioritize socioeconomic support for multicultural families with low levels of education and income.

4.2. Relationships Among Immigrant Mothers' Mental Health, Parental Support, and Adolescents' Self-Esteem in Multicultural Families

This study found significant positive correlations among immigrant mothers' mental health, parental support, and adolescents' self-esteem. Lee and Yoo [36] similarly found that poorer physical and psychological health among married immigrant women was associated with lower adolescent self-esteem, supporting the present finding that better maternal mental health corresponds with higher adolescent self-esteem. However, since previous studies have often treated the physical and mental health of immigrant mothers as a single variable, there is a limitation in making direct comparisons with the mental health of this study. Nevertheless, the current finding is meaningful in that it confirms the influence of mothers on adolescents' self-esteem. In addition, Um's study [41], which focused on multicultural adolescents, reported that parental support was significantly positively correlated with adolescents' self-esteem. Um [41] found that parental support significantly influenced self-esteem ($\beta = 0.06$, $p < 0.001$), consistent with the present study's finding that parental support has a significant impact on self-esteem ($\beta = 0.48$, $p < 0.001$).These results demonstrate the importance of mental health and support for immigrant mothers.

In this way, significant correlations were identified among the major variables. However, the association between immigrant mothers' mental health and adolescents' self-esteem was relatively small. One possible explanation is that in South Korea, the majority of multicultural families have immigrant mothers who often experience emotional difficulties such as depression and anxiety during the process of cultural adaptation, communication problems, and interpersonal relationship difficulties in the host country [20]. Given that mothers in Korean families typically play a more important role in child-raising and education, immigrant mothers may experience increased stress and burden when their parenting values and practices differ from those of their home country.

The cultural adaptation stress of immigrant mothers was found to indirectly affect the development of children's self-concept through parenting efficacy and parental support [28]. The findings suggest that mothers' cultural adaptation stress reduces their parenting efficacy, lowering their parents' support level and ultimately hindering the development of self-concept in adolescent children. In addition, parenting stress has been reported to be higher in vulnerable groups with lower education and income levels [42]. A systematic literature review examining the relationship between household income and child development outcomes found that low socioeconomic status negatively impacts children's cognitive and socio-behavioral development and health [43]. In line with these findings, a meta-analysis study conducted by Ayoub and Bachir [39] reported that mothers from high-income families showed more positive parenting behaviors than those from low-income families and that parental supportive behavior had an effect on increasing children's self-esteem [21].

According to Statistics Korea [44], the standard median income in Korea is approximately KRW 5 million or more for a three-person household and approximately KRW 6 million or more for a four-person household. In this study, although most parents were employed (86.0% of fathers, 66.7% of mothers), 77.3% of households reported an average monthly household income below KRW 4 million. This indicates that most multicultural families in this study were of low socioeconomic status, showing a notable income gap compared to the general population.

Given these findings, the dataset primarily reflects low-income families, which may have limited the variability necessary to detect stronger associations between immigrant mothers' mental health and adolescents' self-esteem. Meanwhile, this study is meaningful in that it identified a strong correlation between parental support and self-esteem and confirmed the mediating effect of parental support between immigrant mothers' mental health and self-esteem. Self-esteem formed through a supportive relationship between parents and their children in early adolescence influences mental well-being in later adolescence [45]. Therefore, further research is needed to confirm the influence of parental support in the future.

4.3. Parental Support as a Mediator Between Immigrant Mothers' Mental Health and Adolescents' Self-Esteem

This study identified a significant mediating effect of parental support on the relationship between immigrant mothers' mental health and adolescents' self-esteem. It was difficult to find previous studies that confirmed the mediating effect of parental support on the same variables as in this study; however, we can discuss them in connection with studies that confirmed the relationship between each variable. A systematic literature review of the relationship between the mental health of immigrant parents and multicultural adolescents in other countries reported that when immigrant parents have mental stress, anxiety, and depression symptoms, it has a negative impact on their children's stress and anxiety symptoms, as well as their self-esteem [21]. In addition, it is generally known that adolescents' self-esteem is affected by their relationship with their parents, and positive interactions with parents, parental support, and encouragement have a significant effect on adolescents' self-esteem [41,46]. Moreover, when parents have a warm and supportive parenting style, their children have been shown to have high self-esteem [21,47]. This finding suggests the need to strengthen parental support systems for multicultural adolescents to achieve stable self-esteem. Therefore, to improve adolescents' self-esteem, a plan to improve mothers' mental health so that they can positively support their children is necessary.

4.4. Limitations and Implications

The limitations of this study are as follows. First, this study has methodological limitations because it analyzed cross-sectional data from 18-year-old multicultural adolescents and their immigrant mothers. Future studies need to verify the longitudinal mediating effect of parental support on adolescents' self-esteem. Second, the mental health of immigrant mothers was assessed through a self-report questionnaire, which may be prone to response bias due to subjective perception. The use of physiological indicators could improve the objectivity of mental health assessments. Third, this study focused on the effects of immigrant mothers' mental health and support on adolescents' self-esteem. Future research will also be needed to analyze the effects of Korean fathers' mental health and support on adolescents' self-esteem. Additionally, further studies should incorporate other potentially influential factors such as peer relationships and teacher support to provide a more comprehensive understanding of the determinants of self-esteem in multicultural adolescents. Fourth, as this study was conducted with multicultural families residing in Korea, its findings may be influenced by cultural and contextual factors unique to the Korean setting, which may limit generalizability to other countries. Lastly, this study has a limitation in that it did not control for factors such as social discrimination or stigma arising from the mother's mental health condition, which could potentially mediate the relationship between maternal mental health and adolescents' self-esteem. Accordingly, future research should explicitly incorporate this variable to clarify its influence. Nevertheless, this study has the strength of generalizing the results by analyzing representative large-scale data from the Multicultural Adolescent Panel Study. Additionally, this study confirmed the mediating effect of parental support on immigrant mothers' mental health and adolescents' self-esteem.

The theoretical and practical implications of this study are as follows. From a theoretical perspective, this study contributes to theoretical models of adolescent development by empirically demonstrating the mediating role of parental support in the relationship between immigrant mothers' mental health and adolescents' self-esteem. This study extends prior research by contextualizing these dynamics within multicultural families.

With regard to practical implications, the findings suggest that programs aiming to enhance adolescents' self-esteem in multicultural families should not only focus on adolescent-centered interventions but also prioritize the mental health of immigrant mothers and strengthen their parenting capacities. Policy makers and practitioners should develop culturally sensitive parent education and mental health support services that empower immigrant mothers in their parenting roles.

5. Conclusions

This study was conducted to identify the mediating effect of parental support on the relationship between immigrant mothers' mental health and adolescents' self-esteem, with the goal of providing foundational data for developing nursing interventions to enhance adolescents' self-esteem.

The findings confirmed that immigrant mothers' mental health significantly influenced their adolescents' self-esteem. Furthermore, parental support was found to partially mediate the relationship between the mothers' mental health and the adolescents' self-esteem. Therefore, to improve adolescents' self-esteem in multicultural families, intervention strategies targeting both parental support and immigrant mothers' mental health are essential.

Additionally, the study identified that parental support had a significant impact on adolescents' self-esteem, with variations depending on their level of education and household income. Based on these findings, this study suggests the development of an educational program aimed at mothers with lower education and income levels to support their children both emotionally and educationally.

Author Contributions: Conceptualization, Y.J. and S.J.; methodology, Y.J. and S.J.; software, S.J.; validation, Y.J. and S.J.; formal analysis, Y.J. and S.J.; investigation, Y.J. and S.J.; data curation, S.J.; writing—original draft preparation, Y.J. and S.J.; writing—review and editing, Y.J. and S.J.; visualization, S.J.; supervision, Y.J. and S.J.; project administration, Y.J. and S.J.; funding acquisition, Y.J. All authors have read and agreed to the published version of the manuscript.

Funding: This work was supported by the research promoting grant from the Keimyung University Dongsan Medical Center in 2024.

Institutional Review Board Statement: The study was conducted in accordance with the Declaration of Helsinki and approved by the Institutional Review Board of Keimyung University (40525-202502-HR-105-01 and 14 March 2025, of approval).

Informed Consent Statement: Not applicable.

Data Availability Statement: The data presented in this study are openly available at the National Youth Policy Institute (https://www.nypi.re.kr/archive, accessed on 4 February 2025).

Conflicts of Interest: The authors declare no conflicts of interest.

References

1. Arnett, J.J. A longer road to adulthood. In *Emerging Adulthood: The Winding Road from the Late Teens Through the Twenties*, 3rd ed.; Oxford University Press: New York, NY, USA, 2024; pp. 1–26.
2. Orth, U.; Erol, R.Y.; Luciano, E.C. Development of self-esteem from age 4 to 94 years: A meta-analysis of longitudinal studies. *Psychol. Bull.* **2018**, *144*, 1045–1080. [CrossRef] [PubMed]
3. Gilbert, W.; Eltanoukhi, R.; Morin, A.J.S.; Salmela-Aro, K. Achievement goals as mediators of the links between self-esteem and depressive symptoms from mid-adolescence to early adulthood. *J. Youth Adolesc.* **2025**, *54*, 103–120. [CrossRef] [PubMed]
4. Gurung, U.N.; Sampath, H.; Soohinda, G.; Dutta, S. Self-esteem as a protective factor against adolescent psychopathology in the face of stressful life events. *J. Indian. Assoc. Child. Adolesc. Ment. Health* **2019**, *15*, 34–54. [CrossRef]
5. Orth, U.; Robins, R.W. Is high self-esteem beneficial? Revisiting a classic question. *Am. Psychol.* **2022**, *77*, 5–17. [CrossRef]
6. Bélanger, D.; Lee, H.-K.; Wang, H.-Z. Ethnic diversity and statistics in East Asia: 'foreign brides' surveys in Taiwan and South Korea. *Ethn. Racial Stud.* **2010**, *33*, 1108–1130. [CrossRef]
7. Choi, Y.; Kim, D.-S.; Ryu, J. Marital dissolution of transnational couples in South Korea. *J. Ethn. Migr. Stud.* **2019**, *46*, 3014–3039. [CrossRef]
8. Seol, D.-H. International marriage migration and national identity. *Econ. Soc.* **2014**, *103*, 278–312.
9. Statistics Korea. Status of International Marriages. 2024. Available online: https://www.index.go.kr/unity/potal/main/EachDtlPageDetail.do?idx_cd=2430 (accessed on 11 May 2025).
10. Statistics Korea. Index Nuri e-National Index. Statistics Korea, 2024. Available online: https://www.index.go.kr/unity/potal/main/EachDtlPageDetail.do?idx_cd=2819 (accessed on 17 April 2025).
11. Lim, Y. Relationship between marriage immigrant mothers' acculturative stress and their adolescent children's career decidedness in South Korea: Mediating roles of parenting and school adjustment. *Sustainability* **2021**, *13*, 14066. [CrossRef]
12. Kim, H.; Han, K.; Won, S. Perceived discrimination as a critical factor affecting self-esteem, satisfaction with physical appearance and depression of racial/ethnic minority adolescents in Korea. *Behav. Sci.* **2023**, *13*, 343. [CrossRef]
13. Metzner, F.; Adedeji, A.; Wichmann, M.L.-Y.; Zaheer, Z.; Schneider, L.; Schlachzig, L.; Richters, J.; Heumann, S.; Mays, D. Experiences of discrimination and everyday racism among children and adolescents with an immigrant background—Results of a systematic literature review on the impact of discrimination on the developmental outcomes of minors worldwide. *Front. Psychol.* **2022**, *13*, 805941. [CrossRef]
14. Park, S.J. Educational manager mothers: South Korea's neoliberal transformation. *Korea J.* **2007**, *47*, 186–213. [CrossRef]
15. Yamamoto, Y. East Asian Parenting and Children's Learning and Education. In *Asian Parenting—Meanings, Characteristics, and Implications*; Chen, X., Ed.; Routledge: New York, NY, USA, 2025.
16. Heo, N. "She has the Japanese style": Parenting by Japanese immigrant women in Korea from the perspective of their children. *Int. J. Environ. Res. Public Health* **2022**, *19*, 1494. [CrossRef]
17. Kim, Y. Ideals and realities in the involvement of Filipino immigrant mothers in their children's education in South Korea. *Ethnicities* **2022**, *22*, 84–107. [CrossRef]

18. Lee, A.-R.; Lee, J.; Son, B.Y. A qualitative study on the multi-cultural adolescents'experience of career barrier. *Korean J. Youth Stud.* **2018**, *25*, 35–64. [CrossRef]
19. Harter, S. *Self-Perception Profile for Adolescents: Manual and Questionnaires*; University of Denver, Department of Psychology: Denver, CO, USA, 2012; pp. 1–47.
20. Ahn, J.A.; Kim, T.; Roh, E.H.; Song, J.E. Health of international marriage immigrant women in South Korea: A systematic review. *J. Immigr. Minor. Health* **2018**, *20*, 717–728. [CrossRef]
21. Bapuji, S.B.; Hansen, A.; Marembo, M.H.; Olivier, P.; Yap, M.B.H. Modifiable parental factors associated with the mental health of youth from immigrant families in high-income countries: A systematic review and meta-analysis. *Clin. Psychol. Rev.* **2024**, *110*, 102429. [CrossRef]
22. Lee, Y.; Lee, M.; Park, S. The mental health of ethnic minority youths in South Korea and its related environmental factors: A literature review. *J. Korean Acad. Child Adolesc. Psychiatr.* **2019**, *30*, 88–99. [CrossRef] [PubMed]
23. Iacono, V.; Beaulieu, L.; Hodgins, S.; Ellenbogen, M.A. Parenting practices in middle childhood mediate the relation between growing up with a parent having bipolar disorder and offspring psychopathology from childhood into early adulthood. *Dev. Psychopathol.* **2017**, *30*, 635–649. [CrossRef]
24. Harries, C.I.; Smith, D.M.; Gregg, L.; Wittkowski, A. Parenting and Serious Mental Illness (SMI): A systematic review and metasynthesis. *Clin. Child Fam. Psychol. Rev.* **2023**, *26*, 303–342. [CrossRef]
25. Metz, D.; Jungbauer, J. "My scars remain forever": A qualitative study on biographical developments in adult children of parents with mental illness. *Clin. Soc. Work. J.* **2021**, *49*, 64–76. [CrossRef]
26. Murphy, G.; Peters, K.; Wilkes, L.M.; Jackson, D. Adult children of parents with mental illness: Losing oneself. Who am I? *Issue Ment. Health Nurs.* **2016**, *37*, 668–673. [CrossRef] [PubMed]
27. Murphy, G.; Peters, K.; Wilkes, L.; Jackson, D. Adult children of parents with mental illness: Navigating stigma. *Child. Fam. Soc. Work.* **2015**, *22*, 330–338. [CrossRef]
28. No, B. The impact of acculturative stress of immigrant mothers on children's self-concept development: Double mediating effects of parental efficacy and parental support. *J. Korea Open Assoc. Early Child Edu* **2024**, *29*, 211–233.
29. Hwang, J.G. *Life Satisfaction, Psychological Health, and Physical Health of Korean Adolescents: Psychosocial Formative Factors*; Korean Spiritual Culture Research Institute: Seongnam-si, Republic of Korea, 1997.
30. Cawte, J. *Cruel, Poor and Brutal Nations: Assessment of Mental Health in an Australian Aboriginal Community by Short-Stay Psychiatric Field Team Methods*; University of Hawaii Press: Honolulu, HI, USA, 1972.
31. The National Youth Policy Institute. *Longitudinal Study of Children and Adolescents from Multi-Cultural Families II*; Research Report 11-R07; The National Youth Policy Institute: Seoul, Republic of Korea, 2011. Available online: https://nypi.re.kr/brdrr/boardrrView.do?menu_nix=4o9771b7&brd_id=BDIDX_PJk7xvf7L096m1g7Phd3YC&cont_idx=317&seltab_idx=0&edomweivgp=R (accessed on 10 May 2025).
32. Park, G.S. The Effects of Acculturative Stress on the Physical and Psychological Health of Marriage Migrant Women—Focusing on the Mediating Effect of Self-Esteem. Ph.D. dissertation, Incheon National University, Incheon, Republic of Korea, 2024.
33. Kim, U.C.; Park, Y.S. Psychological and behavioral pattern of Korean adolescents: With specific focus on the influence of friends, family, and school. *Korean J. Edu Psychol.* **1999**, *13*, 99–142.
34. Hwang, H.B.; Joo, E.S. The effect of parental support on achievement motivation of multicultural youth: Focusing on the mediating effects of national identity and self-esteem. *Welf. Cult. Divers. Stud.* **2023**, *5*, 79–102. [CrossRef]
35. Rogenberg, M. *Society and the Adolescent Self-Image*; Princeton University Press: Princeton, NJ, USA, 1965.
36. Lee, J.T.; Yoo, S.H. The effect of physical and psychological health awareness of married migrant women on adolescents' self-esteem: Focusing on the mediating effect of parental parenting attitudes. *Korean J. Youth Stud.* **2023**, *30*, 291–316. [CrossRef]
37. Baron, R.M.; Kenny, D.A. The moderator-mediator variable distinction in social psychological research: Conceptual, strategic, and statistical considerations. *J. Personal. Soc. Psychol.* **1986**, *51*, 1173–1182. [CrossRef]
38. OECD. *Parental Emotional Support and Adolescent Well-Being: A Cross-National Examination of Socio-Economic and Gender Gaps Based on PISA 2018 Surveys, OECD Papers on Well-Being and Inequalities, No. 20*; OECD Publishing: Paris, France, 2024. Available online: https://www.oecd.org/en/publications/parental-emotional-support-and-adolescent-well-being_2b7a2ac6-en.html (accessed on 11 April 2025).
39. Ayoub, M.; Bachir, M. A meta-analysis of the relations between socioeconomic status and parenting practices. *Psychol. Rep.* **2023**, 1–25. [CrossRef]
40. Barzoki, M.H.; Kiviruusu, O.; Skogberg, N. Self-esteem at the intersection of sex, SES, and immigrant origin. *Curr. Psychol.* **2025**, *44*, 4658–4668. [CrossRef]
41. Um, Y.-J. The relationship between bicultural acceptance attitude and self-esteem among multicultural adolescents: The mediating effects of parental support. *Int. J. Environ. Res. Public Health* **2024**, *21*, 1175. [CrossRef]
42. Gil, P.H.C.; Peixoto, C.D.S.; Piccinini, C.A.; Pizzinato, A. Parental stress associated with international migration processes: A systematic review. *Univ. Psychol.* **2024**, *22*, 1–14.

43. Cooper, K.; Stewart, K. Does household income affect children's outcomes? A systematic review of the evidence. *Child Indic. Res.* **2021**, *14*, 981–1005. [CrossRef]
44. Statistics Korea. Trend of Standard Median Income. 2025. Available online: https://www.index.go.kr/unity/potal/main/EachDtlPageDetail.do?idx_cd=2762 (accessed on 15 May 2025).
45. Carlén, K.; Suominen, S.; Augustine, L. The association between adolescents' self-esteem and perceived mental well-being in Sweden in four years of follow-up. *BMC Psychol.* **2023**, *11*, 413. [CrossRef] [PubMed]
46. Gaur, D.; Gupta, S. The impact of parental support on adolescent's emotional intelligence and self-esteem: A comprehensive literature review. *Int. J. Psychol. Res.* **2024**, *6*, 65–68. [CrossRef]
47. Krauss, S.; Orth, U.; Robins, R.W. Family environment and self-esteem development: A longitudinal study from age 10 to 16. *J. Personal. Soc. Psychol.* **2020**, *119*, 457–478. [CrossRef]

children

MDPI

Review

Emotion and Feeling in Parent–Child Dyads: Neurocognitive and Psychophysiological Pathways of Development

Antonios I. Christou [1,*] and Flora Bacopoulou [2]

[1] Department of Special Education, University of Thessaly, 38221 Volos, Greece
[2] Clinic for Assessment of Adolescent Learning Difficulties, Center for Adolescent Medicine and UNESCO Chair in Adolescent Health Care, First Department of Pediatrics, Medical School, National and Kapodistrian University of Athens, 11527 Athens, Greece; fbacopoulou@med.uoa.gr
* Correspondence: antchristou@uth.gr

Abstract

Although widely used across disciplines, the terms emotion and feeling remain conceptually ambiguous, particularly within developmental science. Emotion is defined as an evolutionarily conserved, biologically embedded system of action readiness and intersubjective communication, shaped by attentional, neural, and physiological reactivity to environmental salience. In contrast, feeling is conceptualized as the consciously experienced, representational outcome of emotional activation, emerging through cognitive appraisal and symbolic processing. Building upon this distinction, the review explores how emotion develops within parent–child dyads through coregulated neurocognitive and psychophysiological mechanisms. Drawing on empirical evidence from eye-tracking studies of visual attention to emotional faces, functional near-infrared spectroscopy (fNIRS) research on social-emotional activation in prefrontal brain regions, and cortisol-based assessments of hormonal synchrony, the paper highlights how emotional attunement and transmission are embedded in early caregiving interactions. The review also emphasizes the moderating role of environmental sensitivity—both in children and parents—in shaping these developmental pathways. By positioning emotion as a dynamic, intersubjective process and feeling as its emergent experiential correlate, this review offers a novel developmental framework for understanding affect and proposes directions for future research on resilience, dysregulation, and intervention.

Keywords: emotion; feeling; parent–child dyads; emotion transmission; environmental sensitivity; emotion regulation; synchrony; developmental neuroscience; psychophysiology

1. Introduction

Emotional development is often complicated by ambiguity in distinguishing 'emotion' from 'feeling,' which are frequently conflated despite being theoretically distinct. Although often used interchangeably, these constructs represent interdependent but distinct processes. Emotion can be conceptualized as an evolutionarily conserved system of action readiness and intersubjective communication, whereas feeling refers to the consciously experienced, representational correlate of emotional activation shaped through appraisal and symbolic processing [1,2]. Clarifying this distinction provides a foundation for tracing how affect is transmitted, regulated, and internalized during child development.

Foundational theories highlight different dimensions of emotion. LeDoux described subcortical circuits that enable rapid survival-oriented responses, positioning emotions

https://doi.org/10.3390/children12111478

as biologically primitive mechanisms [3]. Barrett's theory of constructed emotion, by contrast, emphasized the predictive role of cortical appraisal and conceptual knowledge in shaping differentiated feelings [4]. Tronick's dyadic expansion of consciousness framework extended these debates into the relational domain, underscoring how emotions are co-created through caregiver–infant exchanges [5]. Collectively, these perspectives emphasize the need to integrate biological, cognitive, and relational views of emotional development.

Although the terms "emotion" and "feeling" are often used interchangeably in developmental science, multiple theoretical frameworks emphasize their distinction. Classic and contemporary accounts converge in viewing emotion as an embodied, psychophysiological response to salient stimuli, and feeling as the conscious, subjective awareness of those responses [6–11]. To ensure terminological clarity, Table 1 summarizes the definitional differences between emotion and feeling across neural basis, consciousness, temporal unfolding, measurement, and developmental considerations, drawing on both foundational and recent perspectives.

Table 1. Definitional distinctions between emotion and feeling based on classic and recent theories.

Feature	Emotion	Feeling
Core definition	A rapid, coordinated psychophysiological response to a salient stimulus, encompassing autonomic, hormonal, and behavioral reactions [3,12].	The conscious, subjective experience of an emotional state—the introspective awareness of bodily and neural changes [6–8].
Neural basis	Largely subcortical circuits, including amygdala, hypothalamus, and brainstem, supporting fast survival-oriented responses [9].	Cortical integration of interoceptive and bodily signals in the insula, anterior cingulate, and prefrontal cortices, enabling conscious awareness [8,10].
Consciousness	Can occur outside awareness; emotions involve automatic and unconscious bodily reactions [3,4].	By definition conscious; feelings are the subjective experience of emotion [6,9].
Temporal dynamics	Rapid-onset, short-lived responses aligned with external stimuli, often emerging within milliseconds [3].	Slower to arise, requiring cortical processing, and can persist over time through conscious awareness and reflection [8,13].
Measurement	Inferred from observable indices such as facial/vocal expressions, psychophysiological responses (heart rate, cortisol, fMRI, EEG), and behavior [12].	Primarily assessed via self-report, interviews, or rating scales reflecting subjective experience [4,13].
Ontogeny/Evolution	Emerges early in development and is evolutionarily ancient; even infants and animals display basic emotional responses [3,12].	Develops later with higher cognition, language, and self-awareness; refinement of reported feelings increases across childhood and adolescence [6,14].

Distinguishing Emotion and Feeling: Contemporary Perspectives

Beyond the foundational views of LeDoux, several contemporary frameworks in affective neuroscience and developmental psychology further clarify the emotion–feeling distinction. Neurobiological models such as Damasio's somatic framework define emotions as complex "action programs"—bodily and neural responses triggered by salient stimuli to maintain homeostatic balance—whereas feelings are the conscious mental representations that arise when the brain interprets those bodily changes. In this view, encountering a threat elicits an automatic emotional response (e.g., autonomic arousal, fight-or-flight behavior), and the subjective feeling of fear emerges only when cortical networks integrate the physiological changes into a coherent conscious experience [6,7]. Likewise, affective neuroscience research (e.g., Panksepp's theory) distinguishes between evolutionarily "primary-process" emotions, which are generated by subcortical circuits and can operate without cortical input, and higher-order feelings that depend on cortical representation and self-awareness [15]. For example, decorticate animal studies and cases of human infants with minimal cortex demonstrate that basic emotional reactions (crying in distress, laughter in joy) are present even in the absence of full conscious awareness [15]. These findings suggest that core emotional processes are "built-in" subcortical functions, whereas feelings require additional integrative processes in the brain's cortex to become subjectively accessible.

Developmental perspectives similarly emphasize that emotions precede feelings in ontogeny. Infants express basic affective states from early in life (e.g., crying when distressed, smiling when pleased), but these raw emotions are initially not accompanied by reflective awareness. Only with the gradual maturation of cognitive capacities—such as self-recognition, memory, and language—do feelings (in the sense of conscious, representational experiences of emotion) begin to emerge. Developmental researchers note that while basic emotions like joy, anger, and fear appear within the first year of life, the second year marks a critical transition when toddlers gain self-awareness and symbolic thinking, enabling the first self-conscious feelings to manifest. For instance, classic observations indicate that emotions linked to self-reflection—embarrassment, empathy, pride, shame—only become evident around 15–24 months of age, once children can mentally represent themselves and their internal states. In line with this, contemporary developmental psychology frameworks (e.g., Sroufe's organizational theory) propose that early emotional reactions gradually differentiate into more complex feelings as the child's neural and cognitive systems mature [16]. Collectively, these perspectives converge in portraying emotion as an evolutionarily ancient, automatic and embodied response system, and feeling as its later-developing, conscious and interpretive counterpart. Emotion can thus occur without feeling (e.g., an infant's startle or a conditioned fear response may activate even if the child cannot yet conceptualize "being afraid"), whereas feeling represents the conscious "story" the mind constructs about those emotion signals. Integrating these viewpoints—from Damasio's neurobiological model to Panksepp's cross-species findings and developmental evidence on when children first experience feelings—underscores that emotion and feeling, though deeply interrelated, operate at distinct levels of processing (automatic bodily reaction vs. reflective experiential insight). Recognizing this distinction provides a richer theoretical foundation for examining how parent–child interactions scaffold the progression from raw emotion to organized feeling in development.

Parent–child dyads are now recognized as the primary ecological context within which emotions are scaffolded into coherent feelings. Infants rely on caregivers' facial expressions, vocal prosody, and touch for regulating arousal and assigning meaning to affective states [17]. Attachment theory provides a foundation for understanding this process, showing that secure early relationships facilitate emotion regulation and the internalization of coherent affective states, whereas insecure attachments heighten vulnerability to dysregulation [18–20]. Beyond attachment theory, early relationships can also be conceptualized through an object relations developmental perspective, which focuses on how internalized representations of the caregiver shape the infant's emerging emotional life. As Ainsworth [21] noted, the infant–mother relationship involves both dependency and the gradual organization of object relations, through which the caregiver's consistent responsiveness provides a template for emotional regulation and security. Within this view, the intersubjective experience of early dyadic exchanges—characterized by affective attunement, containment, and repair—forms the experiential matrix from which emotional expression and later feeling states emerge. These early interactions allow the infant to transform raw physiological arousal into organized affective meaning, strengthening the parent–child bond and laying the groundwork for coherent emotional self-representation.

Importantly, caregivers' own mental health—such as maternal depression—can disrupt sensitive attunement and pose additional risk for child emotional dysregulation. The developmental bridge from emotion to feeling is forged within dyadic exchanges. Caregivers help regulate arousal, direct attention, and provide labels and narratives that confer meaning on otherwise raw physiological signals. Micro-analytic studies show that affect is co-constructed through moment-to-moment cycles of attunement, mismatch, and repair; successful repair predicts greater coherence in children's subsequent emotional experience [22]. Attachment theory extends this view: secure relationships offer a "safe haven" and "secure base" that support integration of arousal into organized, self-relevant feeling states, whereas inconsistent, intrusive, or neglectful care undermines modulation and leaves emotions unrepresented or dysregulated [23,24].

From a neurobiological perspective, emotions recruit conserved circuits that orchestrate autonomic, behavioral, and attentional responses, enabling fast adaptation to threat, novelty, or reward. Contemporary models emphasize rapid subcortical pathways that permit swift detection and motor preparation prior to, or independent from, reflective awareness [25]. At the same time, predictive and inferential processes shape how bodily states are categorized and used to guide behavior, highlighting the interactive layering of bottom-up reactivity with top-down expectations [26]. In early development, these functions are evident in cries, smiles, and gaze shifts that signal needs, elicit caregiving, and organize proto-conversations, thereby establishing a communicative platform on which later socioemotional competencies are built [27,28].

Feelings, by contrast, involve the conscious registration and interpretation of affective states. They emerge when interoceptive changes are integrated with memory, language, and conceptual knowledge to produce a subjectively accessible representation of "what it is like" to be in a particular state. Classic neurocognitive accounts propose that feelings arise as somatic changes are mapped onto cortical representations, supporting awareness and reportability of affect [29]. This distinction explains why emotions may occur without conscious recognition (e.g., rapid orienting to threat), whereas feelings require representational capacity, reflective access, and often linguistic scaffolding [30]. Because meaning systems vary across sociocultural contexts, feelings are also culturally shaped—constructed within the emotion concepts and norms available to the child [31].

In this review, emotion is framed as a biologically embedded system of action readiness—rapid, largely automatic, and tuned to environmental salience—whereas feeling denotes the consciously experienced, representational outcome of such activation, constructed through appraisal and symbolic processing [30,31]. In this view, the child's movement from automatic reactivity to conscious feeling is a relational achievement, built through repeated co-regulated encounters that align attention, brain activity, and physiology with language and meaning.

The aim of this review is to provide a developmental framework that distinguishes emotion as an embodied, evolutionarily conserved process and feeling as its consciously experienced correlate, while situating both within parent–child dyads. Evidence is synthesized across multiple modalities: (a) attentional synchrony captured via eye-tracking, (b) neural synchrony examined with hyperscanning methods, and (c) hormonal synchrony assessed through cortisol coupling. By integrating these domains, the review positions emotional development not as an isolated individual process but as an emergent property of dynamic, multilevel caregiver–child interactions. Finally, the review emphasizes the importance of cultural and contextual influences. Cross-cultural research indicates that parental beliefs, caregiving practices, and sociocultural scripts shape how emotions are expressed and scaffolded into feelings [31]. Interventions designed to foster emotional attunement therefore require attention to both individual neurobiological sensitivity and broader sociocultural contexts. Through this synthesis, the review contributes theoretical clarity and outlines future directions for research on resilience, dysregulation, and clinical intervention.

2. Methodological Approach

A comprehensive literature search was conducted to identify peer-reviewed studies that examined the conceptual, neurocognitive, and psychophysiological bases of emotion and feeling within developmental contexts, with particular attention to parent–child dyads. Searches were performed in PubMed, Scopus, PsycINFO, and Web of Science covering the period from January 2000 to June 2025. Search terms combined free-text keywords and Medical Subject Headings (MeSH) related to emotion, feeling, parent–child dyads, synchrony, eye-tracking, functional near-infrared spectroscopy (fNIRS), cortisol, environmental sensitivity, and developmental neuroscience. An example PubMed search string was:

("emotion" OR "affect" OR "feeling") AND ("parent–child dyad" OR "synchrony" OR "attachment") AND ("neurocognitive" OR "neurobiological" OR "psychophysiology") AND ("development" OR "child" OR "infant").

Reference lists of relevant systematic reviews and meta-analyses were also hand-searched to capture additional eligible studies [32,33]. Studies were included if they (a) involved child or adolescent participants up to 18 years of age, (b) reported empirical findings on emotional, neurocognitive, or psychophysiological outcomes in the context of parent–child interactions, and (c) were peer-reviewed and published in English. Exclusion criteria were case reports, editorials, conference abstracts, and studies focused solely on adult populations or purely biomedical outcomes without affective components.

Given the diversity of study designs, methodologies, and outcome measures, a narrative synthesis approach was employed rather than a quantitative meta-analysis. This strategy enabled integration across heterogeneous sources of evidence, ranging from neuroimaging and eye-tracking studies to psychophysiological measures such as cortisol synchrony. Findings were grouped according to key mechanistic domains, including attentional biases and visual scanning, neural coupling and cortical activation, and hormonal and autonomic synchrony. These domains were further embedded within relational frameworks such as attachment theory [34], dyadic regulation models [35], and predictive processing accounts of emotion [36,37].

Parent–child synchrony is shaped not only by biology and individual differences but also by the cultural contexts in which dyads develop. In collectivist societies, caregiving often emphasizes relational harmony, interdependence, and emotional restraint, whereas in individualist contexts, parents may encourage overt expression and autonomous self-regulation. For instance, a recent study comparing Palestinian-Arab (collectivist) and Jewish (more individualist) mother–infant dyads within Israel found that Arab mothers engaged in greater physical proximity and calming behaviors, while Jewish mothers engaged in more face-to-face play and active vocalization. Despite these differences in interactional style, infants in both groups demonstrated effective emotion regulation and secure attachment, suggesting that diverse caregiving strategies can achieve functionally equivalent socioemotional outcomes.

Cultural values also shape how "feelings" are conceptualized and labeled. In some East Asian contexts, feelings are construed relationally (e.g., maintaining group harmony), whereas in Western contexts they are often understood as internal, individualized states. Such differences mean that the trajectory from emotion (automatic physiological and behavioral responses) to feeling (conscious representation) may follow distinct cultural pathways. Over-representation of WEIRD (Western, Educated, Industrialized, Rich, Democratic) samples in synchrony research risks obscuring this variability. Greater cross-cultural research is needed to test whether existing models of dyadic synchrony and emotion–feeling transformation generalize beyond Western contexts, or whether multiple culturally specific routes to healthy emotional development exist.

While the literature reviewed is extensive, several methodological limitations remain. There is considerable heterogeneity in tasks, measurement tools, and cultural contexts, which constrains comparability across studies. Many investigations rely on small sample sizes or focus on specific populations (e.g., children at risk for psychopathology, children with neurodevelopmental disorders), limiting generalizability. Furthermore, cross-sectional designs dominate the field, leaving the developmental trajectories of emotion–feeling distinctions underexplored. These gaps highlight the need for harmonized, longitudinal, and cross-cultural research approaches that can more robustly capture how dyadic processes shape the emergence of emotional experience and conscious feeling across the lifespan [38–41].

In line with a narrative (qualitative) review approach, we broadly surveyed the literature rather than performing a formal meta-analysis. To increase transparency, we provide an overview of the scope of the literature search and synthesis. The initial database searches (across PubMed, Scopus, PsycINFO, and Web of Science for 2000–2025) yielded approximately 600–650 unique articles after removing duplicates. Titles and abstracts were screened for relevance to the topics of emotion, feeling, and parent–child developmental processes, resulting in roughly 150 articles retained for more detailed evaluation. Of these, about 70–80 studies met our inclusion criteria and were ultimately included in the narrative synthesis. These included empirical research spanning modalities (e.g., behavioral observations, eye-tracking, neuroimaging, hormonal assays) as well as theoretical and review papers that informed our conceptual framework. We emphasize that these figures are approximate, as is typical in narrative reviews, which do not adhere to the rigid counting of a systematic review. Nonetheless, providing this range offers readers a sense of the evidence base: on the order of a few hundred studies were surveyed, with a few dozen key sources integrated into our analysis. This narrative synthesis approach allowed us to integrate heterogeneous evidence and draw connections across studies without the constraints of a single quantitative metric. By qualitatively summarizing convergent findings (rather than statistically aggregating them), we aimed to capture the richness of research on parent–child emotional dynamics. Still, we acknowledge potential biases inherent in narrative reviews—for example, the possibility of overlooking some studies or weighting illustrative findings—and thus we strove for comprehensive coverage by hand-searching reference lists and including multiple theoretical perspectives. The estimated numbers of identified, screened, and included articles above further clarify the scope of our review process and enhance the methodological transparency of this work.

To further illustrate the study selection process and align with current reporting expectations, we have included a PRISMA-style flow diagram (Figure 1) summarizing the identification, screening, and inclusion of studies. While our approach is a narrative review rather than a formal systematic review, including this figure provides a clear overview of how studies were identified and selected. The flow chart outlines the number of records identified through database searches, the number remaining after screening and eligibility assessments, and the final set of studies included in the synthesis. Presenting the study flow in this familiar format is intended to enhance methodological transparency and demonstrate the rigor of the review process, even within a qualitative narrative framework.

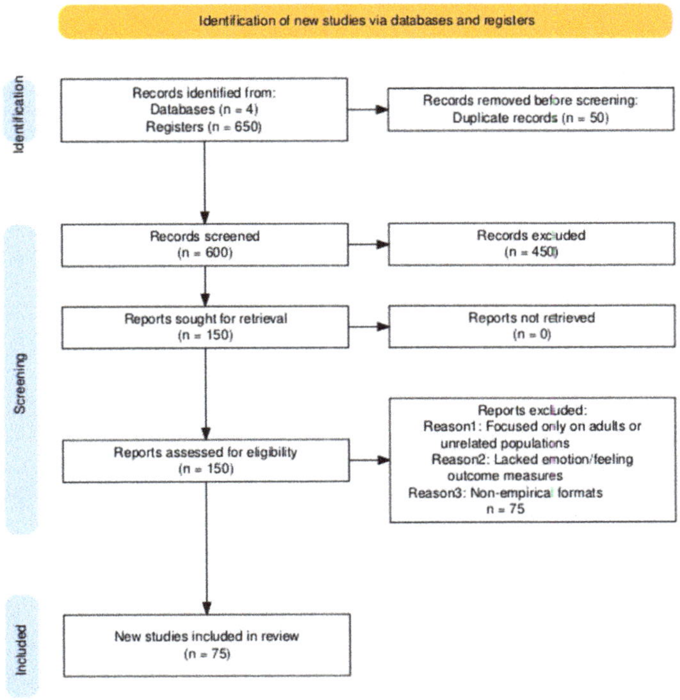

Figure 1. PRISMA-style flow diagram of study selection.

3. Mechanisms of Dyadic Emotion Development

Parent–child dyads provide one of the earliest and most formative contexts in which emotion is scaffolded, regulated, and transmitted. Advances in developmental neuroscience and psychophysiology have enabled increasingly fine-grained accounts of how emotional attunement operates at multiple levels of analysis, from eye gaze to cortical activation to hormonal synchrony. This section synthesizes evidence across these domains, highlighting the multi-layered nature of dyadic emotion development.

3.1. *Attentional Biases and Visual Scanning*

Visual attention plays a central role in the early organization of emotion. Eye-tracking studies have consistently demonstrated that children display selective attentional biases to emotionally salient faces, particularly those expressing anger or fear [42,43]. These biases are not merely intrapersonal phenomena but unfold in the interactive space of the dyad. Parents' attentional patterns shape and moderate how children orient to emotional cues, and congruency in parent–child gaze patterns predicts higher levels of affective attunement. Shared visual focus functions as a pathway of intersubjective communication and provides opportunities for emotion coaching [44,45].

Research by Pérez-Edgar and colleagues has been pivotal in documenting how early attentional biases emerge in infancy and contribute to trajectories of socioemotional functioning. For instance, infants at risk for behavioral inhibition display heightened vigilance to threat-related stimuli, with such attentional tendencies predicting later social withdrawal and anxiety [46,47]. Moreover, these attentional patterns are not fixed but embedded within the broader dyadic system. Quiñones-Camacho et al. emphasize that parent-to-child anxiety transmission unfolds through dynamic social interactions in which parental attention, affective responses, and regulatory strategies shape children's emerging vigilance to threat [48]. From this perspective, attentional coordination between parent and child is one of the central pathways through which emotional dispositions are transmitted intergenerationally.

Recent longitudinal evidence further highlights the bidirectional nature of these processes. Vallorani et al. demonstrated that across the first 24 months of life, infants' temperamental negative affect, maternal anxiety symptoms, and infants' affect-biased attention are dynamically linked [49]. Infant negative affect predicts heightened threat vigilance, which in turn interacts with maternal anxiety to reinforce maladaptive attentional styles, whereas sensitive maternal regulation can attenuate such risk. These findings underscore that the congruence between parent and child gaze does not simply reflect shared focus but constitutes a training ground for attentional flexibility.

Parental sensory processing sensitivity may further amplify these dynamics: highly sensitive parents tend to attune more closely to their children's scanning of negative affective cues, creating additional opportunities for emotional scaffolding and adaptive attention deployment [50]. Conversely, disruptions in attentional alignment—such as reduced parental responsiveness in depression or reinforcement of vigilance in anxious caregiving contexts—may limit opportunities for reciprocal regulation and heighten children's risk for developing rigid attentional biases and anxiety-related psychopathology.

Recent studies further extend this evidence base. Aktar et al. [51] showed that even in infancy, parent–child dyads exhibit positively correlated attentional biases to emotional expressions, with both parents and infants orienting preferentially to fearful faces. Importantly, such alignment emerged even in low-risk families, suggesting that attentional synchrony is a fundamental feature of early dyadic interaction rather than only a marker of risk. In contrast, a 2024 eye-tracking study found that children of mothers with a history of depression displayed faster detection and longer dwell times for sad faces compared to controls, pointing to early attentional biases that may represent prodromal markers of affective vulnerability [52]. Taken together, these findings indicate that while parent–child attentional congruence can scaffold adaptive attention deployment and emotion understanding, it may also, in adverse contexts, reinforce maladaptive vigilance to negative cues.

Crucially, these findings also inform the distinction between emotion and feeling. The attentional coordination that characterizes early dyadic exchanges reflects the operation of emotion as a biologically embedded, intersubjective system of orienting to environmental salience. By contrast, the child's later ability to consciously represent and interpret these affective encounters—as facilitated by parental scaffolding—marks the developmental emergence of feeling. Thus, research on attentional biases and parent–child gaze synchrony demonstrates how emotion initially manifests as shared, embodied orientation processes within dyads, and how the scaffolding of these attentional dynamics provides the experiential substrate from which subjective feeling states are eventually constructed.

3.2. Neural Coupling and Cortical Activation

Beyond attentional processes, parent–child dyads exhibit patterns of neural synchrony that support emotion regulation. Hyperscanning techniques such as functional near-infrared spectroscopy (fNIRS) and EEG hyperscanning have shown correlated prefrontal activation during joint tasks or affectively charged exchanges [53]. Such cortical coupling is not merely epiphenomenal: it has been linked to more adaptive emotion regulation, enhanced perspective-taking, and greater child social competence. For example, synchrony in the medial prefrontal cortex is associated with more effective parental scaffolding, reduced child distress in challenging contexts, and greater readiness to engage in cooperative problem solving [54].

Recent studies further underscore these associations. A longitudinal fNIRS study by Quiñones-Camacho et al. [48] demonstrated that higher parent–child neural synchrony in prefrontal regions during positive play predicted a faster decline in children's internalizing symptoms over 1.5 years, suggesting that neural attunement serves a protective, resilience-building role. Similarly, Liu et al. [55] found that mothers generally exhibited stronger brain-to-brain synchrony with their 3–4-year-old children than fathers, particularly during shared activities such as joint video viewing. Importantly, both maternal and paternal synchrony decreased under conditions of high parenting stress, highlighting stress as a potential disruptor of neural attunement. These findings extend earlier work by showing that neural synchrony is sensitive not only to task context but also to caregiver well-being, and that it functions as a mechanism of resilience in supporting child socioemotional outcomes.

These results are consistent with predictive processing accounts of dyadic interaction [55]. From this perspective, parent and child continuously update internal models of the other's emotional states, minimizing prediction errors via bi-directional neural signaling. Neural coupling thus provides a mechanism by which children learn to anticipate, interpret, and regulate affective states through live feedback with a caregiver. Reduced neural synchrony has been observed in dyads involving parents with psychopathology, highlighting the vulnerability of these mechanisms under stress.

In the context of this review's central distinction, neural synchrony exemplifies emotion as an embodied, biologically instantiated process of intersubjective regulation. Shared cortical activation reflects the dynamic calibration of parent and child to one another's affective states, forming the scaffolding for emotion as an action-oriented, communicative system. Over time, the repeated experience of such coupled neural states contributes to the child's capacity to generate symbolic representations of affect—marking the emergence of feeling as the consciously experienced correlate of these dyadic exchanges. Thus, neural coupling represents both the mechanism through which emotions are co-regulated in real time and the developmental substrate from which children learn to consciously experience, label, and reflect upon their inner affective states.

3.3. Hormonal and Autonomic Synchrony

Physiological coupling provides another channel of emotional coregulation. Cortisol synchrony between parents and children has been consistently observed, particularly under conditions of stress, novelty, or emotional challenge [56–58]. Such biological linkage functions as a mechanism of affect transmission: when parents regulate their stress response effectively, children's reactivity is buffered. Conversely, heightened or dysregulated parental cortisol responses may potentiate child stress and anxiety.

Recent work has nuanced this picture. Xu et al. [59] reported that the developmental impact of cortisol synchrony depends heavily on interactional context: synchrony predicted better child socioemotional adjustment under supportive, low-stress conditions, but showed diminished benefits in unsupportive environments. Similarly, Fleck et al. [60] (2023) found that in mother–adolescent dyads characterized by harmonious interaction, positive cortisol concordance was observed, whereas in high-conflict dyads or when adolescents exhibited borderline traits, synchrony was disrupted or negative. These findings highlight that cortisol alignment is not uniformly adaptive; rather, its meaning depends on whether it occurs in a regulatory or dysregulated caregiving context.

Autonomic indices further illustrate this biobehavioral attunement. Heart rate variability (HRV) synchrony, particularly vagal coupling, has been linked to effective co-regulation during emotionally demanding interactions, with higher synchrony supporting resilience and adaptive soothing [61]. Newer studies emphasize that vagal synchrony operates as a dynamic indicator of dyadic attunement. For example, high parent–child vagal synchrony has been associated with stronger child emotion regulation capacity and lower anxiety symptoms [62]. Conversely, disruptions in these processes—such as in contexts of maltreatment, inconsistent caregiving, or parental psychopathology—are associated with poorer physiological regulation and increased risk for psychopathology in children [63].

These findings underscore that physiological synchrony is both a marker and a mechanism of dyadic emotional functioning, mediating the pathway from caregiving quality to child developmental outcomes. They also reinforce that synchrony is context-dependent: in nurturing relationships, it provides a visceral sense of safety and scaffolds resilience, whereas in adverse contexts, it can transmit distress and dysregulation.

Framed within this review's central conceptual distinction, hormonal and autonomic synchrony highlight emotion as a biological system of action readiness and intersubjective communication. Shared fluctuations in cortisol and vagal tone embody emotion's role as an evolutionarily conserved process that organizes responses to environmental salience and transmits affective states across dyads. Over developmental time, the child's repeated experience of these regulated physiological states, scaffolded by the parent, provides the somatic foundation from which feeling emerges as the conscious awareness of being soothed, distressed, or emotionally aroused. In this sense, physiological synchrony bridges the implicit bodily processes of emotion with the explicit subjective representations that constitute feeling, anchoring the experiential core of affective life in the parent–child relationship.

3.4. Integrative Dyadic Regulation Frameworks

The convergence of attentional, neural, and physiological synchrony supports broader theoretical accounts of dyadic regulation. Attachment theory has long emphasized the role of sensitive responsiveness in shaping secure emotional bonds and long-term socioemotional outcomes [63]. Tronick's Mutual Regulation Model further highlights the inevitability of ruptures in dyadic attunement and the developmental importance of repair processes in fostering resilience and trust [64,65]. Feldman's biobehavioral synchrony framework [66] extends these ideas by positing that moment-to-moment coordination across behavioral, neural, and physiological domains forms the basis for long-term adaptation. In parallel, environmental sensitivity (ES) models [67] add a complementary ecological layer, emphasizing that children differ in their susceptibility to environmental influences and that the quality of dyadic synchrony can amplify or buffer developmental trajectories. From this perspective, highly sensitive children are more strongly shaped by both supportive and adverse caregiving conditions, whereas less sensitive children may be less affected by contextual variation. ES models therefore situate dyadic processes within broader relational and sociocultural contexts, highlighting how individual differences in biological reactivity interact with parental scaffolding to shape emotion–feeling transformations.

To integrate the reviewed evidence, we propose a conceptual model (Figure 2) that maps the interplay between emotion and feeling in parent–child dyads. Emotion is depicted as embodied, implicit processes of synchrony, encompassing attentional, neural, and physiological coordination. Through dyadic scaffolding, these implicit processes are gradually transformed into explicit forms of feeling, reflected in meaning-making, reflective awareness, and subjective experience. Each level of synchrony contributes to specific developmental outcomes: attentional synchrony supports selective attention, emotion recognition, and early regulatory strategies; neural synchrony facilitates cognitive flexibility, perspective-taking, and social cognition; and physiological synchrony underpins affective resilience, empathic responding, and vulnerability to psychopathology. By embedding these mechanisms within the broader parent–child context of attachment, mutual regulation, biobehavioral synchrony, environmental sensitivity, and culture, the model highlights how early intersubjective dynamics channel developmental trajectories toward adaptive or maladaptive outcomes.

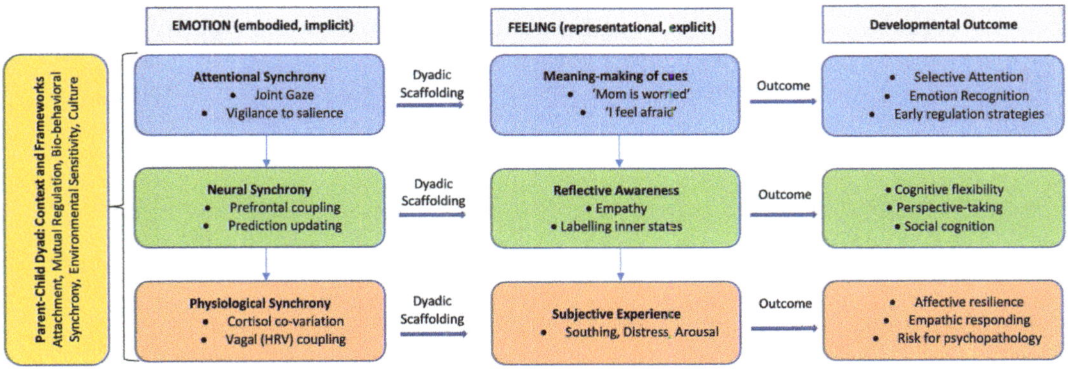

Figure 2. Conceptual model of how emotion (embodied, implicit) and feeling (representational, explicit) interact within parent–child dyads to shape developmental outcomes.

When viewed through the distinction between emotion and feeling, these integrative models illustrate a developmental sequence. At the attentional level, joint gaze and shared vigilance toward emotional cues reveal emotion as a system of orienting and intersubjective signaling; over time, children's internalization of these attentional patterns provides the groundwork for feelings as consciously accessible interpretations of those experiences. At the neural level, cortical coupling embodies emotion as a real-time, embodied process of co-regulation, while recurrent alignment of neural states supports the representational capacities that enable feelings of understanding, empathy, and self-awareness. At the physiological level, cortisol and vagal synchrony illustrate emotion as a biological readiness system, while repeated co-regulation of bodily states fosters the subjective recognition of being soothed or distressed—experiential correlates that constitute feeling.

While attachment, mutual regulation, and bio-behavioral synchrony provide universal frameworks for understanding how dyadic processes scaffold emotional development, environmental sensitivity frameworks highlight that children and parents differ systematically in their susceptibility to these processes. Emerging evidence suggests that such variability—captured in traits like sensory processing sensitivity, callous–unemotional tendencies, and neurodevelopmental profiles—modulates how the transformation from emotion to feeling unfolds. This rationale motivates a closer focus on individual differences in the following section.

4. Individual Differences and Environmental Sensitivity

Although atypical pathways are central to this review, it is equally important to outline normative trajectories of emotion and feeling. Research in developmental psychology and neuroscience shows that even in typically developing children, the capacity to experience, express, and regulate emotions undergoes rapid maturation in the first years of life [16,18,19]. From birth, infants display basic affective responses—distress when uncomfortable and pleasure when soothed—which act as biologically primed signals eliciting caregiving and serving adaptive functions [17]. During the first year, these undifferentiated states become increasingly organized: infants begin to show joy, surprise, anger, and fear, with wariness toward strangers emerging around 6–10 months, marking the transition from diffuse distress/excitement to discrete emotions [16].

By toddlerhood and preschool, children's emotional repertoires expand considerably. The emergence of self-conscious emotions such as embarrassment, empathy, shame, and pride reflects the development of self-awareness, while growing language skills allow children to name and communicate feelings in simple terms [16,18]. By the end of the preschool years, most can anticipate others' emotional reactions and use basic strategies—verbal labeling, seeking comfort, or covering their eyes—to manage fear or frustration. These advances parallel brain maturation, as increasing connectivity among prefrontal, limbic, and associative networks supports greater integration of emotion and cognition [25–27]

Caregiver–child interactions are critical to this progression. Sensitive and consistent caregiving provides external regulation in infancy, helping organize physiological arousal into coherent feeling states [17,18]. Through cycles of attunement, mismatch, and repair, children gradually internalize regulatory strategies and, by early childhood, those with warm, responsive caregiving typically display greater resilience and self-regulation [22–24]. Conversely, less attuned or inconsistent caregiving may complicate modulation of emotions, though normative milestones are generally achieved.

Individual differences temper these processes. Temperament traits evident from infancy shape how emotions are expressed and scaffolded: "easy" infants may regulate with minimal support, whereas more reactive or sensitive infants require greater caregiver involvement [16]. Such variability underscores that multiple healthy pathways exist and that there is no single trajectory of emotional development. What remains consistent, however, is that the first five years represent a critical period in which children move from reflexive, caregiver-managed states to increasingly autonomous and differentiated feelings. By school entry, most can identify basic feelings, empathize with peers, and verbalize experiences such as pride, guilt, or fear—laying the foundation for more complex emotional understanding in later childhood and adolescence [16,18,19].

Although dyadic synchrony provides a powerful scaffold for emotional development, not all children and parents engage with these mechanisms in the same way. Individual differences in temperament, neurocognitive profiles, and broader environmental sensitivity significantly shape how emotional exchanges are experienced and transmitted. This section highlights three key domains of variation: sensory processing sensitivity, callous–unemotional traits, and neurodevelopmental conditions, each of which can moderate the dynamics of parent–child emotional attunement.

4.1. Sensory Processing Sensitivity

Sensory processing sensitivity (SPS) is characterized by heightened reactivity to environmental stimuli, greater depth of processing, and elevated emotional responsiveness [68]. Within parent–child dyads, SPS has been linked to amplified attentional alignment, particularly in contexts involving emotional facial cues. Evidence suggests that children high in SPS display stronger gaze congruency with caregivers during exposure to negative affect, while parents with elevated SPS are more likely to co-orient to their child's scanning patterns [69]. This bidirectional alignment may enhance opportunities for emotional scaffolding but also increase vulnerability to stress in overstimulating contexts [70]. SPS thus exemplifies a differential susceptibility mechanism, whereby heightened sensitivity can function as both a risk and resilience factor depending on environmental quality [71].

From the perspective of emotion and feeling, SPS amplifies the intensity of emotion as embodied synchrony (heightened gaze, physiological reactivity) while also accelerating or complicating the emergence of feeling as subjective awareness. In supportive environments, these children may more readily transform emotional activation into nuanced, reflective feelings, whereas in adverse environments, the same sensitivity may lead to overwhelming or dysregulated feeling states.

4.2. Callous–Unemotional Traits

Callous–unemotional (CU) traits, characterized by reduced empathy, shallow affect, and diminished responsiveness to others' distress, represent another domain of variation with implications for dyadic synchrony. Studies indicate that children with elevated CU traits often exhibit attenuated gaze to emotional faces, reduced physiological synchrony, and weaker neural coupling during affective interactions [72]. These differences may limit the scaffolding opportunities that typically support the transformation of shared emotional states into reflective feelings.

Moreover, while CU traits are often viewed through a deficit lens, some evidence suggests that targeted interventions—particularly those emphasizing warmth, reward sensitivity, and explicit labeling of affective states—can partially restore synchrony and enhance reflective awareness [73,74]. Within the emotion–feeling framework, CU traits represent a condition in which the embodied foundations of emotion (synchrony, orienting, physiological co-activation) are disrupted, making the developmental leap to conscious feeling states less robust.

4.3. Neurodevelopmental Conditions

Neurodevelopmental conditions such as autism spectrum disorder (ASD) and attention-deficit/hyperactivity disorder (ADHD) further illustrate how structural differences in cognition and neurobiology modulate dyadic synchrony. Children with ASD may show atypical attentional alignment, including reduced gaze to faces or difficulties sustaining joint attention, which alters the channels through which emotional scaffolding occurs [75]. Similarly, altered neural coupling in ASD dyads may reflect challenges in prediction error minimization during social exchange [75]. In ADHD, heightened arousal and reduced regulation capacities can disrupt physiological synchrony (e.g., HRV coupling), complicating the establishment of stable co-regulated states [76].

Despite these challenges, interventions that scaffold alternative pathways of synchrony (e.g., multimodal cues, structured routines, or augmented communication strategies) can create new routes for bridging emotion and feeling. This highlights that dyadic scaffolding is flexible and that even when traditional synchrony mechanisms are disrupted, compensatory strategies may still enable the transformation of embodied emotional states into consciously represented feelings.

Taken together, these individual difference factors demonstrate that dyadic synchrony is not a uniform process but a contextually modulated system. Children with heightened sensitivity may thrive under supportive caregiving yet struggle under adversity, while those with CU traits or neurodevelopmental conditions may require tailored interventions to achieve similar developmental outcomes. Viewed through the emotion–feeling distinction, these variations underscore that highly sensitive children may experience amplified emotion that more readily transforms into nuanced or dysregulated feelings depending on context; children with CU traits may experience disrupted emotional scaffolding that weakens the consolidation of reflective feelings; and children with neurodevelopmental conditions may follow atypical synchrony pathways that require compensatory supports to foster the emergence of conscious feeling. Recognizing these patterns is essential for moving beyond one-size-fits-all models of emotion development and toward precision approaches that respect diversity in affective functioning.

5. Developmental Pathways and Risk for Dysregulation

Within parent–child dyads, synchrony across attentional, neural, and physiological systems provides the developmental bridge that allows emotion—an embodied, evolutionarily conserved system of action readiness—to be transformed into feeling, the consciously represented, narrativized correlate of emotional activation. When synchrony processes falter, children may continue to generate emotional reactions at the bodily and attentional levels yet fail to consolidate them into coherent, reflective feeling states. Environmental sensitivity frameworks clarify why disruptions do not affect all children equally: individuals higher in sensitivity (e.g., sensory processing sensitivity) are more responsive to both adverse and supportive contexts, magnifying risk under misattunement and resilience when caregiving is contingent and warm [77–80]. In this section, findings are explicitly parsed as emotion-level (automatic, embodied, synchrony-dependent) versus feeling-level (conscious, representational, language- and concept-dependent) phenomena.

5.1. Disruptions in Attentional Synchrony

Visual attention to emotional faces represents one of the earliest mechanisms through which emotions are organized in parent–child dyads. At the level of emotion, gaze serves as a rapid, embodied orienting response to environmental salience, allowing children to detect signals of safety or threat [81,82]. When caregivers and children fail to achieve congruency in their visual scanning patterns, the emotional signal is left unshared, reducing opportunities for dyadic coordination and intersubjective regulation.

Moving from emotion to feeling, this alignment provides the scaffolding through which raw attentional orienting is transformed into a consciously accessible interpretation of emotional meaning. In secure relational contexts, caregivers' contingent responses and labeling practices help convert gaze-based reactions into felt experiences of comfort, threat, or affiliation [83]. In contrast, inconsistent or intrusive caregiving interrupts this process, leaving children with fragmented or poorly integrated affective experiences.

Notably, environmental sensitivity frameworks shed light on why disruptions in attentional synchrony do not affect all children equally. Children higher in sensory processing sensitivity show amplified responses to dyadic alignment: under supportive conditions, their heightened reactivity facilitates stronger co-orienting and richer emotional scaffolding, accelerating the consolidation of nuanced feeling states. Under adverse conditions, however, the same heightened sensitivity magnifies misalignment, resulting in overwhelming or dysregulated feelings [77–80].

5.2. Neural Dysregulation

Neural synchrony provides another layer of scaffolding through which emotion is shaped into feeling in parent–child dyads. Studies using fNIRS hyperscanning show that prefrontal coupling supports joint action readiness, sustained attention, and early co-regulatory processes during social interactions [84]. At the level of emotion, this shared cortical activation reflects a dynamic system for updating predictions and coordinating responses. When adversity such as parental stress or conflict disrupts this synchrony, the result is a breakdown in the alignment of emotional states between parent and child, leaving the child more vulnerable to unbuffered reactivity [83]. For this synchrony to be consolidated into feeling, cortical integration of interoceptive and contextual signals is necessary. When prefrontal coupling is preserved, it provides the substrate for reflective awareness, enabling children to represent and narrativize their internal states in ways consistent with Barrett's predictive and conceptual models of feeling construction. When coupling is weakened, however, these processes stall, and emotions may remain raw, unprocessed reactions rather than evolving into differentiated, consciously accessible feelings.

Moreover, environmental sensitivity moderates this process. Children higher in sensory processing sensitivity are likely to experience larger swings in neural synchrony: when caregiving is attuned, synchrony is enhanced, promoting more elaborate reflective awareness and nuanced feeling states. In contrast, under misattuned or stressful caregiving, the same heightened sensitivity exacerbates disruptions, leading to stalled representational construction and dysregulated emotional development [78–81].

5.3. Altered Physiological Coupling

Parent–child synchrony is not limited to behavior or neural activity but also extends to the level of physiology, where shared rhythms in cortisol and heart rate variability (HRV) reflect the embodied transfer of arousal and regulatory tone. At the level of emotion, such coupling functions as a biobehavioral channel for transmitting stress and calm across the dyad. When synchrony is disrupted—for example, through mismatched cortisol peaks or reduced vagal concordance—children experience unbuffered emotional reactivity that undermines their capacity for self-regulation [85–88]. For these embodied dynamics to be consolidated into feeling, physiological states must be stabilized within the relational context so that bodily arousal can be integrated into an accessible narrative of safety, distress, or calm. When rhythms align under contingent caregiving, arousal is translated into coherent felt experiences (e.g., "I can calm down with you"), providing a physiological foundation for emotional meaning-making. When alignment fails, arousal remains fragmented and unintegrated, leaving children vulnerable to dysregulated or confusing affective experiences [87,88].

The environmental sensitivity framework highlights how this process is intensified in children and parents high in sensory processing sensitivity. In these dyads, physiological synchrony exerts greater "gain": when caregiving is supportive, heightened sensitivity enhances co-regulation and enriches the child's capacity to build nuanced feelings from emotional arousal. Conversely, when caregiving is inconsistent or stressful, the same sensitivity magnifies dysregulation, exacerbating the risk that emotions remain unprocessed and feelings poorly formed [78–81].

5.4. Developmental Cascade to Psychopathology

When disruptions in attentional, neural, and physiological synchrony converge, children are left with emotional reactions that remain poorly scaffolded and unintegrated. At the level of emotion, such convergent misalignments manifest as hypervigilance, heightened threat sensitivity, and weakened inhibitory control—patterns of raw reactivity that accumulate without the stabilizing influence of dyadic co-regulation [89]. Over time, these unbuffered responses create a developmental cascade in which children are more likely to respond rigidly or impulsively to emotional challenges. The absence of reliable scaffolding impairs the transformation of these embodied reactions into feelings, leaving emotions unrepresented, unlabelled, and uncontained. For some children, this produces internalizing trajectories, where persistent reactivity without reflective containment leads to anxiety or depressive symptoms. For others, the failure of emotional signals to be represented as morally encoded feelings of guilt, empathy, or concern contributes to externalizing trajectories, including aggression and callous–unemotional tendencies [90,91].

Within the environmental sensitivity framework, these divergent pathways are more clearly understood. Children high in sensitivity are particularly susceptible to the quality of their environment: under harsh or inconsistent caregiving, cascades are accelerated, leading to more severe dysregulation; under warm and predictable caregiving, the same heightened responsiveness allows for attenuation or even reversal of these risks [78–81]. This dual potential underscores how environmental conditions shape whether sensitivity operates as a vulnerability factor or as a source of resilience in the transition from emotion to feeling.

5.5. Protective and Compensatory Factors

Even in the presence of risk, protective processes within parent–child dyads can preserve the developmental bridge from emotion to feeling. At the level of emotion, sensitive caregiving stabilizes synchrony across gaze, neural coupling, and autonomic alignment, thereby reducing volatility in embodied responses and supporting co-regulation during stress [92,93]. These stabilizing dynamics ensure that children's raw emotional arousal is contained within a relational context, preventing reactivity from becoming overwhelming. At the level of feeling, caregivers further scaffold the transformation of arousal into coherent experience by providing contingent labeling, narrative elaboration, and reflective dialogue. Through these symbolic and linguistic supports, children learn to interpret bodily states as subjectively meaningful feelings—fear, comfort, pride, or sadness—rather than as diffuse or confusing arousal. This scaffolding is especially beneficial for children high in environmental sensitivity, who show stronger positive returns in supportive contexts: under warm, predictable caregiving, their heightened reactivity facilitates the construction of more nuanced and differentiated feelings (so-called vantage sensitivity) [78–81,92–95].

Psychophysiological synchrony also functions as a protective mechanism when embedded in attuned caregiving. Aligned cortisol rhythms and vagal concordance amplify the translation of embodied arousal into accessible feeling states, acting as a biobehavioral "transducer" that supports resilience [96]. In this way, compensatory systems—whether located in caregiver warmth, sibling bonds, or peer relationships—operate not simply by suppressing emotion but by actively fostering the developmental processes that transform emotion into feeling.

Bringing together from the discussion above, environmental sensitivity operates as a gain-control parameter on the bridge from emotion to feeling. At the emotion level, sensitivity calibrates the magnitude of attentional capture, neural coupling, and physiological concordance; at the feeling level, it magnifies the effects of caregiving on the quality and granularity of conscious emotional representations. Under supportive dyadic conditions, high sensitivity accelerates the transformation of emotional activation into nuanced, reflective feeling; under adverse conditions, it accelerates dysregulated or blunted feeling (e.g., hyperaroused anxiety or reduced felt concern), clarifying apparently paradoxical outcomes within a single framework [79–82]. This account integrates earlier theory—rapid subcortical emotion circuits (LeDoux), predictive/conceptual feeling construction (Barrett), and dyadic scaffolding (Tronick; multilevel synchrony, Feldman)—into a unified, developmentally sensitive model that explains who benefits most from synchrony and when misattunement is most costly.

6. Integrative Developmental Framework

The evidence reviewed across attentional, neural, and physiological domains converges on a central insight: emotion and feeling do not emerge solely within the individual, but within the relational matrix of parent–child interactions. By distinguishing emotion as an embodied, evolutionarily conserved system of action-readiness and feeling as the subjective, representational correlate of this system, a clearer conceptual scaffold is provided for interpreting affective phenomena in development. Crucially, synchrony processes situate the dyad as the crucible of affective growth, building the bridge from raw, embodied reactivity to symbolic, consciously accessible experience. Within this framework, environmental sensitivity becomes a key moderator, determining whether synchrony processes consolidate into resilience or collapse into dysregulation.

Synchrony across attentional, neural, and physiological levels provides the foundation for transforming emotion into feeling. At the level of emotion, shared gaze patterns and attentional alignment function as rapid orienting mechanisms that prepare the child for action and signal salience in the environment [97,98]. At the level of feeling, caregivers translate these reactions into meaning through labeling, narrative, and symbolic scaffolds, allowing children to experience gaze-based orienting as consciously represented affect [99]. Similarly, neural coupling observed in fNIRS and hyperscanning paradigms reflects the co-construction of meaning at the emotion level, where dyads dynamically coordinate cortical activity during joint tasks [54,100,101]. This alignment enables the transition to feeling by providing a cortical substrate for reflective awareness and symbolic representation. Physiological synchrony, indexed by cortisol concordance and vagal tone coordination, represents an embodied channel through which arousal is shared and stabilized [102,103]. Under supportive caregiving, such physiological alignment becomes the basis for felt safety, demonstrating how emotional arousal can be converted into consciously accessible experience. Notably, these synchrony processes integrate dynamically: attentional scaffolds support neural coupling, which in turn sustains physiological co-regulation, creating a multi-level scaffold for the consolidation of emotion into feeling [104,105].

Synchrony mechanisms are not experienced uniformly. Children with high SPS display stronger amplification of synchrony signals, thriving in supportive caregiving environments but showing pronounced dysregulation when caregiving is inconsistent [106–108]. In such children, the movement from emotion to feeling is accelerated under positive conditions, producing nuanced and differentiated affective experiences, but is equally accelerated toward fragmentation under stress. Conversely, children with CU traits show attenuated attention to emotional cues and diminished synchrony across physiological systems [109,110]. In these cases, emotion signals may fail to trigger the embodied arousal necessary for feelings to be consolidated, leading to difficulties in moral encoding and empathic concern. Targeted interventions such as explicit affect labeling and warmth-based parenting can, however, partially restore synchrony and support the emergence of reflective feeling [111,112].

Neurodevelopmental conditions also illustrate how synchrony pathways can diverge. In autism spectrum disorder, atypical gaze and neural coupling patterns may alter the channels through which emotion is scaffolded, yet compensatory strategies—such as multimodal cues or structured routines—can still enable the translation of emotional activation into felt experience [54]. Attachment security further moderates these dynamics: secure relationships stabilize synchrony across levels, while insecure or disorganized attachment undermines the scaffolding of feelings from emotional states [113,114]. Taken together, these findings highlight that the transformation from emotion to feeling depends on the interplay between biological sensitivity, caregiving quality, and attachment context, shaping trajectories of both vulnerability and resilience.

6.1. Implications for Intervention

The emotion–feeling framework underscores that interventions must target the relational processes that bridge embodied reactivity and conscious experience. Parenting programs such as PCIT and Circle of Security enhance attunement and reflective functioning, thereby stabilizing synchrony at the emotion level while strengthening symbolic scaffolds for feeling [115–118]. Parent–Child Interaction Therapy (PCIT) offers a strong evidence base for improving emotional reciprocity and dyadic regulation in parent–child relationships. Originally developed for externalizing disorders, PCIT has since been adapted for children with autism spectrum disorder (ASD) and other developmental disabilities, demonstrating improvements in both behavioral and relational domains. Recent evidence highlights that PCIT not only reduces disruptive behaviors but also strengthens attachment security, caregiver sensitivity, and synchrony during interactional exchanges [119]. Such adaptations emphasize developmental attunement—slowing the pace of interaction, scaffolding communication, and enhancing emotional mirroring—allowing parents to respond more effectively to subtle cues of affect and engagement. These mechanisms make PCIT particularly valuable for neurodevelopmental populations where emotional reciprocity may be limited, underscoring synchrony as a critical pathway through which parent-mediated interventions exert their regulatory effects. Moreover, neuroscience-informed approaches—including HRV biofeedback, mindfulness-based parenting, and gaze-contingency feedback—directly modulate synchrony systems, demonstrating that interventions can be designed to align physiology and behavior in ways that facilitate the transition from arousal into reflective awareness [120–122]. These strategies are particularly critical for highly sensitive children, who stand to benefit disproportionately from supportive scaffolding (vantage sensitivity), and for those with CU traits or neurodevelopmental conditions, where compensatory interventions can restore synchrony and enable feeling construction. At the broader ecological level, policies that reduce parental stress, improve social support, and provide accessible early mental health care indirectly enhance synchrony by increasing caregivers' emotional availability [123]. Developmental timing is also crucial: interventions in infancy emphasize physiological and attentional synchrony, while those in adolescence may focus on scaffolding autonomy, reflective dialogue, and intersubjective negotiation rather than pure physiological alignment [124].

6.2. Limitations

Several limitations of the current literature on parent–child synchrony and affective development should be acknowledged. One concern is publication bias: studies reporting significant synchrony effects (e.g., robust correlations between parent–child physiology or neural activity) are more likely to appear in the published record than those with null or inconsistent findings. This may create an overly optimistic picture of the strength and consistency of synchrony effects. Another important limitation is the over-reliance on WEIRD (Western, Educated, Industrialized, Rich, Democratic) populations. Most studies have been conducted in Western or high-income contexts, raising questions about generalizability. As noted in the cultural variability section, patterns of parent–child interaction and emotion socialization differ across cultural settings, and a "lack" of synchrony in one cultural context may reflect alternative caregiving norms rather than developmental deficits. Finally, many investigations are based on small sample sizes and cross-sectional designs, which limit inferences about developmental trajectories. Future research would benefit from larger, longitudinal, and more culturally diverse samples to evaluate how synchrony processes unfold across development. Highlighting these issues underscores that claims about parent–child emotion–feeling dynamics must be continually tested and refined to ensure they are both robust and inclusive of diverse human experiences.

6.3. Future Research Directions

Looking ahead, several future research directions emerge from this review that can further elucidate the development of emotion and feeling in parent–child dyads. First, there is a clear need for more longitudinal and cross-lagged studies tracking children over time. Most available evidence is cross-sectional, providing snapshots of different ages or dyads. Longitudinal designs—following the same parent–child pairs from infancy through later childhood—would allow researchers to directly observe how early emotional synchrony (or its absence) cascades into later outcomes. Such studies could answer, for instance, when and how initial emotion–feeling integrations (e.g., a toddler learning to label their fear with a parent's help) forecast the child's emotional competence or mental health years down the line. Cross-cultural research is another priority. As noted, feelings are culturally shaped and parenting practices around emotion socialization vary widely. Comparative studies across different cultural or socio-economic contexts will help determine which aspects of the emotion-to-feeling developmental pathway are universal (rooted in biology) and which are culture-specific (shaped by norms and belief systems) [124–126].

In addition, future research should strive to integrate multiple levels of analysis to capture the full complexity of parent–child emotional dynamics. Recent advances (e.g., dual-brain hyperscanning with fNIRS or EEG) make it possible to simultaneously record neural activity in parent and child during real interactions. Applying these tools more widely could illuminate real-time bi-directional processes—for example, how a mother's brain and her toddler's brain become synchronized when sharing an emotional moment, and how such neural coupling might predict the child's emerging capacity for empathy or self-regulation. Likewise, incorporating physiological measures (beyond cortisol and heart rate, to include indices like oxytocin, skin conductance, or respiration) could deepen our understanding of emotion transmission. A multi-method approach—combining behavioral observations, self-reports (when children are old enough), neural data, and physiological data—will provide a more holistic picture of how emotion and feeling co-develop within relationships [127–130].

Another important direction concerns resilience and individual differences. Our review highlighted that some children (for instance, those high in sensory processing sensitivity) are disproportionately influenced by the quality of emotional input—flourishing under supportive conditions and struggling under adversity. Future work should explore the protective factors that enable resilient trajectories even among high-risk groups. For example, are there cases where children with a difficult temperament still develop strong emotion–feeling integration due to exceptionally supportive parenting or other environmental buffers? Unpacking these cases could inform tailored interventions that bolster protective processes. Similarly, investigating gender differences (if any) in emotion–feeling development, or how siblings might differentially negotiate these processes, could add nuance to our understanding of individual variability in normative pathways [130].

Finally, this field is poised to inform and benefit from applied intervention research. The distinction between emotion and feeling underscores that simply managing a child's behavior (emotion expression) is not enough—caregivers and clinicians should also aim to foster the child's understanding and integration of those emotions into feelings. Parent-focused interventions that encourage sensitive attunement, emotion labeling, and contingent responsiveness are likely to help children build robust emotion–feeling bridges. Indeed, preliminary studies with at-risk children show promise: for instance, interventions training parents in warm, explicit emotion communication have partially normalized attention to emotional cues and improved emotional understanding in children with callous–unemotional traits [130]. Future trials could extend such approaches to other groups (e.g., children with autism spectrum disorder who might benefit from augmented multimodal emotional cues) and examine long-term outcomes. In parallel, preventive programs in early childhood—such as attachment-based parenting programs or emotion-coaching curricula in preschools—should be tested for their effectiveness in enhancing emotional synchrony and the early emergence of feelings. Ultimately, an integrative developmental framework can guide interventions to target the relational mechanisms that transform emotion into feeling. By bolstering synchrony in attention, neural responses, and physiology, and by empowering parents to scaffold children's emotional experiences with language and empathy, we can promote healthier emotional development. In summary, future research and practice should jointly focus on filling key knowledge gaps (through longitudinal, cross-cultural, and multi-level studies) and translating insights into strategies that support children's journey from raw emotion to reflective feeling—laying a foundation for emotional well-being and resilience across the lifespan [131].

7. Discussion

The synthesis presented in this review has important clinical and social implications. By distinguishing emotion as an embodied system of action readiness and interpersonal signaling, and feeling as its subjective and symbolic correlate, developmental science can move beyond longstanding conceptual ambiguity to inform applied practice. This distinction matters clinically, as many interventions currently target "emotions" and "feelings" interchangeably, potentially diluting their effectiveness. Recognizing that dyadic synchrony provides the bridge between biological reactivity and subjective experience highlights the parent–child relationship as a central therapeutic leverage point. From a clinical standpoint, this framework underscores the need to design interventions that directly enhance attentional, neural, and physiological synchrony. Eye-tracking-guided parent–child tasks, biofeedback protocols, and parent-focused stress regulation training may amplify attunement and buffer against dysregulation in children at risk for emotional and behavioral difficulties. For populations with neurodevelopmental disorders or callous–unemotional traits, such targeted approaches may prove especially important in fostering adaptive emotional development.

The environmental sensitivity framework further refines these implications. Children differ in how strongly they respond to synchrony processes, with those high in sensory processing sensitivity or related susceptibility traits showing disproportionate outcomes depending on caregiving quality. In supportive environments, their heightened reactivity facilitates richer co-regulation and more differentiated feelings; in adverse environments, the same sensitivity accelerates dysregulation and fragmentation of emotional experience. Clinically, this implies that tailoring interventions to children's sensitivity profiles—whether through vantage sensitivity or differential susceptibility models—can optimize effectiveness by matching strategies to developmental context. Socially, these insights emphasize the broader relevance of relational contexts in supporting resilience. Policies that strengthen early caregiving, reduce parental stress, and promote inclusive technologies can help create environments where children's biological sensitivities are scaffolded into opportunities for growth rather than vulnerabilities for psychopathology. The recognition that environmental sensitivity moderates developmental trajectories also underscores the urgency of addressing inequities in caregiving resources, as these disparities disproportionately affect the most susceptible children.

Overall, the clinical and social significance of the current framework lies in its ability to link basic neurocognitive and psychophysiological research with practical pathways to intervention, prevention, and policy. By treating the dyad as the crucible of affective development, and by recognizing how environmental sensitivity modulates the movement from emotion to feeling, clinicians, educators, and policymakers can adopt a relational and context-sensitive approach to fostering well-being across diverse developmental and cultural settings.

Author Contributions: Conceptualization, A.I.C.; data curation, A.I.C. and F.B.; writing—original draft preparation, A.I.C. and F.B.; writing—review and editing, A.I.C. and F.B. All authors have read and agreed to the published version of the manuscript.

Funding: This research received no external funding.

Institutional Review Board Statement: Not applicable.

Informed Consent Statement: Not applicable.

Data Availability Statement: Not applicable.

Conflicts of Interest: The authors declare no conflicts of interest.

Abbreviations

The following abbreviations are used in this manuscript:

SPS	Sensory Processing Sensitivity
CU traits	Callous-unemotional traits
ADHD	Attention Deficit Hyperactivity Disorder

References

1. Izard, C.E. Emotion theory and research: Highlights, unanswered questions, and emerging issues. *Annu. Rev. Psychol.* **2009**, *60*, 1–25. [CrossRef]
2. Izard, C.E. The many meanings/aspects of emotion: Definitions, functions, activation, and regulation. *Emot. Rev.* **2010**, *2*, 363–370. [CrossRef]
3. LeDoux, J. Rethinking the emotional brain. *Neuron* **2012**, *73*, 653–676. [CrossRef]
4. Barrett, L.F. The theory of constructed emotion: An active inference account of interoception and categorization. *Soc. Cogn. Affect. Neurosci.* **2017**, *12*, 1–23. [CrossRef]
5. Cavelzani, A.; Tronick, E. Dyadically expanded states of consciousness and therapeutic change in the interaction between analyst and adult patient. *Psychoanal. Dialogues* **2016**, *26*, 599–615. [CrossRef]
6. Damasio, A. *The Feeling of What Happens: Body and Emotion in the Making of Consciousness*; Harcourt: New York, NY, USA, 1999.
7. Damasio, A. *Feeling & Knowing: Making Minds Conscious*; Pantheon Books: New York, NY, USA, 2021.
8. LeDoux, J.E.; Brown, R. A higher-order theory of emotional consciousness. *Proc. Natl. Acad. Sci. USA* **2017**, *114*, E2016–E2025. [CrossRef]
9. LeDoux, J. *Anxious: Using the Brain to Understand and Treat Fear and Anxiety*; Viking: New York, NY, USA, 2015.
10. Carvalho, G.B.; Damasio, A. Interoception and the Origin of Feelings: A New Synthesis. *BioEssays* **2021**, *43*, e2000261. [CrossRef]
11. Barrett, L.F. *How Emotions Are Made: The Secret Life of the Brain*; Houghton Mifflin Harcourt: New York, NY, USA, 2017.
12. Ziv, Y.; Arbel, R. Parent–child emotion synchrony: Current knowledge and future directions. *Dev. Rev.* **2022**, *63*, 101016.
13. Hoemann, K.; Gendron, M.; Barrett, L.F. Mixed emotions: Toward a psychological constructionist account. *Emot. Rev.* **2023**, *15*, 97–109.
14. Immordino-Yang, M.H.; Darling-Hammond, L.; Krone, C. Nurturing nature: How brain development is inherently social and emotional, and what this means for education. *Educ. Psychol.* **2022**, *57*, 190–203.
15. Panksepp, J. *Affective Neuroscience: The Foundations of Human and Animal Emotions*; Oxford University Press: New York, NY, USA, 1998.
16. Sroufe, L.A. *Emotional Development: The Organization of Emotional Life in the Early Years*; Cambridge University Press: New York, NY, USA, 1996.
17. Hofer, M.A. Hidden regulators in attachment, separation, and loss. *Monogr. Soc. Res. Child Dev.* **1994**, *59*, 192–207. [CrossRef]
18. Cassidy, J. Emotion regulation: Influences of attachment relationships. *Monogr. Soc. Res. Child Dev.* **1994**, *59*, 228–249. [CrossRef]
19. Fearon, R.P.; Bakermans-Kranenburg, M.J.; van IJzendoorn, M.H.; Lapsley, A.M.; Roisman, G.I. The significance of insecure attachment and disorganization in the development of children's externalizing behavior: A meta-analytic study. *Child Dev.* **2010**, *81*, 435–456. [CrossRef]
20. Bowlby, J. *Attachment and Loss: Vol. 1. Attachment*, 2nd ed.; Original Work Published; Basic Books: New York, NY, USA, 1969.
21. Ainsworth, M.D.S. Object relations, dependency, and attachment: A theoretical review of the infant–mother relationship. *Child Dev.* **1969**, *40*, 969–1025. [CrossRef]
22. Provenzi, L.; Scotto di Minico, G.; Giusti, L.; Guida, E.; Müller, M. Disentangling the dyadic dance: Theoretical, methodological and outcomes systematic review of mother–infant dyadic processes. *Front. Psychol.* **2018**, *9*, 348. [CrossRef]
23. Cooke, J.E.; Kochendorfer, L.B.; Stuart-Parrigon, K.L.; Koehn, A.J.; Kerns, K.A. Parent–child attachment and children's experience and regulation of emotion: A meta-analytic review. *Emotion* **2019**, *19*, 1103–1126. [CrossRef]
24. Brumariu, L.E. Parent–child attachment and emotion regulation. *New Dir. Child Adolesc. Dev.* **2015**, *2015*, 31–45. [CrossRef]
25. Diano, M.; Celeghin, A.; Bagnis, A.; Tamietto, M. Amygdala response to emotional stimuli without awareness: Facts and interpretations. *Front. Psychol.* **2017**, *7*, 2029. [CrossRef]
26. Barrett, L.F.; Simmons, W.K. Interoceptive predictions in the brain. *Nat. Rev. Neurosci.* **2015**, *16*, 419–429. [CrossRef]
27. Hilbrink, E.E.; Gattis, M.; Levinson, S.C. Early developmental changes in the timing of turn-taking: A longitudinal study of mother–infant interaction. *Front. Psychol.* **2015**, *6*, 1492. [CrossRef]
28. Gratier, M.; Devouche, E.; Guellai, B.; Infanti, R.; Yilmaz, E.; Parlato-Oliveira, E. Early development of turn-taking in vocal interaction between mothers and infants. *Front. Psychol.* **2015**, *6*, 1167. [CrossRef]

29. Damasio, A.; Carvalho, G.B. The nature of feelings: Evolutionary and neurobiological origins. *Nat. Rev. Neurosci.* **2013**, *14*, 143–152. [CrossRef]
30. LeDoux, J.E. Thoughtful feelings. *Curr. Biol.* **2020**, *30*, R619–R623. [CrossRef]
31. Friedlmeier, W.; Corapci, F.; Cole, P.M. Emotion socialization in cross-cultural perspective. *Soc. Personal. Psychol. Compass* **2011**, *5*, 410–427. [CrossRef]
32. Davis, M.; West, K.; Bilms, J.; Morelen, D.; Suveg, C. A systematic review of parent–child synchrony: It is more than skin deep. *Dev. Psychobiol.* **2018**, *60*, 674–691. [CrossRef]
33. Birk, S.L.; Stewart, L.; Olino, T.M. Parent–Child Synchrony After Early Childhood: A Systematic Review. *Clin. Child Fam. Psychol. Rev.* **2022**, *25*, 529–551. [CrossRef]
34. Thompson, R.A.; Simpson, J.A.; Berlin, L.J. Taking perspective on attachment theory and research: Nine fundamental questions. *Attach. Hum. Dev.* **2022**, *24*, 543–560. [CrossRef]
35. Hessels, R.S.; Hooge, I.T.C. Eye tracking in developmental cognitive neuroscience—The good, the bad and the ugly. *Dev. Cogn. Neurosci.* **2019**, *40*, 100710. [CrossRef]
36. Wilcox, T.; Biondi, M. fNIRS in the developmental sciences. *Wiley Interdiscip. Rev. Cogn. Sci.* **2015**, *6*, 263–283. [CrossRef]
37. Kervezee, L.; Romijn, M.; van de Weijer, K.N.G.; Chen, B.S.J.; Burchell, G.L.; Tollenaar, M.S.; Tamayo-Ortiz, M.; Philbrook, L.E.; de Weerth, C.; Cao, Y.; et al. Development of 24-hour rhythms in cortisol secretion across infancy: A systematic review and meta-analysis of individual participant data. *J. Clin. Endocrinol. Metab.* **2025**, *110*, e515–e524. [CrossRef]
38. Campbell, M.; McKenzie, J.E.; Sowden, A.; Katikireddi, S.V.; Brennan, S.E.; Ellis, S.; Hartmann-Boyce, J.; Ryan, R.; Shepperd, S.; Thomas, J.; et al. Synthesis without meta-analysis (SWiM) in systematic reviews: Reporting guideline. *BMJ* **2020**, *368*, l6890. [CrossRef]
39. Silvers, J.A. Adolescence as a pivotal period for emotion regulation development. *Curr. Opin. Psychol.* **2022**, *44*, 258–263. [CrossRef]
40. Herd, T.; King-Casas, B.; Kim-Spoon, J. Developmental changes in emotion regulation during adolescence: Associations with socioeconomic risk and family emotional context. *J. Youth Adolesc.* **2020**, *49*, 1545–1557. [CrossRef] [PubMed]
41. Aghaziarati, A.; Nejatifar, S. Emotional development and regulation in children: A review of recent advances. *KMAN Couns. Psychol. Nexus* **2023**, *1*, 118–125. [CrossRef]
42. Xie, W.; Leppänen, J.M.; Kane-Grade, F.E.; Nelson, C.A. Converging neural and behavioral evidence for a rapid, generalized response to threat-related facial expressions in 3-year-old children. *NeuroImage* **2021**, *229*, 117732. [CrossRef]
43. Leppänen, J.M.; Cataldo, J.K.; Bosquet Enlow, M.; Nelson, C.A. Early development of attention to threat-related facial expressions. *PLoS ONE* **2018**, *13*, e0197424. [CrossRef]
44. Pergantis, P.; Bamicha, V.; Doulou, A.; Christou, A.I.; Bardis, N.; Skianis, C.; Drigas, A. Assistive and emerging technologies to detect and reduce neurophysiological stress and anxiety in children and adolescents with autism and sensory processing disorders: A systematic review. *Technologies* **2025**, *13*, 144. [CrossRef]
45. Levy, J.; Goldstein, A.; Feldman, R. Perception of social synchrony induces mother–child gamma coupling in the social brain. *Soc. Cogn. Affect. Neurosci.* **2017**, *12*, 1036–1046. [CrossRef]
46. Pérez-Edgar, K.; Bar-Haim, Y.; McDermott, J.M.; Chronis-Tuscano, A.; Pine, D.S.; Fox, N.A. Attention biases to threat and behavioral inhibition in early childhood shape adolescent social withdrawal. *Emotion* **2010**, *10*, 349–357. [CrossRef]
47. Pérez-Edgar, K.; Reeb-Sutherland, B.C.; McDermott, J.M.; White, L.K.; Henderson, H.A.; Degnan, K.A.; Fox, N.A. Attention biases to threat link behavioral inhibition to social withdrawal over time in very young children. *J. Abnorm. Child Psychol.* **2011**, *39*, 885–895. [CrossRef]
48. Quiñones-Camacho, L.E.; Hoyniak, C.P.; Wakschlag, L.S.; Perlman, S.B. Getting in synch: Unpacking the role of parent–child synchrony in the development of internalizing and externalizing behaviors. *Dev. Psychopathol.* **2022**, *34*, 1901–1913. [CrossRef]
49. Vallorani, A.; Gunther, K.E.; Anaya, B.; Burris, J.L.; Field, A.P.; LoBue, V.; Buss, K.A.; Pérez-Edgar, K. Assessing bidirectional relations between infant temperamental negative affect, maternal anxiety symptoms and infant affect-biased attention across the first 24 months of life. *Dev. Psychol.* **2023**, *59*, 364–376. [CrossRef]
50. Christou, A.I.; Fanti, K.; Mavrommatis, I.; Soursou, G.; Eliadi, E. Parental sensory processing sensitivity predicts children's visual scanning pattern of emotional faces. *J. Psychopathol. Behav. Assess.* **2024**, *46*, 932–942. [CrossRef]
51. Aktar, E.; Venetikidi, M.; Van Bockstaele, B.; Van Giessen, D.; Pérez-Edgar, K. Pupillary Responses to Dynamic Negative versus Positive Facial Expressions of Emotion in Children and Parents: Links to Depression and Anxiety. *Dev. Psychobiol.* **2024**, *66*, e22522. [CrossRef]
52. Kujawa, A.; Klein, D.N.; Pegg, S.; Weinberg, A. Developmental Trajectories to Reduced Activation of Positive Valence Systems: A Review of Biological and Environmental Contributions. *Dev. Cogn. Neurosci.* **2020**, *43*, 100791. [CrossRef]
53. Czeszumski, A.; Eustergerling, S.; Lang, A.; Menrath, D.; Gerstenberger, M.; Schuberth, S.; Schreiber, F.; Rendon, Z.Z.; König, P. Hyperscanning: A valid method to study neural inter-brain underpinnings of social interaction. *Front. Hum. Neurosci.* **2020**, *14*, 39. [CrossRef]

54. Miller, J.G.; Vrtička, P.; Cui, X.; Shrestha, S.; Hosseini, S.M.H.; Baker, J.M.; Reiss, A.L. Inter-brain synchrony in mother–child dyads during cooperation: An fNIRS hyperscanning study. *Neuropsychologia* **2019**, *124*, 117–124. [CrossRef]
55. Liu, Q.; Zhu, S.; Zhou, X.; Liu, F.; Becker, B.; Kendrick, K.M.; Zhao, W. Mothers and fathers show different neural synchrony with their children during shared experiences. *NeuroImage* **2024**, *288*, 120529. [CrossRef]
56. Friston, K.J.; Frith, C.D. Active inference, communication and hermeneutics. *Cortex* **2015**, *68*, 129–143. [CrossRef]
57. DePasquale, C.E. A systematic review of caregiver–child physiological synchrony across systems: Associations with behavior and child functioning. *Dev. Psychopathol.* **2020**, *32*, 1754–1777. [CrossRef]
58. Hibel, L.C.; Granger, D.A.; Blair, C.; Finegood, E.D.; Family Life Project Key Investigators. Maternal–child adrenocortical attunement in early childhood: Continuity and change. *Dev. Psychobiol.* **2015**, *57*, 83–95. [CrossRef]
59. Xu, J.; Zhang, Y.; Wang, H.; Peng, M.; Zhu, Y.; Wang, X.; Yi, Z.; Chen, L.; Han, Z.R. A context-dependent perspective to understand the relation between parent–child physiological synchrony and child socioemotional adjustment. *Dev. Sci.* **2024**, *27*, e13506. [CrossRef]
60. Fleck, L.; Fuchs, A.; Lerch, S.; Möhler, E.; Koenig, J.; Resch, F.; Kaess, M. Adolescent borderline personality traits and dyadic behavior shape mother–adolescent cortisol synchrony. *Borderline Personal. Disord. Emot. Dysregulation* **2023**, *10*, 12. [CrossRef]
61. Lunkenheimer, E.; Hamby, C.M.; Lobo, F.M.; Cole, P.M.; Olson, S.L. The role of dynamic, dyadic parent–child processes in parental socialization of emotion. *Dev. Psychol.* **2020**, *56*, 566–577. [CrossRef]
62. Verhagen, C.; Boekhorst, M.G.B.M.; Kupper, N.; van Bakel, H.; Duijndam, S. Coregulation between Parents and Elementary School-Aged Children in Response to Challenge and in Association with Child Outcomes: A Systematic Review. *Dev. Psychol.* 2024, Advance Online Publication. [CrossRef]
63. Amole, M.C.; Cyranowski, J.M.; Wright, A.G.; Swartz, H.A. Depression impacts the physiological responsiveness of mother–daughter dyads during social interaction. *Depress. Anxiety* **2017**, *34*, 118–126. [CrossRef]
64. Cassidy, J.; Shaver, P.R. (Eds.) *Handbook of Attachment: Theory, Research, and Clinical Applications*, 3rd ed.; Guilford Press: New York, NY, USA, 2016.
65. Tronick, E.; Beeghly, M. Infants' meaning-making and the development of mental health problems. *Am. Psychol.* **2011**, *66*, 107–119. [CrossRef]
66. Feldman, R. The neurobiology of human attachments. *Trends Cogn. Sci.* **2017**, *21*, 80–99. [CrossRef]
67. Pluess, M. Individual differences in environmental sensitivity. *Child Dev. Perspect.* **2015**, *9*, 138–143. [CrossRef]
68. Bülow, A.; Neubauer, A.B.; Soenens, B.; Boele, S.; Denissen, J.J.A.; Keijsers, L. Universal ingredients to parenting teens: Parental warmth and autonomy support promote adolescent well-being in most families. *Sci. Rep.* **2022**, *12*, 16836. [CrossRef]
69. Aktar, E.; Nimphy, C.A.; Kret, M.E.; Pérez-Edgar, K.; Raijmakers, M.E.J.; Bögels, S.M. Attention biases to threat in infants and parents: Links to parental and infant anxiety dispositions. *Res. Child Adolesc. Psychopathol.* **2022**, *50*, 387–402. [CrossRef]
70. Slagt, M.; Dubas, J.S.; Deković, M.; van Aken, M.A. Differences in sensitivity to parenting depending on child temperament: A meta-analysis. *Psychol. Bull.* **2016**, *142*, 1068–1110. [CrossRef]
71. Lionetti, F.; Pluess, M. The role of environmental sensitivity in the experience and processing of emotions: Implications for well-being. *Philos. Trans. R. Soc. B Biol. Sci.* **2024**, *379*, 20230244. [CrossRef]
72. Frick, P.J.; Ray, J.V.; Thornton, L.C.; Kahn, R.E. Annual research review: A developmental psychopathology approach to understanding callous–unemotional traits in children and adolescents with serious conduct problems. *J. Child Psychol. Psychiatry* **2014**, *55*, 532–548. [CrossRef]
73. Díaz-Vázquez, B.; López-Romero, L.; Romero, E. Emotion recognition deficits in children and adolescents with psychopathic traits: A systematic review. *Clin. Child Fam. Psychol. Rev.* **2024**, *27*, 165–219. [CrossRef]
74. Dadds, M.R.; Allen, J.L.; McGregor, K.; Woolgar, M.; Viding, E.; Scott, S. Callous–unemotional traits in children and mechanisms of impaired eye contact during expressions of love: A treatment target? *J. Child Psychol. Psychiatry* **2014**, *55*, 771–780. [CrossRef]
75. Edmunds, S.R.; Fogler, J.; Braverman, Y.; Gilbert, R.; Faja, S. Resting frontal alpha asymmetry as a predictor of executive and affective functioning in children with neurodevelopmental differences. *Front. Psychol.* **2023**, *13*, 1065598. [CrossRef] [PubMed]
76. Mundy, P. A review of joint attention and social-cognitive brain systems in typical development and autism spectrum disorder. *Eur. J. Neurosci.* **2018**, *47*, 497–514. [CrossRef]
77. Redcay, E.; Schilbach, L. Using second-person neuroscience to elucidate the mechanisms of social interaction. *Nat. Rev. Neurosci.* **2019**, *20*, 495–505. [CrossRef]
78. Musser, E.D.; Galloway-Long, H.S.; Frick, P.J.; Nigg, J.T. Emotion regulation and heterogeneity in attention-deficit/hyperactivity disorder. *J. Am. Acad. Child Adolesc. Psychiatry* **2013**, *52*, 163–171.e2. [CrossRef] [PubMed]
79. Shengyao, Y.; Salarzadeh Jenatabadi, H.; Mengshi, Y.; Minqin, C.; Xuefen, L.; Mustafa, Z. Academic Resilience, Self-Efficacy, and Motivation: The Role of Parenting Style. *Sci. Rep.* **2024**, *14*, 5571. [CrossRef]
80. Aktar, E.; Nimphy, C.A.; Van Bockstaele, B.; Pérez-Edgar, K. The Social Learning of Threat and Safety in the Family: Parent-to-Child Transmission of Social Fears via Verbal Information. *Dev. Psychobiol.* **2022**, *64*, e22257. [CrossRef]

81. Phillips, E.M.; Brock, R.L. Interplay between Interparental Relationship Quality and Infant Temperament Predicts Toddler Transdiagnostic Psychopathology. *J. Fam. Psychol.* **2024**, *38*, 1201–1213. [CrossRef]
82. Poerio, G.L.; Kondo, H.M.; Moore, B.C.J. Sensing and Feeling: An Overview. *Philos. Trans. R. Soc. Lond. B Biol. Sci.* **2024**, *379*, 20230242. [CrossRef]
83. Perlstein, S.; Fair, M.; Hong, E.; Waller, R. Treatment of Childhood Disruptive Behavior Disorders and Callous-Unemotional Traits: A Systematic Review and Two Multilevel Meta-Analyses. *J. Child Psychol. Psychiatry* **2023**, *64*, 1372–1387. [CrossRef] [PubMed]
84. Ivanova-Serokhvostova, A.; Fanti, K.; Bonillo, A.; Supèr, H.; Corrales, M.; Pérez-Bonaventura, I.; Pamias, M.; Ramos-Quiroga, A.J.; Torrubia, R.; Nadal, R.; et al. Do Children with High Callous-Unemotional Traits Have Attentional Deficits to Emotional Stimuli? Evidence from a Multi-Method and Multi-Informant Study. *Child Psychiatry Hum. Dev.* 2024, Advance Online Publication. [CrossRef]
85. Fleming, G.E.; Neo, B.; Briggs, N.E.; Kaouar, S.; Frick, P.J.; Kimonis, E.R. Parent training adapted to the needs of children with callous–unemotional traits: A randomized controlled trial. *Behav. Ther.* **2022**, *53*, 1265–1281. [CrossRef]
86. McDonald, R.G.; Cargill, M.I.; Khawar, S.; Kang, E. Emotion Dysregulation in Autism: A Meta-Analysis. *Autism* **2024**, *28*, 2986–3001. [CrossRef]
87. Myruski, S.; Gulyayeva, O.; Birk, S.; Pérez-Edgar, K.; Buss, K.A.; Dennis-Tiwary, T.A. Digital disruption? Maternal mobile device use is related to infant social-emotional functioning. *Dev. Sci.* **2018**, *21*, e12610. [CrossRef] [PubMed]
88. Busuito, A.; Quigley, K.M.; Moore, G.A.; Voegtline, K.M.; DiPietro, J.A. In sync: Physiological correlates of behavioral synchrony in infants and mothers. *Dev. Psychol.* **2019**, *55*, 1034–1045. [CrossRef] [PubMed]
89. Lunkenheimer, E.; Tiberio, S.S.; Buss, K.A.; Lucas-Thompson, R.G.; Boker, S.M.; Timpe, Z.C. Coregulation of respiratory sinus arrhythmia between parents and children: Differences by children's externalizing problems. *Dev. Psychobiol.* **2015**, *57*, 994–1003. [CrossRef]
90. Lunkenheimer, E.; Tiberio, S.S.; Skoranski, A.M.; Buss, K.A.; Cole, P.M. Parent–child coregulation of parasympathetic processes varies by social context and risk for psychopathology. *Psychophysiology* **2018**, *55*, e12985. [CrossRef]
91. Smith, C.G.; Jones, E.J.H.; Charman, T.; Clackson, K.; Mirza, F.U.; Wass, S.V. Anxious parents show higher physiological synchrony with their infants. *Psychol. Med.* **2022**, *52*, 3040–3050. [CrossRef]
92. Stallworthy, I.C.; Elison, J.T.; Berry, D. The infant parasympathetic nervous system is socially embedded and dynamic at multiple timescales, within and between people. *Dev. Psychol.* **2024**, *60*, 1827–1841. [CrossRef]
93. Brandes-Aitken, A.; Hume, A.; Braren, S.; Werchan, D.; Zhang, M.; Brito, N.H. Maternal heart rate variability at 3 months postpartum is associated with maternal mental health and infant neurophysiology. *Sci. Rep.* **2024**, *14*, 18766. [CrossRef] [PubMed]
94. McDonnell, C.G.; Valentino, K.; Comas, M.; Nuttall, A.K. Mother–child reminiscing at risk: Maternal attachment, elaboration, and child autobiographical memory specificity. *J. Exp. Child Psychol.* **2016**, *143*, 65–84. [CrossRef] [PubMed]
95. Schilbach, L.; Redcay, E. Synchrony across brains. *Annu. Rev. Psychol.* **2025**, *76*, 883–911. [CrossRef] [PubMed]
96. Don, B.P.; Simpson, J.A.; Fredrickson, B.L.; Algoe, S.B. Interparental Positivity Spillover Theory: How Parents' Positive Relational Interactions Influence Children. *Perspect. Psychol. Sci.* **2025**, *20*, 639–668. [CrossRef]
97. Porras, M.M.; van Campen, C.A.N.K.; González-Rosa, J.J. Eye Tracking Study in Children to Assess Mental Calculation and Eye Movements. *Sci. Rep.* **2024**, *14*, 18901. [CrossRef]
98. Doherty, E.J.; Spencer, C.A.; Burnison, J.; Čeko, M.; Chin, J.; Eloy, L.; Haring, K.; Kim, P.; Pittman, D.; Powers, S.; et al. Interdisciplinary Views of fNIRS: Current Advancements, Equity Challenges, and an Agenda for Future Needs of a Diverse fNIRS Research Community. *Front. Integr. Neurosci.* **2023**, *17*, 1059679. [CrossRef]
99. Feldman, M.J.; Bliss-Moreau, E.; Lindquist, K.A. The Neurobiology of Interoception and Affect. *Trends Cogn. Sci.* **2024**, *28*, 643–661. [CrossRef]
100. Hoehl, S.; Fairhurst, M.; Schirmer, A. Interactional Synchrony: Signals, Mechanisms and Benefits. *Soc. Cogn. Affect. Neurosci.* **2021**, *16*, 5–18. [CrossRef]
101. Hakim, U.; De Felice, S.; Pinti, P.; Zhang, X.; Noah, J.A.; Ono, Y.; Burgess, P.W.; Hamilton, A.; Hirsch, J.; Tachtsidis, I. Quantification of Inter-Brain Coupling: A Review of Current Methods Used in Haemodynamic and Electrophysiological Hyperscanning Studies. *NeuroImage* **2023**, *280*, 120354. [CrossRef] [PubMed]
102. Berry, D.M.; Jones, S.M.; Barnes, S.P. Maternal sensitivity and the development of adrenocortical functioning from infancy through adolescence. *Dev. Psychopathol.* **2017**, *29*, 1077–1091. [CrossRef]
103. Kalomiris, A.E.; Kiel, E.J. Mother–Toddler Cortisol Synchrony Moderates Risk of Early Internalizing Symptoms. *Infancy* **2018**, *23*, 232–251. [CrossRef]
104. DePasquale, C.E. A systematic review of caregiver–child physiological synchrony across systems: Coordinated connections, common functions, and complementary descriptions. *Dev. Psychopathol.* **2020**, *32*, 1754–1777. [CrossRef]
105. Di Lorenzo, M.G.; Bucsea, O.; Rumeo, C.; Waxman, J.A.; Flora, D.B.; Schmidt, L.A.; Riddell, R.P. Caregiver and Young Child Biological Attunement in Distress Contexts: A Systematic Review and Narrative Synthesis. *Neurosci. Biobehav. Rev.* **2022**, *132*, 1010–1036. [CrossRef]

106. Davies, P.T.; Cao, V.T.; Sturge-Apple, M.L.; Cicchetti, D. Advancing Differential Susceptibility Research: Development and Validation of the Temperamental Sensitivity Q-Scale. *Dev. Psychol.* **2024**, *60*, 2016–2037. [CrossRef]
107. Lionetti, F.; Calcagnì, A.; D'Urso, G.; Spinelli, M.; Fasolo, M.; Pluess, M.; Pastore, M. A Bayesian Approach for Exploring Person × Environment Interaction within the Environmental Sensitivity Meta-Framework. *J. Child Psychol. Psychiatry* **2024**, *65*, 1486–1500. [CrossRef] [PubMed]
108. Costa-López, B.; Ruiz-Robledillo, N.; Moreno, O.; Albaladejo-Blázquez, N.; Hernández, C.; Baryła-Matejczuk, M.; Ferrer-Cascales, R. Sensory processing sensitivity as a predictor of health-related quality of life outcomes via stress and sleep quality. *Sci. Rep.* **2024**, *14*, 22707. [CrossRef] [PubMed]
109. Katz, L.F.; Kerns, S.E.U.; Gurtovenko, K.; Pasalich, D.; Goulter, N.; Dorsey, S.; Pullmann, M.D.; Dawson, A.; Galtieri, L.R.; McMahon, R.J. Integrating Parent Management Training and Emotion Coaching for Young Children with Callous-Unemotional Traits. *J. Appl. Dev. Psychol.* **2025**, *99*, 101808. [CrossRef]
110. Tkalcec, A.; Baldassarri, A.; Junghans, A.; Somasundaram, V.; Menks, W.M.; Fehlbaum, L.V.; Borbàs, R.; Raschle, N.; Seeger-Schneider, G.; Jenny, B.; et al. Gaze Behavior, Facial Emotion Processing, and Neural Underpinnings: A Comparison of Adolescents with Autism Spectrum Disorder and Conduct Disorder. *J. Child Psychol. Psychiatry*, 2025, Advance Online Publication. [CrossRef] [PubMed]
111. Viding, E.; McCrory, E.; Baskin-Sommers, A.; De Brito, S.; Frick, P. An "Embedded Brain" Approach to Understanding Antisocial Behaviour. *Trends Cogn. Sci.* **2024**, *28*, 159–171. [CrossRef] [PubMed]
112. Goagoses, N.; Bolz, T.; Eilts, J. Parenting Dimensions/Styles and Emotion Dysregulation in Childhood and Adolescence: A Systematic Review and Meta-Analysis. *Curr. Psychol.* **2023**, *42*, 18798–18822. [CrossRef]
113. Lu, H.J.; Lansford, J.E.; Liu, Y.Y.; Chen, B.B.; Bornstein, M.H.; Skinner, A.T.; Dodge, K.A.; Steinberg, L.; Deater-Deckard, K.; Rothenberg, W.A.; et al. Attachment Security, Environmental Adversity, and Fast Life History Behavioral Profiles in Human Adolescents. *Dev. Psychopathol.* **2025**, *37*, 1534–1542. [CrossRef] [PubMed]
114. Stuhrmann, L.Y.; Göbel, A.; Bindt, C.; Mudra, S. Parental Reflective Functioning and Its Association with Parenting Behaviors in Infancy and Early Childhood: A Systematic Review. *Front. Psychol.* **2022**, *13*, 765312. [CrossRef]
115. Allen, B.; Timmer, S.G.; Urquiza, A.J. Parent–Child Interaction Therapy as an attachment-based intervention: Theoretical rationale and pilot data with adopted children. *Child. Youth Serv. Rev.* **2014**, *47*, 334–341. [CrossRef]
116. Marvin, R.S.; Cooper, G.; Hoffman, K.; Powell, B. The Circle of Security project: Attachment-based intervention with caregiver–preschool child dyads. *Attach. Hum. Dev.* **2002**, *4*, 107–124. [CrossRef]
117. Cassidy, J.; Brett, B.E.; Gross, J.T.; Stern, J.A.; Martin, D.R.; Mohr, J.J.; Woodhouse, S.S. Circle of Security–Parenting: A randomized controlled trial in Head Start. *Dev. Psychopathol.* **2017**, *29*, 651–673. [CrossRef]
118. Huber, A.; McMahon, C.A.; Sweller, N. Efficacy of the 20-week Circle of Security intervention: Changes in caregiver reflective functioning, representations, and child attachment in an Australian clinical sample. *Infant Ment. Health J.* **2015**, *36*, 556–574. [CrossRef]
119. Papadopoulos, D. A Case Study of Parent–Child Interaction Therapy for a Young Child with Autism Spectrum Disorder: Behavioral and Developmental Considerations. *Psychology* **2020**, *11*, 888–907. [CrossRef]
120. Herhaus, B.; Siepmann, M.; Kahaly, G.J.; Conrad, R.; Petrowski, K. Effect of a biofeedback intervention on heart rate variability in individuals with panic disorder: A randomized controlled trial. *Psychosom. Med.* **2022**, *84*, 199–209. [CrossRef]
121. Bögels, S.M.; Restifo, K. *Mindful Parenting: A Guide for Mental Health Practitioners*; Springer: New York, NY, USA, 2014.
122. Guo, J.; Feng, G. How eye gaze feedback changes parent–child joint attention in shared storybook reading: An eye-tracking intervention study. In *Lecture Notes in Computer Science*; Springer: Berlin/Heidelberg, Germany, 2013; Volume 8010, pp. 30–38.
123. Shonkoff, J.P.; Garner, A.S.; Committee on Psychosocial Aspects of Child and Family Health; Committee on Early Childhood, Adoption, and Dependent Care; Section on Developmental and Behavioral Pediatrics. The lifelong effects of early childhood adversity and toxic stress. *Pediatrics* **2012**, *129*, e232–e246. [CrossRef]
124. Alonso, A.; Cabrera, N.J.; Kerlow, M.A.; Reich, S.M. Mothers' and Fathers' Emotion Socialization: Longitudinal Relations with Toddlers' Social Competence. *Infant Behav. Dev.* **2025**, *78*, 102034. [CrossRef] [PubMed]
125. Christou, A.I.; Fanti, K.; Mavrommatis, I.; Soursou, G. Exploring emotional face processing in children with CU traits using eye-tracking technology: Insights into the role of sex depicted in emotional faces. *Adv. Cogn. Psychol.* **2025**, *21*, 242–252. [CrossRef]
126. Christou, A.I.; Fanti, K.; Mavrommatis, I.; Soursou, G. Parent–Child Eye Gaze Congruency to Emotional Expressions Mediated by Child Aesthetic Sensitivity. *Children* **2025**, *12*, 839. [CrossRef] [PubMed]
127. Christou, A.I.; Fanti, K.; Mavrommatis, I.; Soursou, G.; Pergantis, P.; Drigas, A. Social Affiliation and Attention to Angry Faces in Children: Evidence for the Contributing Role of Parental Sensory Processing Sensitivity. *Children* **2025**, *12*, 524. [CrossRef]
128. Christou, A.I.; Tsermentseli, S.; Drigas, A. The Role of Mobile Games and Environmental Factors in Improving Learning and Metacognitive Potential of Young Students. *Int. J. Interact. Mob. Technol.* **2023**, *17*, 67–84. [CrossRef]
129. Christou, A.I.; Wallis, Y.; Bair, H.; Zeegers, M.; McCleery, J.P. Serotonin 5-HTTLPR genotype is associated with visual scanning patterns of adverse scenes in young children. *Front. Behav. Neurosci.* **2017**, *9*, 118. [CrossRef]

130. Christou, A.I.; Endo, S.; Wallis, Y.; Bair, H.; Zeegers, M.P.; McCleery, J.P. Variation in serotonin 5-HTTLPR short/long genotype modulates resting frontal EEG asymmetries in children. *Dev. Psychopathol.* **2015**, *28*, 239–250. [CrossRef]
131. Christou, A.I.; Wallis, Y.; Bair, H.; Crawford, H.; Frisson, S.; Zeegers, M.; McCleery, J.P. BDNF Val66Met and 5-HTTLPR genotype are each associated with visual scanning patterns of faces in young children. *Front. Behav. Neurosci.* **2015**, *9*, 175. [CrossRef] [PubMed]

children

MDPI

Systematic Review

Socio-Emotional Wellbeing in Parents of Children with Neurodevelopmental Disorders: A Systematic Review

Mª Lourdes Álvarez-Fernández [1,*] and Celestino Rodríguez [2]

1 Department of Psychology, Sociology and Philosophy, University of León, 24071 León, Spain
2 Department of Psychology, University of Oviedo, 33003 Oviedo, Spain; rodriguezcelestino@uniovi.es
* Correspondence: mlalvf@unileon.es; Tel.: +34-987291019

Abstract

Background/Objectives: Neurodevelopmental disorders (NDDs) require contextual approaches emphasizing family roles. Parents of children with NDDs face a complex socio-emotional reality. They may experience high levels of stress, fatigue, depression, and feelings of guilt and uncertainty, and they are often left feeling isolated and unsupported. All of these factors increase their socio-emotional vulnerability and affect their children's wellbeing. A significant part of the available evidence has focused on parents of typically developing children or on a single construct. For these reasons, and considering the impact of the COVID-19 pandemic, the aim of this study was to review interventions targeting the improvement of the socio-emotional wellbeing of parents of children with NDDs, in order to characterise recent research, the specific constructs addressed, and the effectiveness of interventions. **Methods:** No prior protocol/registration. ERIC and Web of Science databases (selected for their broad multidisciplinary coverage in psychology and social sciences) were searched from 2020–2025 (last search: 7 September 2025), limited to English/Spanish publications. Inclusion criteria encompassed parents/primary family caregivers of children with NDDs receiving socio-emotional programs. Two independent reviewers screened the titles/abstracts and full texts, resolving disagreements through discussion. Following PRISMA 2020 guidelines, this systematic review employed narrative synthesis without risk-of-bias assessment and included 16 studies (approximately, 1100 participants). **Results:** The analysis indicated a scarce but growing scientific output, with a complex methodological landscape showing promising preliminary convergence in intervention outcomes. Interventions effects appeared mediated by cultural suitability, accessibility, and contextual alignment. **Conclusions:** Future work should pursue multisystemic approaches engaging diverse societal contexts and agents to optimize child and family wellbeing.

Keywords: family context; parental intervention; socio-emotional variables; wellbeing; neurodevelopmental disorders

1. Introduction

Neurodevelopmental disorders (NDDs), which arise in early years, are characterised by the presence of alterations, deficits, or difficulties in physiological, neurological, and cognitive functioning or development, affecting personal, academic, and social contexts [1,2]. NDDs include autism spectrum disorder, attention deficit and hyperactivity disorder, specific learning disorders, communication disorders, motor disorders, intellectual disabilities, tic disorders, and other unspecified neurodevelopmental disorders [3]. Although prevalence varies between countries, due to a lack of uniform diagnostic criteria, approximately one in six children aged between 3 and 17 years old presents a neurodevelopmental disorder, which is about 17% of the child and adolescent population [4].

NDDs can be studied from two complementary perspectives. One is internal or personal, which focuses on the factors affecting the severity of the disorder, with an emphasis on personal and neuropsychological variables. The other is a contextual perspective, focusing on analysing the external variables that can affect the prognosis and severity along with the child's future development [5–7]. This contextual approach includes research in NDD in the family environment. In the DSM, and in line with family systems theory [8], interactions between members of the family—between parents and between parents and children—are considered key processes that determine the outcome of children's development as well as children's and the family's wellbeing. The nature and quality of family interactions are also influenced by family-level characteristics (such as parental stress) and by child-level characteristics (for example, the needs presented by the child).

Parents of children with NDD face a complex socio-emotional reality, which will vary according to the type of disorder and the specific needs related to it [1,5,9]. While parents do report positive benefits of raising a child with NDD, they have also been shown to have a high risk of suffering high levels of stress and emotional difficulties [10]. To a greater or lesser extent, parenting in these cases, associated with the demands of care and different types of difficulties the children have, seems to have a negative impact on parents, who often find themselves questioning their parenting abilities, feeling ambivalence, and worrying about their children's futures [11]. Parents of children with NDD have higher rates of divorce, and higher levels of social isolation, stigmatisation, and care burden [12]. In such scenarios, one significant challenge for parents is finding sufficient time to deal with their own needs. Parents often do not have time for self-care, a lack that is associated with greater levels of stress, lower perceived social support, worse psychological wellbeing, and exhaustion [13–16]. All of these factors increase socio-emotional vulnerability in the family context, with direct, negative repercussions on children's overall wellbeing [14,16,17].

The scientific literature in the field indicates that parents often feel misunderstood, unsupported, under-appreciated, and ill-prepared to support their children's needs without additional help [18]. In this regard, provision of proactive support at the level of family systems is seen as critical and is increasingly recommended. Parents with effective resources and support can feel empowered to cope with and adapt to their situations, reducing the socio-emotional risks noted above, and strengthening the family as a whole, their children's general wellbeing and therefore their overall health [19].

The Present Study

In summary, it is essential that research also addresses NDD from a contextual perspective, considering the family context, in relation to the impact that it can have on parents, who should in turn be considered active agents in their children's wellbeing. While the family context is essential to any child's development, it is particularly important where there is NDD. Understanding the socio-emotional dimension of parenting in this context is key to comprehensively addressing both family functioning and child development.

In this regard, most interventions in the field of NDD have, nevertheless, continued to adopt an internal or personal approach, aiming their efforts towards personal and neuropsychological variables [16]. From the contextual perspective, a significant part of the available evidence has focused on parents of normotypically developing children or on specific constructs such as parental stress. As a result, the findings to date have been heterogeneous and often not easy to compare.

https://doi.org/10.3390/children13010099

Added to all of this is the impact of the COVID-19 pandemic, which meant a considerable increase in, among other things, families' levels of stress, anxiety, and emotional overload [20]. The suspension of in-person support services, confinement, and greater care demands led to increased parental vulnerability, highlighting the need to reinforce parents' socio-emotional competencies even more [21,22]. This scenario also demonstrated the need for more flexible, accessible, sustainable interventions that incorporated virtual or hybrid formats, maintaining emotional support and guidance for families [21,23,24].

Because of the reasons outlined above, a systematic review is needed allowing the available evidence to be summarised and synthesised. Given the considerable social and emotional impact of the post-COVID period, this review deliberately will focus on studies published between 2020 and 2025 that examined programmes targeting socio-emotional reinforcement aimed at parents, or main family caregivers, of children presenting NDD. This timeframe makes it possible to capture recent research developed in response to new challenges, such as increased parental stress, service disruptions, and the expansion of virtual or hybrid intervention formats. It aims to give an up-to-date picture of interventions in the field, mapping the latest scientific output. In addition, it will look at how participants are characterised (parental predominance, presence of other carers, and types of NDD dealt with, among others), the methodological designs used, the main socio-emotional dimensions examined, and the interventions with the greatest reported benefits.

The resulting synthesis will be a basis for optimising the design of more comprehensive programmes for parents in the future. This will help produce more coherent, evidence-based programmes that effectively respond to families' socio-educational needs and consequently to the overall wellbeing of children with NDD.

2. Method

The literature review followed the criteria in the PRISMA statement [25], with the aim of systematically identifying and examining relevant studies. No prior protocol/registration was established. Following PRISMA 2020 guidelines, this systematic review employed narrative synthesis without risk-of-bias assessment and included 16 studies.

The systematic review included studies that (a) analysed interventions, or the results of interventions, aimed at promoting parents' (or main family carers') socio-emotional variables; (b) had samples of parents or carers whose charges were children or adolescents, under 18 years old; (c) were published in English or Spanish in the ERIC or Web of Science databases; and (d) were published in the previous five years, between 2020 and 2025.

Figure 1 summarises the process for selecting the sample of articles, along with the results, including the reasons for exclusion during the full review of the text. The bibliographic search was performed during the first week of September 2025 in Web of Science and ERIC, as noted above (last search: 7 September 2025). They were selected for their broad multidisciplinary coverage in psychology and social sciences. In Web of Science, the search was also refined by indexed journals, selecting Science Citation Index Expanded (SCI-Expanded) and Social Sciences Citation Index (SSCI). The search used the following Boolean terms in the title, abstract, or key words: ("neurodevelopmental disorders" OR "special educational needs") AND ("parent" OR "caregiver" OR "family") AND ("socioemotional" OR "parental well-being") AND ("intervention" OR "program" OR "support").

In the first stage, all of the possible results were considered, and duplicates between databases and searches were removed. In the second stage, the titles and abstracts were assessed to refine the list, excluding articles that did not refer to the topic of the review or

https://doi.org/10.3390/children13010099

which did not meet the previously established criteria. Lastly, the full texts of the remaining articles were reviewed to produce the final sample.

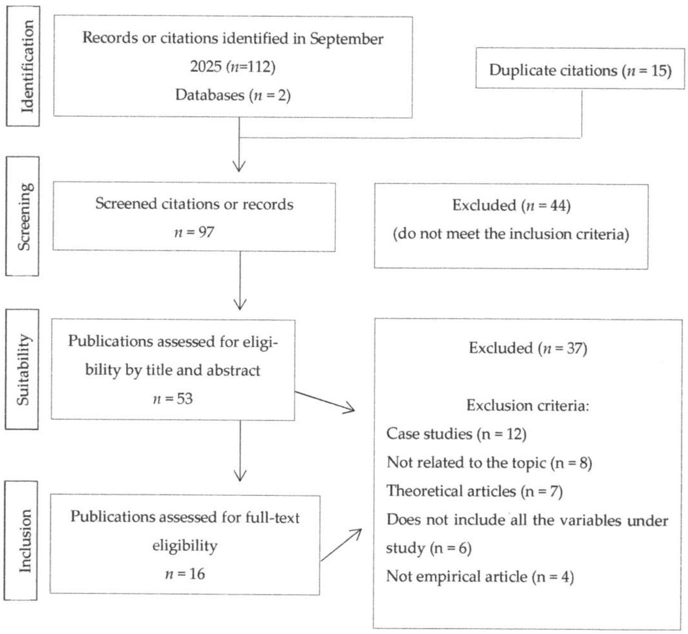

Figure 1. PRISMA Flow diagram of the systematic review. Adapted from [25].

Two independent reviewers screened the titles/abstracts and full texts. Disagreements were resolved through discussion. No snowballing was applied, as the ERIC and Web of Science databases provided 112 relevant records within the restricted timeframe (2020–2025).

2.1. Inclusion and Exclusion Criteria

The criteria for including articles were: (a) that the articles were published between 2020 and 2025. The 2020–2025 timeframe was chosen to focus on recent evidence reflecting post-COVID challenges, providing an updated synthesis amid limited prior reviews on this specific scope; (b) that the samples were parents or, alternatively, other primary family caregivers of children with NDD, and that the children were minors; (c) that they were studies staging interventions focused on promoting parents'/caregivers' socio-emotional variables; and (d) that they were published in English or Spanish.

Studies were excluded if they met the following criteria: (a) studies published as book chapters or conference summaries rather than scientific articles; (b) case studies; and (c) meta-analyses or reviews.

2.2. Data Collection

Following the PRISMA criteria, using the two aforementioned databases in the identification phase, a total of 112 articles were produced by the search terms and publication filters (2020 to 2025). Each of those articles was reviewed against the inclusion and exclusion criteria, with 15 duplicates removed before the screening phase, leaving a total of 97 pre-selected articles.

https://doi.org/10.3390/children13010099

In the screening phase, 44 of the 97 pre-selected articles did not meet the inclusion criteria, as they did not deal with the required variables or were not scientific articles. This left 53 articles for suitability review.

Reviewing the suitability indicated that 37 articles did not meet the inclusion criteria for various reasons: they were cases studies, were not specifically related to the topic, were theoretical articles or meta-analyses, did not include all the variables being studied, or the variables were not clear.

Finally, 16 articles were selected that met all of the criteria, which were subsequently analysed.

3. Results

3.1. Year of Publication, Language, Journal, and Country

Since 2020, based on the review, research on the topic has been scarce. From 2020 to 2022 only a single article was published each year. 2025 saw the most articles, a total of 6, published. All of the articles were published in English in 8 different journals. Only the Journal of Applied Research in Intellectual Disabilities and the Journal of Autism and Developmental Disorders published more than one article on the topic during the last five years. The largest proportion of the studies (31.25%) were conducted in the United States (Table 1).

Table 1. Bibliometric properties of the articles included in the systematic review (N = 16).

Descriptive Variable	Fr	%
Year of publication		
2020	1	6.25
2021	1	6.25
2022	1	6.25
2023	4	25.0
2024	3	18.75
2025	6	37.50
Language		
English	16	100.0
Journal		
Advances in Neurodevelopmental Disorders	1	6.25
Autism	1	6.25
Autism Research	1	6.25
Child: Care, Health and Development	1	6.25
Journal of Applied Research in Intellectual Disabilities	5	31.25
Journal of Autism and Developmental Disorders	5	31.25
Journal of Intellectual & Developmental Disability	1	6.25
Research in Developmental Disabilities	1	6.25
Sample Country		
Canada	2	12.50
USA	5	31.25
United Kingdom	4	25.0
India	1	6.25
Italy	1	6.25
South Africa	1	6.25
Sweden	1	6.25
Turkey	1	6.25
Total	16	100.00

https://doi.org/10.3390/children13010099

3.2. Variables Related to Participants in the Studies Analysed

There was variety in both sample composition and sample size. Mothers predominated, although some studies included fathers or other family members considered to be principal caregivers, reflecting a broader approach to the family context. Sample sizes ranged from small, with 10 participants, to a larger sample of 261 parent–child dyads. Parents' age was only specified in five studies, and the mean age was 39.9. Lastly, in 4 of the studies (25%), the participants came from challenging contexts or were at psychosocial risk.

In relation to the types of NDD the studies addressed, 9 of the interventions considered a variety of NDDs (56.25%), while 6 focused specifically on the autism spectrum (37.5%) and 1 on intellectual disability (6.25%). The age ranges of the children were also very diverse, from studies that looked at broad age ranges (e.g., from 0 to 17 years old) to others that examined narrower ranges (e.g., from 2 to 4 years old). The predominant age range was around 3 to 11 years old, with the largest proportion of studies dealing with parents of preschool or primary school children (Table 2).

3.3. Methodological Characteristics of the Studies Analysed

All of the studies demonstrated a common interest in improving parents' or main family carers' socio-emotional wellbeing. However, each study addressed specific aspects with complementary approaches. 10 of the studies (62.5%) focused specifically on evaluating aspects referring to preliminary efficacy, feasibility, acceptability, and implementation processes of the interventions, some of which were innovative such as online programmes or those based on acceptance and commitment therapies. Other objectives ranged from exploring and describing carers' subjective experiences to identifying risk and protective factors associated with parental stress, or analysing the relationships between variables such as self-compassion, self-efficacy, empowerment, and quality of family life. Consequently, the methodological designs were varied, from quasi-experimental pre–post studies without control groups to controlled randomised trials with parallel groups and pre, post, and follow-up evaluations.

In terms of evaluation instruments, the studies used a wide variety, combining quantitative methods—which included standardised scales and validated questionnaires—and qualitative methods—predominantly semi structured interviews or focus groups, along with emotional journals and self-reports. The most commonly measured variables were parental stress, in 9 studies (56.25%), depression in 5 studies (31.25%), and parental self-efficacy and anxiety, in 4 studies each (25%). The studies measuring aspects such as feasibility and acceptability of interventions did so mainly via checklists, registers of attendance, and ad hoc satisfaction questionnaires.

Finally, it is worth noting that 4 interventions (25%) were designed with the additional consideration of being applied in very specific situations of psychosocial risk, such as in populations with cultural or linguistic barriers to accessing services, or in rural communities with limited economic resources.

All of the information noted above related to the focus or objective of each study, the participants, methodological design, measures, and evaluation instruments are classified and specified in the table below (Table 2).

A high methodological heterogeneity was observed, which was addressed through a thematic narrative synthesis. This approach made it possible to identify convergences in the effectiveness of the interventions, moderated by factors such as cultural adequacy and format accessibility (Tables 2–4).

https://doi.org/10.3390/children13010099

Table 2. Focus and methodological characteristics of each study.

Authors (Year)	Objective	Participants	Methodological Design	Measures (Instruments)
Ahmed et al. (2023) [4]	Evaluate the feasibility of a short, asynchronous, online intervention focused on promoting self-compassion.	50 parents (48 mothers, 2 fathers; mean age: 42.1 years), with children aged between 3 and 17 years old with: Down syndrome, ASD, ADHD, intellectual disability, overall developmental delay, others (spina bifida, cerebral palsy, apraxia, oppositional defiant disorder).	Pre-post design, without control group.	- Self-compassion (SCS scale). - Overall wellbeing (WEN-WBS). - Depression and stress (DASS-21). - Feasibility (Bowen's model: 5 dimensions).
Bergman et al. (2023) [26]	Evaluate the feasibility and preliminary results of a group intervention based on Acceptance and Commitment Therapy.	94 parents (85 mothers, 9 fathers) of children with various disorders (ASD, autism spectrum disorder, ADHD, among others), with children aged 2 to 17 years old.	Pre, post, and follow up design, without control group.	- Parental stress (PSS). - Anxiety and depression (HADS). - Experiential avoidance in parenting (PAAQ). - Mindfulness (MAAS). - Strengths and difficulties in the children (SDQ). - Satisfaction, credibility, and usefulness of the intervention (CEQ; SEF & PEF).
Boule et al. (2023) [27]	Examine the emotional experience during a group support program for wellbeing.	104 parents (mainly mothers: 92 versus 8 fathers) of children up to 7 years old with intellectual disability and developmental difficulties.	Qualitative longitudinal study with repeated measures based on emotion journals and self-reports.	Emotional experience (online emotion journal).
Buyuk & Ozmen (2025) [28]	Evaluate the effectiveness of an empowerment programme based on reducing stress, improving self-efficacy and family empowerment.	69 mothers of children with ASD aged 6 to 14 years old: - Experimental group: 34. - Control group: 35.	Randomised controlled trial with two non-blinded parallel groups. - Experimental group: 4 training sessions and 2 individual motivational interviews. - Control group: standard practice. Pre and post design	- Parental self-efficacy (PSES). - Carer overload (ZCBS). - Perceived stress (PSS-14). - Family empowerment (FES).
Fante et al. (2025) [29]	Explore the impact of ASD on quality of life, and how a multidisciplinary intervention with parental participation influences quality of life and the process of adaptation.	31 parents (16 mothers and 15 fathers: 42.55 years old), with children diagnosed with level 2 or 3 ASD severity, aged 5 to 11 years old.	Qualitative transversal study based on semi-structured interviews, with inductive (bottom up) thematic analysis without a control group.	Quality of life: semi structured interview about quality of life, parents' experiences, perception of the intervention, difficulties, and available resources.

https://doi.org/10.3390/children13010099

Table 2. *Cont.*

Authors (Year)	Objective	Participants	Methodological Design	Measures (Instruments)
Gore et al. (2022) [30]	Explore experiences after attending a group intervention programme, as well as the group processes and mechanisms from the carers' perspectives.	35 family carers (90% mothers; mean age 36.9 and 38.8 years old) of children aged 2 to 4 years old presenting overall developmental delay, Down syndrome, ASD, or other genetic conditions.	Qualitative study based on individual interviews and focus groups about the experience held after the intervention.	Interviews and focus groups about: - Emotional wellbeing and resilience. - Feelings of belonging and group social support. - Parental self-efficacy. - Coping with stress. - Self-care. - Strategies to deal with challenging behaviours and improve family emotional balance.
Ibrahim et al. (2025) [31]	Analyse changes in mental health, mindful parenting, and parenting practice after participation in a community cognitive-behavioural group therapy programme.	77 parent–child dyads (mean age: 42.47 years old): verbally capable autistic children aged 8–13 years old.	Quasi-experimental pre-post study, without a control group.	- Stress and anxiety (DASS-21). - Mindful parenting (BMPS). - Parenting practices and family adjustment (PAFAS).
Ingersoll et al. (2024) [32]	Compare effectiveness of 2 parent-mediated distance intervention models (self-guided and with therapeutic support) in fidelity to the intervention, wellbeing, and engagement with the programme.	64 parents (mean age: 35.27 years old) of autistic children aged 1.5 to 8 years old.	Randomised controlled trial with 3 parallel groups. Pre and post evaluation and follow up.	- Parental self-efficacy (PSOC). - Knowledge about the intervention. - Perceived positive impact (FIQ). - Parental stress (PSI-SF). - Acceptability and satisfaction (STP). - Perceived obstacles (BTPS). - Technological fluency (CEW). - Expectations (CEP-Q).
Lodder et al. (2020) [20]	Evaluate feasibility, acceptability, and initial impact of a programme aimed at improving mental health and how it helps in protecting against stigmatisation.	17 parents of children with ASD up to 10 years old: - Experimental group: 9. - Control group: 8.	Randomised controlled trial with mixed quantitative and qualitative measures. Pre, post, and follow-up evaluations.	- Mental health (MHI-5). - Stigma (PCSS). - Self-esteem (Rosenberg's scale). - Self-compassion (SCS-SF). - Positive meaning in the role of carer, self-blame, perceived social support (MOS). - Social isolation (UCLA). - Feasibility (retention and attendance rates, Fidelity of implementation, opinions about randomisation). - Acceptability (participation in focus groups, satisfaction comments, quantitative indicators).

https://doi.org/10.3390/children13010099

Table 2. *Cont.*

Authors (Year)	Objective	Participants	Methodological Design	Measures (Instruments)
Ondrušková et al. (2023) [33]	Evaluate implementation process of a group intervention.	261 parent–child dyads (children aged 2.5 to 5 years old presenting moderate to severe intellectual disability, with challenging or problematic behaviours): - Experimental group: 155. - Control group: 106.	Evaluation of process within a multi-centre randomised controlled trial.	- Fidelity (checklist adapted from the i-Basis Intervention Fidelity Rating Scale). - Dose and reach (attendance data). - Adaptations (systematic record of adaptations). - Acceptability (semi-structured individual topic interviews and parental satisfaction questionnaire).
Proctor et al. (2024) [34]	Evaluate the impact of a group intervention for reinforcing skills, focused on empowerment, peer support, social inclusion, exchange of knowledge and defensive skills.	37 parents who participated in 17 parent groups, with children under 10 who had developmental difficulties. A rural setting in the south of India.	Qualitative study based on focus groups held 6 months after the intervention, analysed via hybrid thematic analysis (deductive and inductive).	- Experiences of peer support, social inclusion, knowledge exchange, and exchange of defensive skills (discussion guide in focus groups).
Safer-Lichtenstein et al. (2023) [35]	Evaluate feasibility and acceptability of 2 parental interventions.	60 carers (mainly mothers) of children aged 0 to 5 years old with developmental delays. Split into two intervention groups: - Group 1: 30. - Group 2: 30. Spanish speakers residing in the United States.	Randomised controlled trial with a mixed approach. Pre, post, and follow-up evaluations.	- Parental satisfaction (PSQ). - Parental stress (PS-4-SF). - Childish behaviour (CBCL). - Acculturation (VIA). - Session attendance. -Assessment of the experience, challenges, value (focus groups).
Schelbusch et al. (2024) [36]	Evaluate feasibility, acceptability, and possible impact of a short wellbeing programme based on acceptance and commitment therapy.	10 carers (9 mothers and 1 grandmother; Mean age: 41.27 years old) of children with developmental difficulties aged between 4 and 11 years old. Participants were residents in a rural community with limited resources in South Africa.	Quasi-experimental pilot study. Pre and post evaluation without a control group.	- Psychological Flexibility (AAQ-II). - Depression (PHQ-9). - Anxiety (GAD-7). - Perceived social support (MSPSS). - Positive and negative impact of the disability on the family (FICD). - Parental wellbeing (McConkey). - Feasibility and acceptability (ad hoc feedback and post-session satisfaction form).

https://doi.org/10.3390/children13010099

Table 2. *Cont.*

Authors (Year)	Objective	Participants	Methodological Design	Measures (Instruments)
Schwartzman et al. (2021) [37]	Evaluate the efficacy of an intervention to increase resilience and reduce parental stress, and explore collateral effects on family, marriage, and child functioning.	35 parents of children with ASD aged between 4 and 11 years old.	Randomised controlled trial with two groups. Pre, post, and follow-up evaluations.	- Resilience (CD-RISC-25). - Stress, anxiety, and depression (DASS-21). - Parental stress (PSI-4-SF). - Mindful attention (MAAS). - Life orientation (LOT-R). - Acceptance and action (AAQ-II). - Self-compassion (SCS). - Family empowerment (FES). - Marriage quality (QMI). - Strengths and difficulties (SDQ). - Social responsiveness (SRS-2). - Disruptive behaviour (ABC-2).
Sutherland et al. (2025) [38]	Examine the experiences of participants and facilitators in a systematic family support programme, and the processes involved in the perceived changes.	8 parents (mainly mothers) and 9 family facilitators trained for the programme. Children aged 8 to 13 years old with ASD or intellectual disability.	Qualitative study evaluating processes and experiences, based on semi-structured interviews and focus groups, with thematic analysis applied to the participants' and facilitators' experiences and perspectives after the intervention.	- Semi-structured interviews.
Yu et al. (2025) [39]	Evaluate feasibility, acceptability, and preliminary effects of family intervention aimed at promoting health and wellbeing.	30 parents (mostly mothers) of children with intellectual disability and developmental difficulties, aged 6 to 17 years old. Hispanic families, with cultural and linguistic barriers to accessing services, in the United States.	Pilot study of intervention with a mixed approach. Pre-post evaluation.	- Self-efficacy in health (Self-Rated Abilities for Health Practices). - Social support (MSPSS). - Dietary behaviour (NCI Dietary Screener). - Physical activity (CHAMPS and PAQ-C). - Quality of life (PROMIS). - Index of unhealthy eating, screen time, depression, and stress (CESD-10, PSS-10). - Body mass index (BMI).

Note. ASD = Autism Spectrum Disorder; ADHD: Attention Deficit/Hyperactivity Disorder.

https://doi.org/10.3390/children13010099

Table 3. Summary of the main characteristics of each intervention.

Authors (Year)	Intervention Characteristics
Ahmed et al. (2023) [4]	Short online intervention, 4 weeks, asynchronous (allowing access to the programme in line with participants' other day to day commitments). Weekly modules lasting about 12 min (weekly reminders to finish modules): (1) Psychoeducation in self-compassion, (2) self-kindness, (3) shared humanity, and (4) mindfulness. Each module includes short psychoeducation about the topic being dealt with and a written experiential activity adapted to reflect parental experiences. Various activities: reflection exercises, writing about painful parenting events, and practices to promote self-compassion, self-kindness, recognition of shared humanity, and mindfulness.
Bergman et al. (2023) [26]	Group coping intervention based on Acceptance and Commitment Therapy (ACT Navigator) 5 group sessions each lasting 3.5 h and 1 reinforcement session lasting 2.5 h: (1) Where am I? Parenting a child with a disability; psychoeducation about parental stress, grief, the importance of rest; coping strategies; acceptance as an alternative to control and avoidance. (2) What is important for me? Impact of language on suffering; healthy distance from internal experiences; mindfulness in everyday tasks, play, and activity; valuable areas of life; accepting the child; self-compassion. (3) What can hold me back? Working on values: "Navigator for parenting and life"; identifying and managing internal and external barriers; unwritten rules that act as barriers; triggers in challenging parenting situations. (4) What do I need to do? The observer's perspective and changing perspective; mindfulness and experiential acceptance in difficult situations; committed action that matters. (5) What do I promise myself? Creating an energetic balance: changing or accepting daily activities; engaging with parenting values; self-care; mindfulness in pleasant situations; self-compassion; psychologically flexible parenting. Closed groups of between 8 and 16 parents. Actively experiential methods: exercises, metaphor, dramatization, imaginary presentations, psychoeducation, mindfulness
Boule et al. (2023) [27]	Early Positive Approaches to Support (E-PAtS). Group intervention lasting 8 weeks involving psychoeducational strategies and emotional support, with weekly 2–2.5 h group sessions in-person or online: (1) how to deal with available support and services, (2) parental self-care, (3) sleep, (4) communication, (5) adaptive behaviours, (6 & 7) challenging behaviours, and (8) close and reflection. Intervention co-implemented by a mental-health specialist and a trained parent. Use of emotion journals to record and reflect on parents' own emotions before and after each session.
Buyuk & Ozmen (2025) [28]	Parental empowerment programme in two parts: (1) training in empowerment for parents (4 in-person group sessions lasting 45 min each), and (2) motivational interviews (2 individual sessions). The topics addressed include the importance of play and communication, problems and managing them in nutrition, sleep, safety, self-care, and strategies for coping with parental stress. The sessions used interactive methods: structured presentations, guided discussion, and question and answer sessions. The motivational interview was performed by a certified researcher to ensure adherence and competence.
Fante et al. (2025) [29]	Mainly clinical intervention, but with activity in the home agreed with the family, based on TEACCH. Involving specialists from different areas (clinical psychologists, paediatricians, child neuropsychologists, speech therapists) in constant collaboration with the families. Variable duration, with individual, weekly 2–4 h sessions (the number of sessions is not specified: ongoing intervention). Parental training with an emphasis on active parental participation in all stages of diagnosis and rehabilitation, active collaboration between parents and specialists, parental training, psychological support, and generalisation of learning in the home. Topics: personalised TEACCH strategies, behavioural management, developing skills, parental and family support, training and support, social inclusion.

https://doi.org/10.3390/children13010099

Table 3. *Cont.*

Authors (Year)	Intervention Characteristics
Gore et al. (2022) [30]	Early Positive Approaches to Support (E-PAtS). Group intervention, co-facilitated by a specialist and a family carer to offer early support to families. 8 weekly sessions lasting about two and a half hours, with groups of between 4 and 8 families. Combines practical exercises, group discussions, and psychoeducation. Subjects covered: access to services and training in assertiveness skills; carer's wellbeing, promoting self-care and emotion management; helping the child sleep; communication and interaction with the child; development of adaptive skills; managing challenging behaviour (2 session); and incorporating knowledge and planning for the future.
Ibrahim et al. (2025) [31]	Community intervention based on cognitive behavioural therapy (CBT), with a strong parental participation component in 2 different directions: intervention for children and intervention for parents. The intervention for parents offers 3 possible formats: (1) 9 weekly forty-five-minute sessions, (2) 18 thirty-minute sessions, or (3) 2 two-hour sessions spaced each three weeks for 9 weeks. Regardless of format, the program begins with a 2-h informative session. Online version is available (applied during the COVID-19 pandemic).
Ingersoll et al. (2024) [32]	ImPACT Online: parent-mediated intervention programme, based on the Naturalistic–Developmental–Behavioural Intervention (NDBI). 2 possible formats: (1) Self-directed (over 6 months, 12 online interactive readings each lasting 75 min, depending on the pace of each participant). The readings cover: benefits of parent-mediated intervention, social communication, preparing the home for success, and other strategies (concentrating on the child, tailoring communication, creating opportunities, teaching new habits, and modelling interaction). (2) Self-directed + remote assistance from a therapist (includes 24 thirty-minute remote coaching sessions over 6 months: 2 sessions per week provided by a clinical specialist).
Lodder et al. (2020) [20]	Psychosocial intervention protecting against stigma (SOLACE programme). Eight weeks of weekly sessions (hybrid format: in-person sessions (1, 4, and 8) and online (2, 3, 5, 6, and 7)). The programme is based on psychoeducational strategies, cognitive restructuring, and techniques centred on compassion for reducing internalisation of stigma and protecting parents' mental health. It includes group activities, discussion, and shared experiences to encourage identification with other parents and social support. Topics covered: myths and stereotypes about autism, managing stigma, positive meaning in care, resilience, self-esteem, social support, self-care and acceptance, as well as strategies for dealing with automatic negative thoughts related to stigma.
Ondrušková et al. (2023) [33]	Stepping Stones Triple P (SSTP) programme, parent-mediated. A psychoeducational programme based on the social learning model, comprising 6 in-person group sessions lasting 2.5 h and 3 individual thirty-minute calls over 9 weeks, given by trained therapists. Teaches behavioural strategies and management strategies to improve parents' confidence and reduce challenging behaviours, promoting a positive parent–child relationship.
Proctor et al. (2024) [34]	Parental intervention programme with a group approach for reinforcing parenting skills. 8 group sessions lasting 2 h each. Uses a participative methodology where the facilitators guide, but the parents share and direct. Focus: parent empowerment and self-efficacy; peer support, connection between families facing similar challenges; social inclusion; sharing knowledge about resources, rights, and wellbeing related to disabilities; defensive skills and being advocates of children with disabilities; others such as health and community integration.
Safer-Lichtenstein et al. (2023) [35]	2 parental interventions (initially in-person but due to COVID-19, an online format was adopted): - Psychoeducation, stress reduction and mindfulness (MBSR). - Behavioural training for parents (BPT). 10 group support sessions, each lasting about 90 min, weekly over 10 weeks. Psychoeducation content + parental behavioural training or + mindfulness-based stress reduction techniques (MBSR).

https://doi.org/10.3390/children13010099

Table 3. *Cont.*

Authors (Year)	Intervention Characteristics
Schelbusch et al. (2024) [36]	The Well-Beans for Caregivers programme (an adaptation of a wellbeing module for carers from the WHO Caregiver Skills Training (CST) programme). 3 in-person group sessions each lasting 2 h, over 3 weeks: - Session 1: introduction to acceptance and commitment, with emphasis on identifying personal values and the importance of accepting difficult emotions; activities to learn to be present and observe thoughts without judgement. - Session 2: techniques for coping with stressful thoughts and feelings related to caring for the child; exercises to improve psychological flexibility and manage emotional stress. Session 3: reinforcing commitment with actions in line with identified values; strategies for self-care, and construction of social support networks that strengthen resilience. The intervention is facilitated by a tiered model of training and supervision that includes mental health specialists and non-specialists. It is based on Acceptance and Commitment Theory (ACT). The sessions include stories, live exercises, and group discussions to help carers manage stress and improve their mental wellbeing. Strategies are applied to facilitate understanding, accessibility, and cultural adaptation, such as simplified language, use of illustrations, and the possibility of mixing local idioms with English.
Schwartzman et al. (2021) [37]	AMOR programme (Acceptance, Mindfulness, Optimism, Resilience Method). Facilitated by specialists in psychology 8 weekly group sessions lasting about 90 min each, which combine teaching, group discussion, behavioural practice, and weekly homework. Meditation exercises, reviewing homework, teaching new resilience strategies based on cognitive-behavioural therapy, full attention, self-compassion, and optimistic thinking. Content: managing stress, changing mentality about stress, gratitude, mindfulness, acceptance, facing grief and loss, optimism (in two sessions), self-compassion, and review to prioritise resilience.
Sutherland et al. (2025) [38]	Positive Family Connections Programme. Facilitated by trained family carers, supervised by psychologists. 6 online group sessions lasting 2 h with groups of 6–8 families (up to 2 carers per family). Topics covered: strengthening family relationships and wellbeing through peer support and promotion of healthy family processes.
Yu et al. (2025) [39]	Family PODER: an intervention culturally adapted for Latin American families. 10 weekly virtual individual sessions with a trained promotor, each lasting about 1 h, plus 3 group sessions reinforcing the content, two in-person and one virtual as an adaptation to overcome logistical obstacles. Individual session content: wellbeing and managing stress; balanced nutrition and food preparation; social support and healthy decision-making. The group sessions involve interactive activities to reinforce the learning, including practical demonstrations.

Table 4. Socio-emotional variables addressed, principal related results, and percentages of effectiveness and adherence to the interventions.

Intervention	Aspects Addressed to Improve Socio-Emotional Wellbeing	Main Related Results	Effectiveness (%)	Adherence (%)
Ahmed et al. (2023) [4]	- Self-compassion - Emotional wellbeing	- Reduced parental stress - Increased self-compassion	~60–65%	>80%
Bergman et al. (2023) [26]	- Parental stress - Self-care	- Improved emotional acceptance - Reduced parental stress	>70%	80–85%
Boule et al. (2023) [27]	- Parental self-care - Communication	- Improved self-care - Improved family life	65–75%	>75%

https://doi.org/10.3390/children13010099

Table 4. Cont.

Intervention	Aspects Addressed to Improve Socio-Emotional Wellbeing	Main Related Results	Effectiveness (%)	Adherence (%)
Buyuk & Ozmen (2025) [28]	- Stress management - Communication - Empowerments	- Increased parental self-efficacy - Reduced stress	70%	70–75%
Fante et al. (2025) [29]	- Behavioural management - Social abilities	- Reduction in disruptive behaviours - Improved social skills	>70%	75–80%
Gore et al. (2022) [30]	- Self-care - Adaptive skills	- Improved access to services - Promoted self-care - Improved adaptive skills	65–70%	>70%
Ibrahim et al. (2025) [31]	- Stress - Parenting skills	- Improved parenting abilities - Improved stress management	>70%	70–80%
Ingersoll et al. (2024) [32]	- Social communication - Behavioural management	- Improved social communication - Reduction in disruptive behaviours	75–85%	80%
Lodder et al. (2020) [20]	- Resilience - Stigma - Social support	- Increased resilience - Reduced stigma - Improved social support	65–70%	70%
Ondrušková et al. (2023) [33]	- Behavioural management - Parenting strategies	- Improved parenting strategies - Improved confidence	70–80%	>75%
Proctor et al. (2024) [34]	- Empowerment - Peer support	- Strengthened active participation - Strengthened social networks - Benefits in defensive skills	65–70%	75%
Safer-Lichtenstein et al. (2023) [35]	- Stress - Emotional wellbeing	- Reduced parental stress	>70%	70–75%
Schelbusch et al. (2024) [36]	- Self-care - Resilience	- Increased resilience - Reduced anxiety	70%	80%
Schwartzman et al. (2021) [37]	- Social support - Family wellbeing	- Strengthened social support - Strengthened family wellbeing	65–70%	75%
Sutherland et al. (2025) [38]	- Coping - Resilience	- Improved emotional wellbeing	70–80%	80–85%
Yu et al. (2025) [39]	- Stress - Emotional wellbeing - Parent empowerment - Social support	- Improved stress management	70–75%	70–75%

3.4. Description of the Interventions in the Reviewed Studies

Firstly, looking at the format of the interventions, 10 were implemented in groups (62.5%), 3 were individual (18.75%), and 3 were mixed modality (18.75%). In terms of how they were delivered, 7 were in-person (43.75%), 4 were online or virtual (25%), and 2 were in a hybrid format (12.5%). In addition, 1 intervention that was initially designed to be delivered in person was adapted to an online format due to the COVID-19 lockdown, and another intervention could be applied in both formats.

Two of the interventions (both online) were self-directed (12.5%), 7 were facilitated by specialists in mental health, psychology, or associated areas (43.75%), and the remained were co-facilitated by specialists and parents or family carers (43.75%).

The interventions lasted between 2 and 18 sessions, with the most common duration being 6 to 10 sessions. Sessions lasted from 30 min for individual sessions to up to 3.5 h in intensive group sessions. The session content, related to direct care for parents/main family carers, focused on a variety of topics: parental self-care, stress management, parenting skills, self-compassion, parental empowerment, reduction in stigma, and aspects related to physical wellbeing. From a methodological perspective, the interventions used cognitive-

https://doi.org/10.3390/children13010099

behavioural therapy, acceptance and commitment therapy, psychoeducation, experiential interventions, mindfulness, and parent-mediated behavioural strategies.

Specific information about the main characteristics of each intervention reviewed is provided in detail in the table below (Table 3).

3.5. Principal Results and Findings from the Analysed Studies

The table below (Table 4) summarises the aspects that the interventions were identified as working on, related to parental wellbeing at the socio-emotional level, along with the main related results. It also shows a combination of specific numeric data and qualitative data in relation to percentages of effectiveness and adherence to the interventions.

There was a convergence in terms of efficacy, with most interventions reporting, for example, significant reductions in parental stress and parents' emotional health, along with increased active participation and social networks from the participants. In addition, there was over 70% adherence reported, which reinforces the idea that these interventions are viable and accepted.

Interventions such as [4,26,37] stand out for applying techniques centred on self-compassion, mindfulness, and based on Acceptance and Commitment Therapy (ACT), achieving consistent effects in improving parents' wellbeing and excellent adherence (between 80–85%). On the other hand, programmes such as [27,38,39]—which combined professional facilitation, active participation from trained parents and community promotors, in online and in-person formats—demonstrated outstanding results in self-efficacy, emotional regulation, and social support, with high scores in satisfaction and adherence above 70%. The interventions focusing on training behavioural skills and social communication, such as [32,33], stand out for their positive effects on behavioural management and improvements in family communication, again with good adherence (>75%).

The evidence indicates that the effectiveness of the interventions in this review is mediated by cultural suitability, the format, and the relevance to the specific needs of each family context. Because of that, interventions incorporating a multidimensional, adaptive focus achieve better overall results. Parental self-efficacy was strengthened through empowerment programs and Acceptance and Commitment Therapy interventions, which fostered more effective coping strategies. Social support acted as a key mediator in reducing stress and feelings of isolation, with better outcomes observed in group-based or parent co-facilitated interventions. Improvements in parental self-efficacy stemmed from specific skill training and peer emotional validation, which significantly reduced perceived burden. Social support, particularly in group-based programs, emerged as a key resilience mechanism, moderated by contextual factors such as service accessibility and cultural barriers.

4. Discussion

This systematic review looked at studies published between 2020 and September 2025 on interventions focused on improving or promoting socio-emotional wellbeing in parents (or main family carers) of children with NDD. The review confirms that, although scientific output has been scarce, it is growing, particularly from 2023 onwards. This has perhaps been largely driven by the negative impact of the COVID-19 pandemic on these families, because lockdowns and suspension of support services led to them facing an increased care load and more stress.

The participants in the interventions were largely mothers. This is another confirmation of the fact that mothers tend to take on the bulk of primary care in the family context, with greater levels of stress according to the literature in the field [10,11]. This situation underscores why mothers have been the main focus of the interventions' attention. The re-

https://doi.org/10.3390/children13010099

view also showed the wide range of sample sizes and greater attention to autism spectrum disorder and intellectual disability. The main ages of children covered by the interventions was between 3 and 11 years old, which is perhaps justified by the high prevalence of these disorders and their early diagnostic visibility [3].

The methodological designs and aspects of the interventions analysed in this review also reflect a wide diversity, from quasi-experimental pre-post designs without control groups, to randomised controlled trials with parallel groups, combining quantitative, qualitative, and mixed approaches. On the one hand, this picture shows the growing maturity of this line of research and the richness and complexity of the field. On the other hand, it reflects the rapid changes and urgent adaptations forced by the COVID-19 pandemic [31]. That said, it is worth noting that a significant majority of the studies used quasi-experimental pre–post designs without control groups, with a quantitative approach, prioritising the evaluation of feasibility and the preliminary effectiveness of the interventions.

Turning to the characteristics of the interventions themselves, in-person, group formats, facilitated by specialists, or co-facilitated by trained parents, predominated over self-directed formats. Nonetheless, there was evidence of an increased tendency towards online or hybrid formats, again driven by the impact of COVID-19. Both formats, online and hybrid, have been shown to be viable, increasing the flexibility available to interventions, and facilitating participation in rural environments or places with limited resources, although challenges remain such as those related to accessibility and technological and social obstacles, which need to be addressed to ensure equity [34].

The number of sessions and how long they last varied according to the formats and modalities, the types of facilitation and the methodological approach of the interventions. With regard to the latter, the approaches mainly combined psychoeducation, cognitive-behavioural therapy, acceptance and commitment therapy, experiential intervention, mindfulness, and parent-mediated behavioural strategies. They addressed topics within socioemotional wellbeing, linked to parental self-care, stress management, parenting competencies, communication and social skills, managing challenging behaviours, self-compassion, parental empowerment, reduction in stigma, and aspects of physical wellbeing. The most common methodological approach was psychoeducation to address parental self-care and stress, the socioemotional variables that were most commonly present in the interventions in this review.

On this point, it is worth noting that the review found promising preliminary convergence across the 16 interventions analysed, despite their methodological diversity, with significant reductions in parental stress, improvements in emotional health, and greater active participation or improvements in parents' social networks. More specifically, the interventions based on acceptance and commitment therapy, mindfulness, and self-compassion stood out for their consistency. These types of experiential techniques may be more accessible than others for families in challenging situations [4,26,37]. Co-facilitated interventions exhibited high percentages of satisfaction [27,38,39], and those that included parent-mediated behavioural strategies or that addressed family communication achieved high percentages of adherence. In this regard, the scientific evidence about the benefits of peer-directed self-help groups is sound. The support they provide has been shown to be essential in reducing feelings of isolation, stigmatisation, and internalisation of self-stigma [20,27]. Creating safe spaces for exchanging experiences and mutual validation promotes feelings of belonging, normalisation, and empowerment [30,33].

In short, the evidence suggests promising preliminary effectiveness of these interventions, but this effectiveness is also mediated by cultural suitability, accessibility, and whether they are aimed at specific contextual needs [34–36,39]. In low-resource settings,

https://doi.org/10.3390/children13010099

short asynchronous online programs [4,32] proved most feasible. Peer co-facilitation should be prioritized when professional access is limited [27,30].

5. Conclusions

Interventions aimed at the parents or family carers of children with NDD should be considered an area of particular interest, owing to the socio-emotional challenges these families face [20,30]. The present systematic review has allowed us to take a detailed snapshot of the current scientific picture in the field, and shows that these types of interventions are key tools in helping families face that challenge, indirectly contributing to the children's wellbeing and quality of life [14]. That said, there are some considerations that should be borne in mind that may offer greater robustness and soundness to this field of research, related for example, to more robust methodological designs, longitudinal follow-up of interventions to consolidate knowledge of their impact and sustainability, and the balance between scientific validity and practical applicability, among other aspects.

The findings of our systematic review have notable implications, especially given the scarcity of research over recent years, although it is growing. This scarcity makes it even more important to analyse the socio-emotional impact on parents, mostly mothers, who face high levels of stress, anxiety and depression, overload, and social isolation, aggravated by the COVID-19 pandemic, which underscores the urgency of family context approaches [21]. For this reason, various practical implications at the family, educational, political, and social level are discussed below.

Firstly, at the family level, we should bear in mind that raising a child with NDD produces socio-emotional maladjustment in parents that may lead to less adaptive parenting styles, increasing the burden of care and stigmatisation. Consequently, it is essential to develop accessible, culturally appropriate family programmes that equip parents with skills for self-care, stress management, and empowerment [40]. In this regard, interventions should be multidimensional, as well as directly addressing child wellbeing.

Secondly, on an educational level, parents' socio-emotional state is also a priority. Children with NDD present difficulties and vulnerabilities that affect school and family contexts. This is why education professionals must be trained in socio-emotional competencies to help prevent parental exhaustion and to promote group interventions. Seeking family involvement is essential, and it needs to be quality involvement, through two-way communication between school and the home [19].

On a political level, the most important implication is related to the promotion of inclusive policies in line with socio-emotional care in all of the environments surrounding children with NDD and their parents, considering their day-to-day challenges. It would be useful to design early detection programmes and access to services that combine educational, social, family, and mental health work, encouraging co-facilitation by skilled, trained parents to reduce stigma and social isolation and to optimise community resources, with particular attention to vulnerable family situations [41]. These interventions must be within comprehensive systems of family care in order to maximise their impact on quality of life and social inclusion [30,34,42,43].

Finally, in the mental health sphere, there should be better collaboration with schools to offer integrated support to students with NDD and their families through specific programmes [44]. In addition, parents and educators need good quality training in early detection and the application of evidence-based interventions [5,45–48].

Despite these practical implications, the review does have a series of limitations that need to be considered when interpreting the results. In the first place, the sample of articles included for the review was small, as there were only a limited number of studies published on the topic in the time period selected, and the search was limited to only

https://doi.org/10.3390/children13010099

two databases. On the other hand, no protocol/registration was established prior to the search nor was a risk-of-bias assessment conducted. In addition, the selected studies also included interventions that were not limited solely to developing or strengthening socio-emotional variables, to a single modality, format, or specific intervention characteristics, cultural contexts, family scenarios, participants or NDD, or specific age ranges, which may limit how representative and generalisable the findings are. These are aspects that future research may address specifically in a variety of ways, with the present systematic review being seen as a first approach. Finally, in accordance with the implications noted above, it would be interesting for future studies to address the same research objective, but from a multisystemic perspective. Consequently, the present review emphasises the need for future interventions to address parental socio-emotional wellbeing with the involvement of different contexts and agents in society, with the same ultimate aim of improving the overall wellbeing of children with NDD.

Author Contributions: Conceptualization, M.L.Á.-F.; methodology, C.R. and M.L.Á.-F.; investigation, C.R. and M.L.Á.-F.; resources, C.R. and M.L.Á.-F.; writing—original draft preparation, M.L.Á.-F.; writing—review and editing, M.L.Á.-F. All authors have read and agreed to the published version of the manuscript.

Funding: This research was funded by the Spanish Ministry of Science and Innovation (MCIN/AEI/10.13039/501100011033/FEDER, UE), and conducted within the project PID2021-1244011NB-I00.

Institutional Review Board Statement: Not applicable.

Informed Consent Statement: Not applicable.

Data Availability Statement: The original contributions presented in this study are included in the article. Further inquiries can be directed to the corresponding author.

Conflicts of Interest: The authors declare no conflicts of interest.

References

1. Chua, J.Y.X.; Shorey, S. The effect of mindfulness-based and acceptance commitment therapy-based interventions to improve the mental well-being among parents of children with developmental disabilities: A systematic review and meta-analysis. *J. Autism Dev. Disord.* **2022**, *52*, 2770–2783. [CrossRef] [PubMed]
2. Zablotsky, B.; Black, L.I.; Maenner, M.J.; Schieve, L.A.; Danielson, M.L.; Bitsko, R.H.; Blumberg, S.J.; Kogan, M.D.; Boyle, C.A. Prevalence and trends of developmental disabilities among children in the United States: 2009–2017. *Pediatrics* **2019**, *144*, e20190811. [CrossRef] [PubMed]
3. American Psychiatric Association. *Diagnostic and Statistical Manual of Mental Disorders Fifth Edition Text Revision DSM-5-TR*; American Psychiatric Publishing: Arlington, VA, USA, 2022. Available online: https://www.appi.org/dsm-5-tr (accessed on 22 October 2025).
4. Ahmed, A.N.; Raj, S.P. Self-compassion intervention for parents of children with developmental disabilities: A feasibility study. *Adv. Neurodev. Disord.* **2023**, *7*, 277–289. [CrossRef] [PubMed]
5. Abín, A.; Pasarín-Lavín, T.; Areces, D.; Rodríguez, C.; Núñez, J.C. The emotional impact of family involvement during homework in children with neurodevelopmental disorders: A systematic review. *Children* **2024**, *11*, 713. [CrossRef]
6. Cueli, M.; Martín, N.; Canamero, L.M.; Rodríguez, C.; González-Castro, P. The impact of children's and parents' perceptions of parenting styles on attention, hyperactivity, anxiety, and emotional regulation. *Children* **2024**, *11*, 313. [CrossRef]
7. Wolf, M.; Gotlieb, R.J.M.; Kim, S.A.; Pedroza, V.; Rhinehart, L.V.; Tempini, M.L.G.; Sears, S. Towards a dynamic, comprehensive conceptualization of dyslexia. *Ann. Dyslexia* **2024**, *74*, 303–324. [CrossRef]
8. Trivette, C.M.; Dunst, C.J.; Hamby, D.W. Influences of family-systems intervention practices on parent-child interactions and child development. *Top. Early Child. Spec. Educ.* **2010**, *30*, 3–15. [CrossRef]
9. Zerihun, T.; Kinfe, M.; Koly, K.N.; Abdurahman, R.; Girma, F.; Team, W.; Hanlon, C.; de Vries, P.J.; Hoekstra, R.A. Non-specialist delivery of the WHO Caregiver Skills Training Programme for children with developmental disabilities: Stakeholder perspectives about acceptability and feasibility in rural Ethiopia. *Autism* **2024**, *28*, 95–106. [CrossRef]
10. Hastings, R.P. Do children with intellectual and developmental disabilities have a negative impact on other family members? The case for rejecting a negative narrative. *Int. Rev. Res. Dev. Disabil.* **2016**, *51*, 167–197. [CrossRef]

https://doi.org/10.3390/children13010099

11. Hamilton, V.E.; Matthews, J.M.; Crawford, S.B. Development and preliminary validation of a parenting self-regulation scale: "Me as a Parent" (MaaP). *J. Child Fam. Stud.* **2015**, *24*, 2853–2864. [CrossRef]
12. McMahon, S.M.; Wilson, C.E.; Sharry, J. Parents Plus parenting programme for parents of adolescents with intellectual disabilities: A cluster randomised controlled trial. *J. Appl. Res. Intellect. Disabil.* **2023**, *36*, 871–880. [CrossRef] [PubMed]
13. Anderson, L.L.; Kardell, Y.; Hall, S.; Magaa, S.; Reynolds, M.; Crdova, J. A research agenda to support families of people with intellectual and developmental disabilities with intersectional identities. *Intellect. Dev. Disabil.* **2024**, *62*, 162–173. [CrossRef] [PubMed]
14. Dodds, R.L.; Walch, T.J. The glue that keeps everybody together: Peer support in mothers of young children with special health care needs. *Child Care Health Dev.* **2022**, *48*, 772–780. [CrossRef] [PubMed]
15. Lunsky, Y.; Albaum, C.; Baskin, A.; Hastings, R.P.; Hutton, S.; Steel, L.; Wang, W.; Weiss, J.A. Group virtual mindfulness-based intervention for parents of autistic adolescents and adults. *J. Autism Dev. Disord.* **2021**, *51*, 3959–3969. [CrossRef]
16. Ericson, S.; Hesla, M.W.; Stadskleiv, K. Gaining super control: Psychoeducational group intervention for adolescents with mild intellectual disability and their parents. *J. Intellect. Disabil.* **2022**, *26*, 350–364. [CrossRef]
17. Maughan, A.L.; Lunsky, Y.; Lake, J.; Mills, J.S.; Fung, K.; Steel, L.; Weiss, J.A. Parent, child, and family outcomes following Acceptance and Commitment Therapy for parents of autistic children: A randomized controlled trial. *Autism* **2024**, *28*, 367–380. [CrossRef]
18. Douglas, S.N.; Meadan, H.; Ostrosky, M.M. Effects of parent-delivered aided language modeling during shared storybook reading. *J. Early Interv.* **2017**, *38*, 177–188.
19. Finn, L.L. Improving interactions between parents, teachers, and staff and individuals with developmental disabilities: A review of caregiver training methods and results. *Int. J. Dev. Disabil.* **2020**, *66*, 390–400. [CrossRef]
20. Lodder, A.; Papadopoulos, C.; Randhawa, G. SOLACE: A psychosocial stigma protection intervention to improve the mental health of parents of autistic children—A feasibility randomized controlled trial. *J. Autism Dev. Disord.* **2020**, *50*, 4477–4491. [CrossRef]
21. Lake, J.K.; Volpe, T.; St. John, L.; Thakur, A.; Steel, L.; Baskin, A.; Durbin, A.; Chacra, M.A.; Lunsky, Y. Mental health and COVID-19: The impact of a virtual course for family caregivers of adults with intellectual and developmental disabilities. *J. Intellect. Disabil. Res.* **2022**, *66*, 677–689. [CrossRef]
22. Murthy, S.; Harris, S.P.; Hsieh, K. Formal support and service needs of family caregivers of adults with intellectual and/or developmental disabilities in India. *J. Appl. Res. Intellect. Disabil.* **2024**, *37*, e13235. [CrossRef]
23. Apanasionok, M.M.; Paris, A.; Griffin, J.; Hastings, R.P.; Finch, E.; Austin, D.; Flynn, S. Digital psychological wellbeing interventions for family carers of children and adults with intellectual and developmental disabilities: A systematic review. *J. Appl. Res. Intellect. Disabil.* **2025**, *38*, e70081. [CrossRef] [PubMed]
24. Swanson, S.E.; Duijff, S.N.; Campbell, L.E. Care4Parents: An evaluation of an online mindful parenting program for caregivers of children with 22q11.2 deletion syndrome. *Adv. Neurodev. Disord.* **2025**, *9*, 195–212. [CrossRef]
25. Page, M.J.; McKenzie, J.E.; Bossuyt, P.M.; Boutron, I.; Hoffman, T.; Mulrow, C.D.; Shamseer, L.; Tetzlaff, J.M.; Akl, E.A.; Brennan, S.E.; et al. The PRISMA 2020 statement: An updated guideline for reporting systematic reviews. *Res. Methods Rep.* **2021**, *74*, 790–799.
26. Bergman, T.H.; Renhorn, E.; Berg, B.; Lappalainen, P.; Ghaderi, A.; Hirvikoski, T. Acceptance and commitment therapy group intervention for parents of children with disabilities: Navigator ACT, an open feasibility trial. *J. Autism Dev. Disord.* **2023**, *53*, 1834–1849. [CrossRef]
27. Boule, M.; Rivard, M.; Mello, C. Parents' emotional journey throughout their participation in a well-being support group intervention. *J. Appl. Res. Intellect. Disabil.* **2025**, *38*, e70107. [CrossRef]
28. Büyük, D.Ş.; Özmen, D. Effectiveness of a parent empowerment program for parents of children with autism: A randomized controlled trial. *Child Care Health Dev.* **2025**, *51*, e70148. [CrossRef]
29. Fante, C.; Musetti, A.; De Luca Picione, R.; Dioni, B.; Manari, T.; Raffin, C.; Capelli, F.; Franceschini, C.; Lenzo, V. Parental quality of life and impact of multidisciplinary intervention for children with autism spectrum disorders: A qualitative study. *J. Autism Dev. Disord.* **2025**, *55*, 310–322. [CrossRef]
30. Gore, N.; Bradshaw, J.; Hastings, R.; Sweeney, J.; Austin, D. Early Positive Approaches to Support (E-PAtS): Qualitative experiences of a new support programme for family caregivers of young children with intellectual and developmental disabilities. *J. Appl. Res. Intellect. Disabil.* **2022**, *35*, 889–899. [CrossRef]
31. Ibrahim, A.T.; Lee, V.; Vashi, N.; Roudbarani, F.; Modica, P.T.; Pouyandeh, A.; Sellitto, T.; Ameis, S.H.; Elkader, A.; Gray, K.M.; et al. Parent outcomes following participation in cognitive behavior therapy for autistic children in a community setting: Parent mental health, mindful parenting, and parenting practices. *Autism Res.* **2025**, *18*, 570–582. [CrossRef]
32. Ingersoll, B.; Frost, K.M.; Straiton, D.; Ramos, A.P.; Howard, M. Relative efficacy of self-directed and therapist-assisted telehealth models of a parent-mediated intervention for autism: Examining effects on parent intervention fidelity, well-being, and program engagement. *J. Autism Dev. Disord.* **2024**, *54*, 3605–3619. [CrossRef] [PubMed]

https://doi.org/10.3390/children13010099

33. Ondrušková, T.; Oulton, K.; Royston, R.; Hassiotis, A. Process evaluation of a parenting intervention for preschoolers with intellectual disabilities who display behaviours that challenge in the UK. *J. Appl. Res. Intellect. Disabil.* **2024**, *37*, e13263. [CrossRef] [PubMed]
34. Proctor, K.; Patel, M.; Krishna, D.; Venkatachalapathy, N.; Brien, M.; Langlois, S. A capacity-building intervention for parents of children with disabilities in rural South India. *Res. Dev. Disabil.* **2024**, *150*, 104766. [CrossRef] [PubMed]
35. Safer-Lichtenstein, J.; McIntyre, L.L.; Rodriguez, G.; Gomez, D.; Puerta, S.; Neece, C.L. Feasibility and acceptability of Spanish-language parenting interventions for young children with developmental delays. *Intellect. Dev. Disabil.* **2023**, *61*, 307–325. [CrossRef]
36. Schlebusch, L.; Chambers, N.; Rosenstein, D.; Erasmus, P.; WHO CST Team; de Vries, P.J. Supporting caregivers of children with developmental disabilities: Findings from a brief caregiver well-being programme in South Africa. *Autism* **2024**, *28*, 199–214. [CrossRef]
37. Schwartzman, J.M.; Millan, M.E.; Uljarevic, M.; Gengoux, G.W. Resilience intervention for parents of children with autism: Findings from a randomized controlled trial of the AMOR method. *J. Autism Dev. Disord.* **2021**, *52*, 7387–7413. [CrossRef]
38. Sutherland, D.; Flynn, S.; Griffin, J.; Hastings, R.P. Programme recipient and facilitator experiences of Positive Family Connections for families of children with intellectual disabilities and/or who are autistic. *J. Appl. Res. Intellect. Disabil.* **2025**, *38*, e70003. [CrossRef]
39. Yu, A.P.L.; Suarez-Balcazar, Y.; Errisuriz, V.L.; Parra-Medina, D.; Mirza, M.; Zhang, M.; Lee, P.-C.; Zeng, W.; Brown-Hollie, J.P.; Mendoza, E.Y.; et al. PODER Familiar: A culturally tailored health intervention for Latino families of children with intellectual and developmental disabilities. *J. Appl. Res. Intellect. Disabil.* **2025**, *38*, e70048. [CrossRef]
40. Haraguchi, H.; Inoue, M. Evaluating outcomes of a community-based parent training program for Japanese children with developmental disabilities: A retrospective pilot study. *Int. J. Dev. Disabil.* **2024**, *70*, 251–263. [CrossRef]
41. Rangel, E.; Rieth, S.; Mejia, Y.; Cervantes, L.; Vazquez, B.B.; Brookman-Frazee, L. Community-led adaptations of a promotora-delivered intervention for Latino families of youth with developmental disabilities. *J. Child Fam. Stud.* **2024**, *33*, 3812–3850. [CrossRef]
42. Gaidhane, A.; Telrandhe, S.; Holding, P.; Patil, M.; Kogade, P.; Jadhav, N.; Khatib, M.N.; Zahiruddin, Q.S. Effectiveness of family-centered program for enhancing competencies of responsive parenting among caregivers for early childhood development in rural India. *Acta Psychol.* **2022**, *229*, 103669. [CrossRef]
43. Gordon-Brown, S.; Flynn, S.; Finch, E.; Hastings, R.P.; Austin, D. Experiences of peer mentors in digital wellbeing interventions: Supporting family carers of individuals with intellectual and developmental disabilities. *J. Appl. Res. Intellect. Disabil.* **2025**, *38*, e70102. [CrossRef]
44. Stone-Heaberlin, M.; Blackburn, A.; Qian, C. Caregiver education programme on intellectual and developmental disabilities: An acceptability and feasibility study in an academic medical setting. *Child Care Health Dev.* **2023**, *50*, e13178. [CrossRef]
45. Jacob, B.; Izar, R.; Tran, H.; Akers, K.; Aranha, A.N.F.; Afify, O.; Janks, E.; Mendez, J. Medical student program to learn from families experiencing developmental disabilities. *Int. J. Dev. Disabil.* **2024**, *70*, 160–171. [CrossRef]
46. Passmore, A.H.; Hughes, M.T. Using eCoaching to support mothers' pretend play interactions at home. *Early Child. Educ. J.* **2024**, *52*, 207–219. [CrossRef]
47. Chaidi, I.; Drigas, A. Parents' involvement in the education of their children with autism related research and its results. *Int. J. Emerg. Technol. Learn.* **2020**, *15*, 194–203. [CrossRef]
48. Postma, A.; Ketelaar, M.; van Nispen Tot Sevenaer, J.; Downs, Z.; van Rappard, D.; Jongmans, M.; Zinkstok, J. Exploring individual parent-to-parent support interventions for parents caring for children with brain-based developmental disabilities: A scoping review. *Child Care Health Dev.* **2024**, *50*, e13255. [CrossRef]

https://doi.org/10.3390/children13010099

MDPI AG
Grosspeteranlage 5
4052 Basel
Switzerland
Tel.: +41 61 683 77 34

Children Editorial Office
E-mail: children@mdpi.com
www.mdpi.com/journal/children

www.ingramcontent.com/pod-product-compliance
Lightning Source LLC
Chambersburg PA
CBHW061558210926
51850CB00009B/2147
* 9 7 8 3 7 2 5 8 7 3 2 0 3 *